Myles Professional Studies for Midwifery Education and Practice

Concepts and Challenges

Myles Professional Studies for Midwifery Education and Practice

Concepts and Challenges

JAYNE E. MARSHALL, FRCM PFHEA PHD MA PGCEA ADM RM RN

Foundation Professor of Midwifery and NMC Lead Midwife for Education
School of Allied Health Professions
College of Life Sciences
George Davies Centre
University of Leicester
Leicester
UK

Foreword by

Professor Emeritus Diane M. Fraser

ELSEVIER

Edinburgh London New York Oxford Philadelphia St Louis Sydney 2019

ISBN: 978-0-7020-6860-7

Printed in Poland
Last digit is the print number: 9   8   7   6   5   4   3   2   1

Content Strategist: Alison Taylor
Content Development Specialists: Katie Golsby and Carole McMurray
Content Coordinator: Kirsty Guest
Project Manager: Anne Collett
Design: Renee Duenow
Illustration Manager: Paula Catalano
Marketing Manager: Deborah Watkins

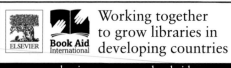

CONTENTS

Given the vast amount of information that can be accessed electronically, it might be questioned why a book about professional studies for midwives is necessary. The answer lies in 'professional studies' – the reader is expected to interact with the text. Each chapter, as appropriate, describes historical contexts then details current practices and legislation. Chapters then point the reader to an anticipated future direction for midwifery education and practice. The reader is therefore provided with a wealth and depth of information before being challenged to consider what this means for them and their practice.

This book can be used merely to increase one's knowledge about a topic, as each chapter contains factual information of relevance to students as well as experienced midwives working in practice or academia. The factual information is well referenced, presented clearly and is supported by annotated further reading, lists of key points and useful websites. However, the reader is not allowed to merely absorb information but is expected to engage with the many scenarios and activities created by the chapter authors. Where situations appear more complex, helpful strategies for reflection and action are provided.

Each chapter stands alone and for this reason some details and figures are presented in more than one chapter, for example revalidation is explained in Chapters 2 and 15. In others the authors refer the reader to different chapters where content is complementary, e.g. Chapters 4 (philosophy), 5 (reflection) and 6 (ethics). Many textbooks are accused of being England biased. The editor of this book has effectively drawn upon the expertise of midwives working, or having worked, globally, in particular Australia, Canada, Slovenia and Zambia. The variations in ways of working in the four countries of the United Kingdom (UK) are detailed. The influences of the International Confederation of Midwives (ICM) and the European Union (EU) directives on midwives' practice are explained as is the uncertainty for the UK once it is no longer a member of the EU.

The first two chapters explore what it means to 'be a midwife' and the standards and regulations expected of midwife professionals. Midwives' aspirations and the realities of practice are discussed and set alongside the need for midwives to build resilience in an often short-staffed maternity service. The third chapter addresses what might be considered an obvious requirement for healthcare practitioners, 'effective communication'. However, many complaints from childbearing women and their families arise from poor communication about their care. The chapter authors provide a range of theories and tools to help midwives improve their communication skills and also highlight the strengths and dangers in the explosion of social media.

Chapter 7 provides helpful case studies and examples to illustrate how the law has been applied in the maternity services. The section on female genital mutilation is particularly pertinent given the recent prosecution of a mother in the UK. Chapters 8 and 9 look at the scope of practice, including extended/advanced practice, whilst ensuring safety of mothers and babies. Chapter 9 also lists some useful tips for midwives who might be experiencing fear in their practice as midwives. Contrasts between safety in developing and developed countries are highlighted through safe motherhood and white ribbon alliance initiatives. Chapter 10 goes on to discuss employer-led models of midwifery supervision now that supervision is no longer a statutory requirement in the UK.

Different uses of terminology can be confusing and explanations about mentorship, preceptorship, coaching and assessment are discussed in Chapter 11. Clear understanding of these terms is likely to be even more important in the UK when the NMC removes the requirement for each student to work regularly with a named mentor. Research terminology is explained in Chapter 12 to demonstrate the hierarchy of evidence which underpins the science and art of midwifery practice.

The final three chapters, which can also stand alone, will benefit the reader if all are read in a similar time frame. The immense change in healthcare practice, education and research means that midwives cannot afford to stand still. These chapters challenge midwives to not just keep up to date with their professional development but to seek ways to innovate and consider a variety of career pathways. Transformational leadership and effective management are essential if the future needs of mothers and their families are to be met and enhanced.

Throughout the book the text is illustrated with excellent case studies, figures, tables and diagrams which will enhance learning and stimulate further critical enquiry. This book will be invaluable to students throughout their midwifery programme and will assist midwives in determining and realizing their career trajectory.

Diane M. Fraser, PhD, MPhil, BEd, MTD, RM, RGN
Professor Emeritus of Midwifery, University of Nottingham,
February 2019

Dr Kuldip Kaur Bharj, OBE PhD MSc BSc (Hons) FHEA MTD DN RM RN
Visiting Associate Professor
The University of Leeds
Leeds
UK

Professor Michelle Butler, PhD MSc BSc RM RN
Executive Dean
Faculty of Science and Health
Dublin City University
Dublin
Ireland

Dr Val Collington, PhD MSc DipN MTD, FHEA RM RN
Education Consultant and former Deputy Dean (KUSGUL)
Faculty of Health, Social Care and Education
Kingston University and St George's, University of London
London
UK

Lynne Cornford-Wood, MSc PGCEA ADM RM RN
Senior Lecturer (retired)
Department of Midwifery
School of Allied Health, Midwifery and Social Care
Faculty of Health, Social Care and Education
Kingston University and St George's, University of London
London
UK

Professor Hannah G Dahlen, FACM PhD Grad Cert (Pharm) MCommN BN (Hons), RM, RN
Professor of Midwifery
School of Nursing and Midwifery
Western Sydney University
Sydney
New South Wales
Australia

Dr Gina Finnerty, PhD BEd ADM, RM, RN
Senior Lecturer
Department of Family Care & Mental Health
Faculty of Education and Health
University of Greenwich
London
UK

Professor Jan Fook, PhD MSW BSW FAcSS
Professor and Head of Social Work
Department of Social Work
University of Vermont
Vermont
USA

Jane Forman, FHEA MSc PGCEA BSc RM RN
Senior Lecturer
Department of Midwifery
School of Allied Health, Midwifery and Social Care
Faculty of Health, Social Care and Education
Kingston University and St George's, University of London
London
UK

Lindsay J Gillman, FHEA MSc BSc (Hons) PGCEA RM RN
Associate Professor
Department of Midwifery
School of Allied Health, Midwifery and Social Care
Faculty of Health, Social Care and Education
Kingston University and St George's University of London
London
UK

Dr Julie M Harrison, PhD PGCEA BSc (Hons) ADM RM RN
Senior Lecturer (retired)
Department of Midwifery
School of Allied Health, Midwifery and
    Social Care
Faculty of Health, Social Care and Education
Kingston University and St George's,
    University of London
London
UK

Sima Hay, FHEA PGCAP MSc RM RN
Senior Lecturer
Department of Midwifery
School of Allied Health, Midwifery and
    Social Care
Faculty of Health, Social Care and Education
Kingston University and St George's,
    University of London
London
UK

Lesley Kay, SFHEA PhD MSt PGCME BSc (Hons) RM BA (Hons)
Associate Professor
Department of Midwifery
School of Allied Health, Midwifery and
    Social Care
Faculty of Health, Social Care and Education
Kingston University and St George's
    University of London
London
UK

Michelle Knight, PGCLTHE RM BSc
Lead Midwife: Normality / Honorary
    Lecturer (Kingston University and
    St George's, University of London)
Epsom and St Helier University Hospitals
    NHS Trust
Carshalton
UK

Carmel Lloyd, MEd, PGDip, PGCEA, ADM, RM RN
Head of Education and Learning and NMC
    Lead Midwife for Education
Royal College of Midwives
London
UK

Claire McKellow, FHEA SEDA MA BSc (Hons) RM RN
Senior Lecturer
Department of Midwifery
School of Allied Health, Midwifery and
    Social Care
Faculty of Health, Social Care and Education
Kingston University and St George's,
    University of London
London
UK

Professor Jayne E. Marshall, FRCM, PFHEA PhD MA PGCEA ADM RM RN
Foundation Professor of Midwifery and
    NMC Lead Midwife for Education
School of Allied Health Professions
College of Life Sciences
George Davies Centre
University of Leicester
Leicester
UK

Crecious Mutinta Muleya, MSc BSN RM RN
Midwifery Lecturer
Department of Midwifery, Women and
    Child Health
School of Nursing Sciences
University of Zambia
Lusaka
Zambia

Petra Petročnik, MSc (UK) RM
Senior Lecturer
Department of Midwifery
Faculty of Health Sciences
The University of Ljubljana
Ljubljana
Slovenia

Leontia Pillay SFHEA MSc PGCEA ADM RM RN
Senior Lecturer (retired)
Department of Midwifery
School of Allied Health, Midwifery and
    Social Care
Faculty of Health, Social Care and Education
Kingston University and St George's,
    University of London
London
UK

Lai Yen Polenz, MSc PGCEA ADM RM RN
Senior Lecturer (retired)
Department of Midwifery
School of Allied Health, Midwifery and
    Social Care
Faculty of Health, Social Care and Education
Kingston University and St George's,
    University of London
London
UK

Sarah Purdy, FHEA PGCert MA RM RN
Senior Lecturer
Department of Midwifery
School of Allied Health, Midwifery and
    Social Care
Faculty of Health, Social Care and Education
Kingston University and St George's,
    University of London
London
UK

Jessica Read, MSc BSc (Hons) RM RN
Regional Maternity Lead for London
NHS England London Region
London
UK

Lyndsey Smith, MSc RM
Consultant Midwife
Kingston Hospital NHS Foundation Trust
Galsworthy Road
Kingston-upon-Thames
UK

ACKNOWLEDGEMENTS

It is with pride and joy that I initiated and led the development of *Myles Professional Studies for Midwifery Education and Practice: Concepts and Challenges* and as a consequence have further contributed to the education and training of midwives about the very essence of being a professional in the 21st century. True to the title, the journey from start to finish has indeed been a challenge at times, but with great effort, determination and eventual relief, my ambition to edit a book that is predominantly written by midwifery academics and practitioners associated with my former employer, Kingston University and St George's, University of London, has been finally realized.

I am so very grateful to the many individuals whose support and assistance have made this possible, each in different ways.

- To the authors and co-authors of the chapters for their invaluable contributions in sharing their specific knowledge and experience for the benefit of the future midwife.
- To Emily Handford, my personal assistant at Kingston University and St George's, University of London, who strived in supporting me to acquire the manuscripts from the authors.
- To Dawn Aubrey (former Senior Lecturer in Midwifery at Kingston University and St George's, University of London) and Georgina Sims (Associate Professor, Head of Department of Midwifery and Lead Midwife for Education at Kingston and St George's, University of London) for the contributions they made in the initial stages of the development of Chapter 1 and Chapter 11, respectively
- To Alison Taylor, Veronika Watkins, Katie Golsby and Anne Collett from Elsevier for their endless support, patience and perseverance in seeing this project through
- To Paul, who put up with my frustrations, read through many draft manuscripts and always had faith in me to complete the project.

I am deeply indebted to you all.

Jayne E. Marshall
Foundation Professor of Midwifery, University of Leicester,
NMC Lead Midwife for Education and Visiting Professor,
Kingston University and St George's, University of London
January 2019

This book is dedicated to my late parents Mabel *and* Colin Marshall, *who both inspired me to follow my ambition to become the professional academic midwife I am today, always seeking out opportunities to develop myself as well as others.*

They were my *first teachers and mentors, but very importantly, the most honest of friends, who always gave me sound advice: I miss them greatly.*

Mabel Marshall: 1923–1998
Colin Marshall: 1922–2009

Background and Rationale for the Book's Development

It is well recognized that maternity services throughout the world are under constant review, with the call to improve care and safety for childbearing women, their babies and their families. This often impacts on midwifery practice and subsequently midwifery education. In addition, it has to be recognized that professions exist to serve society, and as society changes, so must the professions. This is true of the midwifery profession.

To be effective in their role, midwives are required to be knowledgeable of both the physiological processes and the increasing complexities surrounding childbirth; be good leaders, team members and responsible role models; be able to think critically and creatively and make appropriate decisions; use and advance the science of midwifery; participate in interprofessional collaborations to optimize childbirth/neonatal outcomes; grapple with increasing ethical dilemmas related to the constant advancement of technology; and demonstrate they are caring, compassionate, competent, good communicators, courageous, committed *and professional*. Without any doubt, taking all these factors into consideration, midwifery, like society, continues to undergo transformation.

Inspired by an earlier text, Professional Studies for Midwifery Practice, which was published in 2000, this new text aims to meet the demands of midwifery education and practice in the 21st century. The former book was written by midwife academics and practitioners from Nottingham, United Kingdom (UK), and edited by Professor Emeritus Diane Fraser, former Head of Midwifery Education at the University of Nottingham, and was totally reflective of midwifery practice in the UK. It is therefore fitting that the foreword to *Myles Professional Studies for Midwifery Education and Practice: Concepts and Challenges* has been written by Diane.

The aim of *Myles Professional Studies for Midwifery Education and Practice: Concepts and Challenges* is to address the many challenges midwife educationalists and practitioners face in preparing future generations of midwives to be safe, competent and confident in providing appropriate care to a diverse and increasingly complex and multicultural childbearing population. Each chapter has been written by midwife academics from the former School of Midwifery (now Department of Midwifery) at Kingston University and St George's, University of London, with knowledge, expertise and interest in the specific subject area, in collaboration with international colleagues and midwives from clinical practice. This has ensured the content is grounded in sound reasoning and safe practice based on the fundamental role of the midwife. Coming under the internationally renowned 'Myles family' brand, this new addition is aimed not only at student midwives as a resource for them to assimilate specific knowledge and understanding of the professional issues, concepts and challenges facing the 21st century midwife but also at registered practising midwives as a textual aid to support their continuing professional development.

How to Use the Book

Each of the 15 chapters is designed to be read independently and used as stand-alone content according to the specific learning needs of the reader, and thus they can be read in any order. However, there is some degree of progression in how the chapters are presented. The earlier chapters explore what it means to become a professional, including the fundamental elements that enable midwives to develop into autonomous and accountable practitioners, such as effective communication skills, having understanding of the conceptual and philosophical basis of midwifery and appreciating the value of using reflection and intuition to guide professional practice and decision-making.

As it is widely appreciated that childbirth is associated with high litigation costs, delivering contemporary maternity and neonatal care can be extremely challenging for midwives as they should always ensure that supporting women's choice is finely balanced with safety and risk. Chapters that explore these issues, including the extent that midwives should be cognizant of ethical and legal aspects associated with childbirth (as well as within midwifery education), are included in the book for midwives to explore more extensively and in true context.

It is vital that midwives fully understand their scope of practice, professional boundaries and responsibilities in ensuring their knowledge and skills remain contemporary as new developments in maternity and neonatal care arise, some practices of which may become an integral part of the role of the midwife. Consequently, the later chapters address not only the importance of continuing professional development, professional revalidation and the various career options open to midwives but also the role that research/evidence-based practice, leadership and management, and change and innovation play in advancing all aspects of midwifery education and practice.

Strengths and Limitations

During the development of the book, notable changes occurred within the midwifery profession in the UK, and these have been captured in the contents (e.g. major professional regulatory reform, the demise of statutory supervision and the emergence of employer-led supervision as well as introduction of new standards for student supervision and assessment). This will be the first time that such detail has been presented in a professional studies book, which will add to the originality and its contemporary appeal. However, at the time of publication, the UK Nursing and Midwifery Council is developing new standards for pre-registration midwifery education and thus the final detail was not available to include in this book. Nevertheless, an attempt has been made to 'future-proof' the composition of these new standards in order to raise awareness, stimulate debate and guide the reader into considering new approaches in educating and supporting future student midwives and newly qualified midwives, such as adopting coaching principles.

Format of the Book

The format of the chapters is consistent throughout the book, in that all chapters contain learning outcomes at the outset, with key points clearly stated at the end that act as a summary and revision aid. Theoretical concepts and models provide the basic structure of each chapter. Real-life case scenarios and reflective activities, as well as figures and tables, aim to illustrate the application of the theoretical components more effectively and draw comparisons across an international context, stimulating enquiry and a desire for new knowledge. Furthermore, annotated reading lists and significant websites provide additional resources for the reader to use, particularly those insatiable for further learning opportunities. Although this book aims to address the many issues student midwives and midwives may have regarding their professional practice, it is anticipated that it may also raise further questions and initiate debate to further inform contemporary midwifery education and practice.

Jayne E. Marshall
Leicester 2019

CHAPTER 1

Becoming a Midwife: The History and Socialization Into Professional Practice

Kuldip Kaur Bharj　▪　Jayne E. Marshall

LEARNING OUTCOMES

By the end of this chapter the reader will:

- have an understanding of the historical developments in midwifery that have shaped contemporary midwifery education and practice
- appreciate the controversies surrounding the social context in which childbirth takes place
- be cognizant of what a profession is and what professionalism actually means
- understand the value of shaping a professional identity in becoming a midwife
- be aware of the factors contributing to effective socialization of midwives into the workplace

Overview

This chapter explores the ways in which midwives become socialized into the maternity services. It provides an overview of the history of the changing social context of childbirth and how developments in midwifery education have served in raising the societal profile of the midwife. Having an understanding of what constitutes a profession and having an understanding of how professionalism is defined are key elements to *becoming a midwife*. In addition to examining the role that the various workplace settings play in the process of a midwife's socialization, the factors that shape professional identity in becoming a midwife will also be debated. Within the chapter are activities for the reader to undertake to assist them in contextualizing the theory that is presented and support them in being an effective health professional within contemporary maternity services.

Introduction

Recruitment to midwifery education programmes in recent years has been characterized by a marked interest in midwifery as a profession, and Higher Education Institutions (HEIs) saw an increase in applications; however, the number of applicants to midwifery programmes in England has fallen each year since 2013. It is likely, however, that the media interest in birth and midwifery, epitomized by popular television programmes such as *Call the Midwife* and *One Born Every Minute,* bringing midwifery to the notice of a wider audience, has inspired viewers to consider midwifery as a career (Royal College of Midwives [RCM] 2012). Whilst it is recognized that such programmes popularize childbirth and midwifery, it is debatable as to what extent such depictions are realistic or desirable. Furthermore, it can be questioned that in some instances the media portrayals serve only to fuel misconceptions about the role of the midwife and the nature of childbirth (Boden 2012).

On entry to the profession, students embark on a process of *professional socialization*, which is the means whereby individuals internalize the characteristics, attributes, attitudes and values of a given profession that results in the formation of a sense of identity and commitment to a professional field. It begins on recruitment into professional education programmes and continues with the entry into the workforce (Mackintosh 2006). Given the social nature of the process, it is influenced by the culture of the organizations in which it takes place; that is, both education institutions and maternity care settings. These concepts will be explored throughout this chapter, beginning with a brief overview of the historical context of midwifery practice and delivery of maternity care, as this is well documented elsewhere in other texts.

The History of the Social Context of Midwifery

Contemporary maternity services are seen as essential public health services, playing a key role in improving health and reducing inequalities. According to the NHS England (2016: 8) *Better Births* report, the overall vision for the maternity services in England

> *is for them to become safer, more personalised, kinder, professional and more family friendly; where every woman has access to information to enable her to make decisions about her care; and where she and her baby can access support that is centred around their individual needs and circumstances.*

The premise behind this vision, as in other countries, is that maternity services should be flexible and individualized, designed to fit around the needs of the woman, her baby and her family's journey through pregnancy, childbirth and parenthood. Women and their partners should be supported and encouraged to experience childbirth as a physiological phenomenon. Medical intervention may be required but only in instances where it will be of benefit to the woman and/ or her baby. Midwifery and obstetric care should always be based on the best available evidence to ensure good clinical and psychological outcomes for the woman and her baby. However, this has not always been the case in the history of midwifery as the controversies around the place of birth and medicalization of childbirth have demonstrated.

SHIFT OF PLACE OF BIRTH

In the early 1900s, most women in the United Kingdom (UK) were attended by female friends and relatives during childbirth, with the place of birth predominantly in the home (Oakley 1984). However, in the latter part of the 20th century, birth was transformed from a social, domestic event into a highly technological, medical procedure where care was provided and managed by health care professionals within a hospital setting (Macfarlane and Campbell 1994), propelled by the philosophy that hospitals were places of greater safety (Oakley 1986; Towler and Bramall 1986; Donnison 1988). As childbirth became more hospitalized, it became *'doctors' business'* (Doyal 1995), based on the assumption that they were superior in knowledge to midwives (Oakley 1986; 2000; Donnison 1988). As a consequence, the role of midwives became subordinate to that of doctors, giving doctors a competitive advantage by reducing midwives' power and status. Many midwives and women opposed these moves, but even the lack of evidence that hospital births were safer than home births made little difference to the prevailing ideology; maternity care remained hospital centred and has continued to be so into the 21st century.

MEDICALIZATION OF CHILDBIRTH

Much has been written about the growth of power of the medical profession, with the increased involvement of obstetricians in childbirth and the role this played in its medicalization (Stacey 1988; Wraight et al 1993). With hospitalization, childbirth was increasingly treated like an illness, subjected to greater use of technology and intervention (Oakley 1984; Arney 1985; Devries 1989; Kitzinger 1990). The process of childbirth, once a *normal* event, became viewed as *pathological* and *a risk*; and its associated dangers meant it was normal only in retrospect (see Chapter 9). With this prevailing ideology, childbirth required a medical expert to oversee the event (Murphy-Lawless 1998; Kent 2000) and consequently the hospital setting for birth was regarded as appropriate because emergency facilities were readily available (Maternity Services Advisory Committee 1982, 1984; Oakley 1984).

Doctors took control of negotiating the demarcation between normal and abnormal, exerting professional dominance over midwives and women, thereby disempowering them (Oakley 1984), a process that was aided and abetted by patriarchal ideology, underpinned by oppressive discourses (Pateman 1989; Starhawk 1990), bound within which were concepts of power and knowledge. With doctors' knowledge professed to be superior (Oakley 2000), women and midwives found themselves increasingly dependent on medical science and technology, with a widespread view emerging that *'doctor knows best'*. The dominant values and beliefs that underpinned the medical model were supported and reinforced by many social groups, including midwives. Midwives had become socialized into this model of care and, arguably, over time became technocrats and managers of labour using intervention and invasive techniques, consequently at the expense of eroding their competence in physiological childbirth (Oakley 1984; Bryar 1995).

THE EMERGENCE OF WOMAN-CENTRED CARE

Towards the latter half of the 20th century, there was resistance to medical control from both midwives and women's organizations, such as the National Childbirth Trust (NCT) and the Association for Improvements in Maternity Services (AIMS). These organizations campaigned for accessible maternity services and individualized midwifery care, urging increased choice and greater control over childbirth for women, reduced medical intervention and increases in natural childbirth (Kitzinger 1990; Durward and Evans 1990). Although schemes to improve maternity care were pioneered (Flint et al 1989), it was the publication of the *Winterton Report* (Department of Health [DH] 1992) and *Changing Childbirth* (DH 1993) (the latter for which women had been consulted for the very first time to give their views and accounts of childbirth) which created the cornerstone of change. *Changing Childbirth* made far-reaching recommendations, placing the woman at the centre of care, proposing continuity and choice of care and making the place of birth and women's right to unbiased information central tenants of maternity services (DH 1993), this ideology becoming accepted in the maternity services as *woman-centred care* (Pope et al 2001), on the basis of which a range of innovative, woman-centred service models have subsequently developed.

The issues of choice, control and continuity have been the subject of much debate, but the recommendations advocated in *Changing Childbirth* have only paid lip service to the needs of women using the maternity services (Kirkham and Stapleton 2001). Inadequate national financial structure and lack of information for women about their choices have meant the concept of choice, control and continuity remains rhetoric for some women (Hunt and Symonds 1995; Kirkham and Stapleton 2001; Stapleton et al 2002).

The juncture of the 20th and 21st centuries saw a number of government directives to modernize the National Health Service (NHS) (DH 1997, 1999, 2000, 2006), leading to a major restructuring programme, bringing dramatic changes to the way health and social care were planned and delivered. Models emerged, shifting services from hospitals into the community, opening up the competition and giving service users more choice, control and a voice in the way services were planned and delivered. The focus on childbirth continues with the concepts of safety and quality at the heart of the NHS's maternity services (Vincent 2010; Berwick 2013; Vincent and Amalberti 2016).

The focus on improving maternity services is not surprising given the evidence that midwifery makes a difference to the lives of women and their newborn babies worldwide by contributing to the reduction in maternal and infant mortality and recognizing that midwives are essential in providing high-quality maternal and neonatal care in all settings (Homer et al. 2014; Renfrew et al. 2014a; ten Hoope-Bender et al. 2014; Van Lerberghe et al. 2014). The National Maternity Review (NHS England 2016), culminating in the publication of *Better Births*, articulated the aforementioned vision recommending that maternity services must provide safe and personalized care, continuity of carer, better postnatal and perinatal mental health care and multiprofessional and across-boundary working with a fair payment system. Furthermore, the report highlighted the pivotal role that midwives and other health professionals play in providing woman-centred care and consequently their need to be supported and valued to reduce attrition, which also supports the advice from Ball et al (2002) RCM (2016a).

SOCIETY-CHANGING DEMOGRAPHICS

The standard of midwifery practice and the quality of maternity care are critical in the reduction of global maternal and neonatal mortality, with midwives playing a key role in achieving this. It is an expectation that newly qualified midwives are knowledgeable, skilled and competent to deliver safe and compassionate midwifery care to childbearing women, their newborn babies and their families across the continuum from pre-pregnancy to during pregnancy, during childbirth, postpartum and during the early weeks of life and contexts. As Renfrew et al (2014b) state, the core characteristics of the midwife include optimizing normal biological, psychological, social and cultural processes of reproduction and early life, timely prevention and management of complications, consultation with, and referral to, other services, respecting women's individual circumstances and views, and working in partnership with women to strengthen the woman's own capabilities to care for themselves and their families. These characteristics are further endorsed within the professional framework developed by the International Confederation of Midwives (ICM) that determines the role and scope of a midwife's practice within the country in which they practise (see Chapter 8).

It has been highlighted that midwives continue to experience unprecedented change as a result of ongoing maternity services developments, including scientific and technological advances, the emergence of woman-centred care and focus on safety and quality. Adding to the complexities of their role is accommodating the changing and diverse demographical profile of childbearing women. Official figures indicate that the proportion of births in England and Wales to women born outside the UK has continued to rise (Office for National Statistics (ONS) 2017). Many of these women do not speak English as their first language and may require additional support to access maternity services. Furthermore, the most disadvantaged and vulnerable women and babies in society are the most likely to die or suffer from ill health (Knight et al 2017). As a result, the midwifery role can be powerful in supporting these women and managing diversity. The development of specialist midwifery roles and services (e.g. public health, substance misuse, homelessness, diabetes, obesity) contributes to improving outcomes and experiences of care and reducing inequalities.

Organizational Culture and Woman-Centred Care

Midwives have been working for many decades within a complex and demanding environment (Yoshida and Sandall 2013; Young et al 2015) characterized by its masculinized organizational culture and coupled with the oppressive medical model of childbirth. Consequently, Scamell (2016) purports that midwives are often in conflict with organizational prescriptions and their personal philosophies of providing women-centred care. For example, many midwives endeavour to support women to give birth naturally through harnessing holistic, compassionate and personalized care; however, they are often working in settings which are shaped by a culture of fear, risk management and governance structures. The dilemma midwives may find themselves in could be likened to street-level bureaucrats, which Lipsky (1980: 4) affirms

> are constantly torn by the demands of service recipients to improve effectiveness and responsiveness and by the demands of citizen groups to improve the efficacy and efficiency of government services.

In addition, to negotiate work pressures, street-level bureaucrats also modify their own expectations, values, attitudes and behaviours. The context in which midwives work is polarized in that the way in which they wish to work is inhibited by the organizational culture. As a consequence, there are many midwives who are becoming frustrated with working within the constraints of the organizations and workloads, and those who are unable to give women the best care in the way advocated by the government proposals are either leaving the profession or working independently (RCM 2016a). Midwives who continue to work within the environment where there is conflict between ideals and practice are likely to experience stress and/or burnout on the one hand and emotional labour on the other.

Nonetheless, the midwifery profession has continued to work in partnership with women, influencing the development of new service models, including small group practices based on the social enterprise model, to promote normality in childbirth, focus on specific inequalities and meet the diverse needs of vulnerable women and those from disadvantaged backgrounds. However, the growth of maternity care providers other than the NHS providers, such as the voluntary sector, private sector and social enterprise, has been slow to develop to provide childbearing women with a *real* choice in the services they want and need. Notwithstanding this, midwives have seized the opportunity to use care pathways and managed maternity care networks, ensuring that they work in partnership with the multiprofessional team in determining that the care childbearing women receive is always safe and of high quality.

Key Developments in Midwifery Education

The ICM aims to strengthen midwifery worldwide through midwifery education ensuring midwives have the requisite qualifications to be registered and/or legally licensed to practise midwifery and use the title *midwife* and demonstrate competency in the practice of midwifery (ICM 2017) (see Chapter 2). Pre-registration midwifery education and training equips midwifery students with the competencies for entry into the profession so that they can work as qualified midwives, and has developed over time to meet the health and social care needs of the childbearing woman, her baby and her family. However, wide inconsistencies exist in the nature and content of education programmes, including regulation of practice and professional midwifery associations between countries (Fullerton et al 2013). The potential impact of these inconsistencies is that the preparation of practitioners and the provision of maternal and neonatal care is likely to differ across and between countries. Globally, educators are challenged in providing learning opportunities to ensure that future practitioners acquire necessary competencies to deliver maternal and neonatal care advocated by the ICM (2018) and within the model developed in the *Lancet* series (Renfrew et al 2014a).

THE MOVE TO HIGHER EDUCATION AND BECOMING AN ALL-GRADUATE PROFESSION

In the UK, the Nursing and Midwifery Council (NMC) (2007) determined that all pre-registration midwifery education programmes in the UK should be at degree level by 2008, with the ultimate aim of the profession becoming all graduate. A decade earlier, in the mid-1990s, midwifery education transferred from the NHS to the higher education sector, along with nurse education. Such a move served in raising the societal profile of midwives and the midwifery profession as well as providing academic staff and students with access to a wider range of educational and research resources to support their studies and continuing professional development. However, the severance from the NHS has created *a distance* between academic and clinical midwives that requires effort on both parts to ensure the partnership is always effective and conducive to student learning.

The length of study is currently 4600 hours, which is divided between theory and practice, of which at least 50% has to be undertaken in practice (NMC 2009). This is usually completed in 3 years based on a 45-week year, albeit a small number of programmes are 4 years in length and follow a traditional shorter academic year. A much reduced number of HEIs offer shortened programmes into midwifery for registered nurses on the adult part of the professional register, some of which are at postgraduate level. All midwifery education programmes, regardless of level, have to comply with the NMC (2009) pre-registration midwifery education standards.

The role of the midwives has evolved quite rapidly in this century; however, the NMC standards have not kept pace with the changes and new standards have been developed and will be published in 2020 for full adoption by 2021. However, it is the responsibility of all HEIs to ensure their pre-registration midwifery education programmes prepare midwives who are competent and safe to deliver appropriate care that women, their newborn babies and their families deserve and need. Whilst waiting for the revised standards, many HEIs have drawn upon *The Code* (NMC 2018), contemporary health policy and other evidence such as Renfrew et al (2014a) to inform their curricula delivery.

Becoming a Midwife and Shaping a Professional Identity

Understanding the tenets of the midwifery profession is a vital component of being socialized into the profession (i.e. *becoming a midwife*). The place of birth and the model by which maternity care is delivered can influence the extent that midwives fulfil their midwifery role and protect their professional identity. Becoming a midwife is achieved through successful completion of the theoretical *and* practical components of a midwifery education programme by the student satisfying the professional statutory regulatory body's education standards as well as the approved education institution's/HEI's academic regulations. In the UK, this would be the NMC and the higher education sector, respectively. During this process, it is expected that the student will develop into a midwife who will uphold the profession's standards. More discussion about the professional regulation of midwifery can be found in Chapter 2.

DEFINING A PROFESSION

A profession is an occupation that is based on a specialized body of knowledge and skills, where entry is restricted to individuals who demonstrate their competence in the subject area and practice is undertaken in accordance with specific rules of self-regulation and ethical codes of conduct, which ultimately benefit those whom the professional serves.

PROMOTING PROFESSIONALISM

The four chief nursing officers in the UK have launched a framework (Fig. 1.1) around enabling professionalism in midwifery and nursing that is supported by the NMC (2017). Professionalism is determined by the autonomous evidenced-based decision-making by members of an occupation who share the same values and line of work and is vital to delivering safe and high-quality care to childbearing women, their babies and their families. The framework embraces *The Code* (NMC 2018) through the attributes or prerequisites of midwifery and nursing practice:

- accountable (practise effectively)
- a leader (promoting professionalism and trust)
- an advocate (prioritizing people)
- competent (preserving safety).

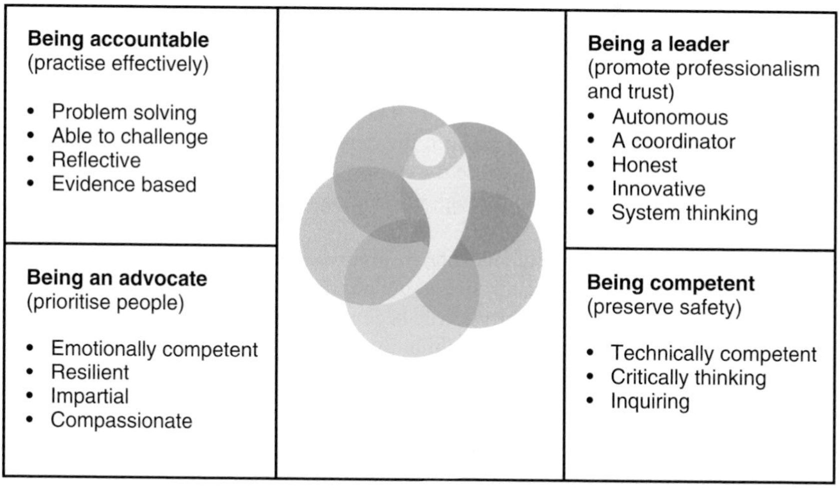

Being accountable
(practise effectively)

- Problem solving
- Able to challenge
- Reflective
- Evidence based

Being a leader
(promote professionalism and trust)

- Autonomous
- A coordinator
- Honest
- Innovative
- System thinking

Being an advocate
(prioritise people)

- Emotionally competent
- Resilient
- Impartial
- Compassionate

Being competent
(preserve safety)

- Technically competent
- Critically thinking
- Inquiring

Fig. 1.1 Enabling professionalism framework (NMC 2017).

It is acknowledged that organizational and environmental factors are crucial in supporting and enabling professional practice and behaviours. The NMC (2017) defines an environment that promotes professionalism as one that:

- recognizes and encourages midwifery leadership
- encourages autonomous innovative practice
- enables positive interprofessional collaboration
- enables practice learning and development
- provides appropriate resources.

However, employers need to provide the systems and conditions for midwives to continually develop and practise safe care, which is becoming increasingly challenging where services are under-resourced and societal health and social care needs are becoming more complex and demanding. The framework of enabling professionalism (NMC 2017) explores how various strategies can support and promote professional practice and behaviour within the workplace as well as identifying the ways in which the individual midwife should uphold their professional practice, such as raising concerns when issues arise that could compromise safety, quality and experience.

Now undertake Activity 1.1.

ACTIVITY 1.1 ■

With Fig. 1.1 as a guide, determine the factors (positive and negative) that affect the professionalism within the environments in which you learn and work.
Provide examples of how the following may (or may not) contribute to promoting professionalism:
- leadership
- autonomous, innovative practice
- interprofessional collaboration
- practice learning and development
- resources.

To what extent can you/do you contribute to promoting professionalism in your role and practice area?

Many students enter the midwifery profession with the goal of facilitating a healthy birth outcome for the childbearing woman, her baby and her family, but how this goal is translated into practice is not entirely clear until they begin their education as a student midwife. Becoming a student midwife is the first step in their socialization into professional practice, the goal of which is the development of professionalism. The overarching aim of midwifery education is more than teaching students how to perform the requisite clinical skills, and includes how to educate them to think like a midwife, to see the context of health care through the lens of midwifery and to develop professionalism through responding to the effects of both theoretical and clinical experiences.

This process requires the student midwife to internalize new knowledge, skills, attitudes, behaviours, values and ethical standards and assimilate these as part of their own professional identity. Professional socialization of the midwife begins during formal midwifery education programmes and will continue as they practise within the real world.

Socialization Into the Work Setting

Socialization is complex, diverse and unpredictable, and it has both positive and negative consequences (Dinmohammadi et al 2013). Positive outcomes are the acquisition of a professional identity and the ability to cope with professional roles, combined with professional and organizational commitment. Negative forms of socialization can cause undesired consequences, such as frequent turnover of staff, continuance of ritualized practice and bureaucratic views, role ambiguities, lack of critical thinking, increased attrition and gradual desensitization in relation to the needs of childbearing women, their babies and their families.

MODELS OF PROFESSIONAL SOCIALIZATION

A number of models of professional socialization in nursing have emerged (Bandura 1977; Benner 1984; Cohen 1981) that midwifery educationalists and clinicians can use to effect successful socialization into the work setting. The well-known stages of nursing proficiency (Benner 1984) as seen in Table 1.1 demonstrate how learning theories can be applied to adult skill acquisition through five stages: *novice, advanced beginner, competent practitioner, proficient practitioner* and *expert practitioner*.

The *first stage* (*novice*) begins when the student midwife begins their midwifery education programme. They generally have little background on which to base their behaviour in the practice setting and so will depend rather rigidly on rules and expectations that are established for them as their practical skills are limited. Progressing to the *second stage* (*advanced beginner*), the student midwife will have established that a particular order exists in the practice setting and their performance is slightly competent. Whilst they are able to base their actions on their knowledge of theoretical principles, at this stage they may experience difficulty in formulating priorities, believing that many approaches are equally important. As the student midwife acquires more experience, about 2–3 years in the practice setting, they reach the *third stage* (*competent practitioner*), where for most of the time they feel competent, organized and efficient in their practice such that they are able to coordinate several complex demands at the same time. A competent midwife is able to recognize that situations can change quickly and it is essential to plan their work schedule to ensure that midwifery care is provided, even when emergencies or unexpected events occur. The *fourth stage* (*proficient practitioner*) occurs when the midwife has been in practice for 3–5 years, and is able to see midwifery situations holistically rather than in parts and easily recognize priorities for care. These midwives would usually be leaders of their practice area, having a wealth of knowledge and experience with confidence to be flexible and adaptable to the needs of others. The *fifth stage* (*expert practitioner*) is reached after extensive practice experience and is assigned to those midwives who perform intuitively, without conscious thought, automatically grasping the needs of the childbearing woman, such that their expertise appears to come naturally.

In comparison, Cohen's (1981) model of basic student socialization, as seen in Table 1.2, has four stages based on developmental theory in which a positive outcome in each of the sequential stages is necessary for successful socialization to occur. However, unlike the model of Benner (1984), this model has so far not been tested for its validity.

The *first stage* (*unilateral dependence*) is where, because of their lack of knowledge and experience, student midwives rely on external limits and rules established by those in authority, such as their

TABLE 1.1 ■ **Stages of Nursing Proficiency**

Stage	Behaviours
1. Novice	Has little background and limited practical skills; relies on rules and expectations of others for direction
2. Advanced beginner	Has slightly competent skills; uses theory and principles much of the time; experiences difficulty establishing priorities
3. Competent practitioner	Feels competent, organized; plans and sets goals; thinks abstractly and analytically; coordinates several tasks at the same time
4. Proficient practitioner	Views patients holistically; recognizes subtle changes; sets priorities with ease; focuses on long-term goals
5. Expert practitioner	Performs flexibly; grasps patient needs automatically; responses are integrated; expertise comes naturally

From Benner (1984).

TABLE 1.2 ■ **Model of Basic Socialization**

Stage	Key Behaviours
1. Unilateral dependence	Reliant on external authority; limited questioning or critical analysis
2. Negative/independence	Cognitive rebellion; diminished reliance on external authority
3. Dependence/mutuality	Reasoned appraisal; begins integration of facts and opinions following objective testing
4. Interdependence	Collaborative decision-making; commitment to professional role; self-concept now includes professional role identity

From Cohen (1981).

lecturers and mentors/practice supervisors, and are less likely to question others. In the *second stage* (*negative/independence*), the student midwives' critical-thinking abilities increase and they begin to question authority figures and rely more on their own judgement, known as *cognitive rebellion* (Cohen 1981). The *third stage* (*dependence/mutuality*) is where the student midwife develops a more reasoned appreciation of others' ideas and learns to test concepts, facts, ideas and models more objectively. As a result, the student midwife develops more sophisticated critical-thinking skills and becomes impartial, accepting some ideas and rejecting others. In the *fourth stage* (*interdependence*), the student midwives' needs for independence and sharing with others (mutuality) are drawn together as they develop the ability to make decisions in collaboration with others. Student midwives successfully socialized into midwifery practice complete this stage with a self-concept that includes a midwifery role identity that is both personally and professionally acceptable and compatible with their other life roles. Such student midwives are usually highly self-directed, often seeking out learning opportunities to maximize their knowledge before completing their midwifery education programme.

Now undertake Activity 1.2.

ACTIVITY 1.2 ■

Using one of the models of professional socialization and the stage at which you are at in your midwifery studies/midwifery career, decide which of the behaviours identified in the model best describe the extent of your professional socialization.

- Give examples from practice that would serve in providing evidence that you have indeed acquired this level of professional socialization.
- How will you prepare/what will you need to demonstrate to get to the next stage of the chosen model?
- How will you know that you have achieved this?

THE STUDENT EXPERIENCE

Despite the initial attraction of being recruited into the midwifery profession as a student midwife, the RCM (2014) report that an increasing number of students choose not to stay and consequently attrition rates appear to be rising. The reasons for student attrition are complex and multifactorial but may include a variety of '*personal*' reasons such as family circumstances, stress and the overwhelming clinical and academic demands of the programme (Green and Baird 2009; Hughes 2013). The '*wrong career choice*' has also been cited by some students. However, Hughes (2013) suggests that academically able and goal-orientated students enter a programme with expectations of practice environments which focus on normality and midwives who act as advocates and empower women, but instead encounter a discrepancy between this ideology and the reality. Students' experience of practice environments is that they are inadequately funded and provide limited services, have staff shortages and have an increasing number of complex births (RCM 2011, 2016a).

Miles (2008) identifies the skilled *presentation of self* that students need to project to ensure a favourable reception from midwives, balancing being reticent and unassuming with being assertive enough to gain knowledge and skills. Such complex manipulation of this relationship reflects the notion of Goffman's (1959) *presentation of self* where individuals attempt to control the impression they are making on others. With use of an analogy where *social interactions* are regarded as *a performance*, all actors in a scene are required to collude in the *reality*; thus students play their subservient role and midwives assume and exert power. In their doing so, the status quo is maintained, which confirms and perpetuates the reality of the situation.

Box 1.1 provides strategies for the student midwife to actively participate in their own professional socialization so as to successfully develop their own professional identity (Black 2014).

Now undertake Activity 1.3.

ACTIVITY 1.3 ■

Recall your first day in the following environments:
- university
- maternity unit
- birthing centre
- woman's home.

Make a list of the feelings you had about how you would *fit in* to each of the different settings.
- How did you prepare for your first day?
- What socialization strategies did you use?
- Which strategies have worked so far?
- How do you anticipate continuing the development of your own professional identity as a graduate midwife/lifelong learner?

Draw up an action plan of the strategies that you may use to achieve this, using *SMART* objectives (*S*pecific, *M*easurable, *A*chievable, *R*ealistic and *T*imely) to assist you in achieving your goal.

Becoming a Midwife: The Reality

The transition from student to health care practitioner is recognized as a stressful time as the new registrant faces the challenges of clinical decision-making, autonomous practice, developing a professional identity and dealing with new working environments and colleagues. Being a student may well have buffered student midwives from the realities of working life as a midwife and the

---

BOX 1.1 ■ Strategies for Active Participation in Professional Socialization

- Actively involve yourself in the learning process.
- Keep your goal in mind: you are temporarily uncomfortable but will ultimately get something you want (e.g. degree, promotion, sense of self-confidence, personal growth).
- Keep your perspective. It is your choice to undertake studies.
- Set aside preconceived ideas, prejudices and habits. Give yourself and the university/practice placement experience a chance.
- Open up your creative side and your abstract thinking and be willing to engage in hypothetical thinking. Everything may not be available in the practice placement setting to be of value.
- Be receptive to feedback, even if it is critical.
- Get a mentor/buddy for emotional support: another student, a midwife, an older friend, a relative or a member of the academic team.
- The university academic team are an important resource. They want to help but you need to ask for their guidance.

Adapted from Black (2014).

responsibilities of what is commonly referred to as *'practising under your own PIN'* (Professional Identification Number), a phrase that denotes the autonomy and responsibility of a practising registered midwife (Cescutti-Butler and Fisher 2016). The term *reality or transition shock* derived by Kramer (1974) when studying newly qualified nurses has been used to describe the phenomenon whereby they felt ill-prepared and shocked by the experience of clinical practice despite years of preparation as a student and has since been applied to other professional and occupational groups. The transition to qualified status in midwifery has been described as *tempestuous* (Hobbs 2012), and the metaphor relating to *sinking or swimming* has been used to describe this phase for new midwives (Hughes and Fraser 2011; Fenwick et al 2012). Studies from the United States of America, Ireland, and Australia indicate that this is not an issue confined to UK midwives (Fenwick et al 2012). The sense of responsibility that comes with that of being a registrant has been described as *overwhelming*, and is particularly acute when the newly registered midwife finds themselves as the only practising midwife in complex situations or in busy ward areas (Reynolds et al 2014).

SUPPORT AND PRECEPTORSHIP

Although newly registered practitioners are considered autonomous and accountable at the point of registration, it is recognized that they require support to develop further their competence and confidence, particularly in respect of developing their decision-making skills. This requirement is acknowledged and addressed by a period of practice referred to as *preceptorship*, during which time individuals are supported in their new role (see Chapter 11). Such a period of transition is a concept that exists across many professions, but has been increasingly directed towards health care (Foster and Ashwin 2014). Social relationships and support amongst peers and colleagues are not only significant for individuals in terms of health and emotional well-being but are vital in the development of clinical decision-making skills, an essential evolving component of midwifery practice. A lack of access to such support is likely to leave individuals professionally and socially isolated (Young 2012). A period of internship, *employed* within the maternity services during the final stage of the midwifery programme, may help the student midwife in making the transition to registered practising midwife with more confidence.

CONFORMING AND BEING ACCEPTED

Midwives beginning their first position may feel a need to gain acceptance from their colleagues; even if they are taking up employment in maternity units where they have previously undertaken clinical practice as a student midwife, they re-establish themselves in their new identity as a midwife, team member and co–worker so as to join the group. *Conformity* describes the strategic behaviour used by an individual to belong to a favoured group of people. However, such behaviour may not be as a result of a willingness or desire to belong, but may evolve from a fear of the consequences of *not* conforming and *not* being accepted (Grabowska 2016). Midwives who demonstrate non-conformity may be regarded as deviant and disruptive to the established social order of their working environment, consequently becoming scapegoats. However, *service and sacrifice* have been identified by Kirkham (1999) as core dispositions amongst midwives and included not taking breaks or days off and working overtime. Newly registered midwives continued with this disposition of service, working long hours and going without breaks to engender respect from colleagues and aid their integration into a team, rather than not conforming and being regarded as a deviant (Hobbs 2012). Furthermore, Begley (2002) highlights that many newly qualified midwives readily adapt and rapidly transition to registered midwife, but in so doing can appear to forget their recent experiences as student midwives and treat more junior students with the degree of irritation and intolerance that midwives may have previously demonstrated towards them. Consequently, this *'reinforcing'* cycle continues.

BULLYING AND BUILDING RESILIENCE

Bullying is an under-reported, widespread problem within the NHS and is evident within midwifery. The reasons for it may be multifactorial, associated with the working culture and tensions between a medical model and a social model of care resulting in conflict and lack of respect (Astrup 2015). Such interdisciplinary rivalry and disputes may impact on a working and clinical environment with serious and possibly fatal consequences for women and their families (Kirkup 2015). The disruptive intergroup behaviours exhibited amongst midwives categorized as *horizontal violence* which Leap (1997) acknowledges as including a lack of support for colleagues, failure to help out, negative comments and criticism, innuendo and backstabbing result in a hostile and intimidating working environment in which the new midwife registrant may be particularly vulnerable if their questions are perceived as challenging to more senior colleagues (Astrup 2015). For the individual, the consequences of being targeted may result in being unable to function effectively in their role, feeling unable to express themselves freely and enduring the impact of unfair criticism or inappropriate workloads (Ovayolu et al 2014).

A recent survey by the RCM (2016b) identified that a third of midwives had experienced bullying from colleagues in the previous year, with a significant number citing managers and service users as sources of harassment, intimidation and bullying. Respondents clearly described maternity units that are overworked and understaffed, organizations that relied on the goodwill of the staff to cope with the demands of the service. Hunger and dehydration were common phenomena as staff missed breaks. Those who became ill, that necessitated time off work felt under intense pressure to return and thought that managers were often unsupportive, focusing on mistakes rather than recognizing good work, consequently resulting in a *blame culture*. The burnout and stress experienced by midwives clearly impacts on their health and family life and ultimately may lead them to leave midwifery (RCM 2016b).

The ability to withstand the adverse workplace conditions in midwifery was examined by Hunter and Warren (2014), who highlighted that those midwives who were able to remain positive and motivated displayed self-knowledge and self-awareness, and the use of strategies to *switch off* and leave behind the stresses of daily work, through social support, distraction or physical activity. An additional theme identified was that of building *resilience* over time in both self and colleagues so as to foster a sustainable working environment. For the new registrant midwife this may be an additional aspect of the role that they need to develop or become an essential component that is nurtured during pre-registration midwifery education programmes. The emotional capabilities of midwives are valued by not only childbearing women and student midwives but also other colleagues. Furthermore, Byrom and Downe (2010) emphasize that a culture of mutual respect, empathy and fairness results in the empowerment of both women and staff with the creation of a *virtuous circle*, whereby one effective action leads to the creation of more effective actions that are integral to a satisfying and inspiring working environment.

Conclusion

This chapter has provided an overview of the changes in the social context of childbirth, including a number of challenges which could potentially provide a caustic environment for both childbearing women and maternity care professionals. Providing opportunities for midwives to develop their competence and acquire a greater understanding of professional and political drivers which shape maternity services are likely to equip them with the tools to bring about changes to promote an environment in which women can give birth safely and midwives can practise with confidence and with enthusiasm. Considering the ways in which socialization is an ongoing process which begins in the formal education programmes and continues in the practice learning environment, it is essential that student midwives are supported in developing their own professional identity from both the HEIs' and the maternity service providers' perspective. Activities within this chapter provide the reader with opportunities to put the theory into context, and the inclusion of models of professional socialization should help in supporting student midwives and newly qualified midwives to develop their own professional identity in the workplace and with transitioning into their future role as practising midwives and beyond.

KEY POINTS

- Professional socialization is a means whereby individuals internalize the attributes, attitudes and values of a given profession that results in the formation of a sense of identity and commitment to a professional field.
- Professional socialization is influenced by the culture of the organizations in which it takes place.
- The professional socialization of midwives has been influenced by working for many decades within a complex and demanding environment characterized by its masculinized organizational culture, coupled with the oppressive medical model of childbirth.
- The *Enabling Professionalism in Nursing and Midwifery Practice* framework (NMC 2017) can be used by midwives to uphold the principles of *The Code* (NMC 2018) in the delivery of high-quality midwifery and neonatal care.
- Models of professional socialization can be used to support student midwives' development and transition into the midwifery profession.
- Building *resilience* over time in both self and colleagues is essential to foster a sustainable working environment and should be an essential component of pre-registration midwifery education curricula.
- A culture of mutual respect, empathy and fairness results in the empowerment of both women and staff and supports the creation of a satisfying and inspiring working environment.

References

Arney, W. R. (1985). *Power and the profession of obstetrics*. Chicago: University of Chicago Press.

Astrup, J. (2015). Bullying: the writing's on the wall. *RCM midwives: The Official Journal of The Royal College Of Midwives, 18*, 37–41.

Ball, L., Curtis, P., & Kirkham, M. (2002). *Why do midwives leave?* Sheffield: University of Sheffield, Women's Informed Childbearing and Health Research Group.

Bandura, A. (1977). *Social learning theory*. Englewood Cliffs: Prentice-Hall.

Begley, C. (2002). 'Great fleas have little fleas': Irish student midwives' views of the hierarchy in midwifery. *Journal of Advanced Nursing, 38*(3), 310–317.

Benner, P. (1984). *From novice to expert: Excellence and power in clinical nursing practice*. Menlo Park: Addison-Wesley.

Berwick, D. (2013). *A promise to learn: a commitment to act; Improving the Safety of Patients in England National Advisory Group on the Safety of Patients in England*. Available at: https://www.gov.uk/government/uploads/system/uploads/attachment_data/file/226703/Berwick_Report.pdf.

Black, B. P. (2014). *Professional nursing: Concepts and challenges*. St. Louis: Elsevier.

Boden, G. (2012). Childbirth as entertainment. *AIMS Journal, 24*(4). Available at: https://www.aims.org.uk/journal/item/childbirth-as-entertainment.

Bryar, R. M. (1995). *Theory for midwifery practice*. Basingstoke: Macmillan.

Byrom, S., & Downe, S. (2010). 'She sort of shines': Midwives' accounts of 'good' midwifery and 'good' leadership. *Midwifery, 26*(1), 126–137.

Cescutti-Butler, L., & Fisher, M. (2016). *The hands-on guide to midwifery placements*. Chichester: John Wiley and Sons.

Cohen, H. (1981). *The nurse's quest for a professional identity*. Menlo Park: Addison-Wesley Publishing Co.

Department of Health. (1992). *Health Committee second report, session 1991-92: Maternity services. Winterton report*. London: Her Majesty's Stationery Office.

Department of Health. (1993). *Changing childbirth: Report of the Expert Maternity Group*. London: Her Majesty's Stationery Office.

Department of Health. (1997). *The new NHS: Modern and dependable*. London: Her Majesty's Stationery Office.

Department of Health. (1999). *Making a difference*. London: The Stationery Office.

Department of Health. (2000). *The NHS plan. A plan for investment, A plan for reform*. London: The Stationery Office.

Department of Health. (2006). *Our health, our care, our say: A new direction for community services*. White paper. Cm 6737. London: The Stationery Office.

Devries, R. G. (1989). Caregivers in pregnancy and childbirth. In Chalmers, I., Enkin, M., & Keirse, M. J. N. C. (Eds.), *Effective care in pregnancy and birth* (pp. 143–161). Oxford: Oxford University Press.

Dinmohammadi, M., Peyrovi, H., & Mehrdad, N. (2013). Concept analysis of professional socialization in nursing. *Nursing Forum, 48*(1), 26–34.

Donnison, J. (1988). *Midwives and medical men: A history of the struggle for the control of childbirth*. London: Historical Publications.

Doyal, L. (1995). *What makes women sick: Gender and the political economy of health*. Basingstoke: Macmillan.

Durward, L., & Evans, R. (1990). Pressure groups and maternity care. In Garcia, J., Kilpatrick, R & Richards, M. (Eds.), *The Politics of maternity care: Services for childbearing women in twentieth-century Britain*. Oxford: Clarendon Press.

Fenwick, J., Hammond, A., Raymond, J., Smith, R., Gray, J., Foureur, M., Homer, C., & Symon, A. (2012). Surviving, not thriving: a qualitative study of newly qualified midwives' experience of their transition to practice. *Journal of Clinical Nursing, 21*(13–14), 2054–2063.

Flint, C., Poulengeris, P., & Grant, A. (1989). The 'Know your Midwife Scheme' – a randomised trial of continuity of care by a team of midwives. *Midwifery, 5*(1), 11–16.

Foster, J., & Ashwin, C. (2014). Newly qualified midwives' experiences of preceptorship: A qualitative study. *MIDIRS Midwifery Digest, 12*(3), 301–305.

Fullerton, J. T., Thompson, J. B., & Johnson, P. (2013). Competency-based education: The essential basis of pre-service education for the professional midwifery workforce. *Midwifery, 29*(10), 1129–1136.

Goffman, E. (1959). *The presentation of self in everyday life*. New York: Anchor Books.

Grabowska, C. (2016). Conformity and conflict in maternity services. In Lindsay, P., & Peate, I. (Eds.), *Introducing the social sciences for midwifery practice* (pp. 71–86). Abingdon: Routledge.

Green, S., & Baird, K. (2009). An exploratory, comparative study investigating attrition and retention of student midwives. *Midwifery, 25*(1), 79–87.

Hobbs, J. A. (2012). Newly qualified midwives' transition to qualified status and role: assimilating the 'habitus' or reshaping it? *Midwifery, 28*(3), 391–399.

Homer, C. S., Friberg, I. K., Bastos Dias, M. A., ten Hoope-Bender, P., Sandall, J., Speciale, A. M., & Bartlett, L. A. (2014). The project effect of scaling up midwifery. *The Lancet, 384*(9948), 1146–1157.

Hughes, H. A. (2013). Factors influencing attrition rates in midwifery students. *Nursing Standard, 27*(26), 42–48.

Hughes, A. J., & Fraser, D. M. (2011). Sink or swim: the experience of newly qualified midwives in England. *Midwifery, 27*(3), 382–386.

Hunt, S. C., & Symonds, A. (1995). *The social meaning of midwifery*. Basingstoke: Macmillan.

Hunter, B., & Warren, L. (2014). Midwives' experiences of work place resilience. *Midwifery, 30*, 926–934.

International Confederation of Midwives. (2017). *Definition of the midwife*. Available at: https://www.internationalmidwives.org/assets/files/definitions-files/2018/06/eng-definition_of_the_midwife-2017.pdf.

International Confederation of Midwives. (2018). *Essential Competencies for midwifery practice*. Available at: https://www.internationalmidwives.org/our-work/policy-and-practice/essential-competencies-for-midwifery-practice.html.

Kent, J. (2000). *Social perspectives on pregnancy and childbirth for midwives, nurses and the caring professions*. Buckingham: Open University Press.

Kirkham, M. (1999). The culture of midwifery in the National Health Service in England. *Journal of Advanced Nursing, 30*(3), 732–739.

Kirkham, M., & Stapleton, H. (Eds.). (2001). *Informed choice in maternity care: An evaluation of evidence-based leaflets*. NHS Centre for Reviews and Dissemination, report 2. York: University of York.

Kirkup, B. (2015). *The report of the Morecambe Bay Investigation, Preston, Lancashire*. London: The Stationery Office. Available at: https://www.gov.uk/government/uploads/system/uploads/attachment_data/file/408480/47487_ MBI_Accessible_v0.1.pdf.

Kitzinger, J. (1990). Strategies of the early childbirth movement: a case study of the National Childbirth Trust. In Garcia, J., Kilpatrick, R. & Richards, M (Eds.), *The politics of maternity care: Services for childbearing women in twentieth-century Britain* (pp. 95–115). Oxford: Clarendon Press.

Knight, M., Nair, M., Tuffnell, D., Shakespeare, J., Kenyon, S., & Kurinczuk, J. J. (Eds.). Mothers and Babies: Reducing risk through Audits abd Confidential Enquiries across the UK (MBRRACE-UK). (2017). *Improving mothers' care - lessons learned to inform maternity care from the UK and Ireland confidential enquiries into maternal deaths and morbidity 2013–15.* Oxford: National Perinatal Epidemiology Unit, University of Oxford.

Kramer, M. (1974). *Reality shock: Why nurses leave nursing.* St. Louis: Mosby.

Leap, N. (1997). Making sense of 'horizontal violence' in midwifery. *British Journal of Midwifery, 5*(11), 689.

Lipsky, M. (1980). *Street-level bureaucracy, dilemmas of the individual in public services.* New York: Russell Sage Foundation.

Macfarlane, A., & Campbell, R. (1994). *Where to be born? The debate and the evidence* (2nd ed.). Oxford: National Perinatal Epidemiology Unit.

Mackintosh, C. (2006). The socialisation of pre-registration student nurses: A longitudinal qualitative descriptive study. *International Journal of Nursing Studies, 43*(8), 953–962.

Maternity Services Advisory Committee. (1982). *Maternity care in action part I: Antenatal care.* London: Her Majesty's Stationery Office.

Maternity Services Advisory Committee. (1984). *Maternity care in action part II: Care during childbirth (intrapartum care).* London: Her Majesty's Stationery Office.

Miles, S. (2008). Make or break: the importance of good mentorship. *British Journal of Midwifery, 16*(11), 704–711.

Murphy-Lawless, J. (1998). *Reading birth and death, a history of obstetric thinking.* Cork: Cork University Press.

National Health Service England. (2016). *Better births: Improving outcomes of maternity services in England. A five year forward view for maternity care.* Available at: https://www.england.nhs.uk/wp-content/uploads/2016/02/national-maternity-review-report.pdf.

Nursing and Midwifery Council. (2007). *Review of pre-registration midwifery education: Decisions made by the Midwifery Committee. Circular 14/2007.* London: Nursing and Midwifery Council.

Nursing and Midwifery Council. (2009). *Standards for pre-registration midwifery education.* London: Nursing and Midwifery Council.

Nursing and Midwifery Council. (2017). *Enabling professionalism in nursing and midwifery practice.* London: Nursing and Midwifery Council. Available at: https://www.nmc.org.uk/globalassets/sitedocuments/other-publications/enabling-professionalism.pdf.

Nursing and Midwifery Council. (2018). *The code: Professional standards of practice and behaviour for nurses, midwives and nursing associates.* London: Nursing and Midwifery Council.

Oakley, A. (1984). *The captured womb: A history of the medical care of pregnant women.* Oxford: Blackwell.

Oakley, A. (1986). *From here to maternity: becoming a mother.* Harmondsworth: Penguin.

Oakley, A. (2000). *Experiments in knowing: Gender and method in social sciences.* London: Polity Press in association with Blackwell Publishers.

Office for National Statistics. (2017). *Births by parents' country of birth, England and Wales: 2016. Annual statistics on live births.* Available at: https://www.ons.gov.uk/peoplepopulationandcommunity/birthsdeathsandmarriages/livebirths/bulletins/parentscountryofbirthenglandandwales/2016.

Ovayolu, O., Ovayolu, N., & Karadag, G. (2014). Workplace bullying in nursing. *Workplace Health and Safety, 62*(9), 370–374.

Pateman, C. (1989). *The disorder of women.* Cambridge: Polity Press.

Pope, R., Graham, L., & Patel, S. (2001). Woman-centred care. *International Journal of Nursing Studies, 38*, 227–238.

Renfrew, M. J., McFadden, A., Bastos, M. H., Campbell, J., Channon, A. A., Cheung, N. F., et al. (2014a). Midwifery and quality care: findings from a new evidence-informed framework for maternal and newborn care. *The Lancet, 384*, 1129–1145.

Renfrew, M. J., Homer, C. S. E., Downe, S., McFadden, A., Muir, N., Prentice, T., et al. (2014b). *Midwifery: an executive summary for the Lancet's series.* Available at: http://www.thelancet.com/pb/assets/raw/Lancet/stories/series/midwifery/midwifery_exec_summ.pdf.

Reynolds, E. ,K., Cluett, E., & Le-May, A. (2014). Fairy tale midwifery—fact or fiction: the lived experiences of newly qualified midwives. *British Journal of Midwifery, 22*(9), 660–668.

Royal College of Midwives. (2011). *The Royal College of Midwives survey of student midwives.* London: Royal College of Midwives.

Royal College of Midwives. (2012). Headlines: series success. *RCM midwives: The Official Journal of the Royal College of Midwives, 15*(2), 7.

Royal College of Midwives. (2014). The next generation. *RCM midwives: The Official Journal of the Royal College of Midwives, 17*(2), 17.

Royal College of Midwives. (2016a). *Why midwives leave – revisited*. London: Royal College of Midwives.

Royal College of Midwives. (2016b). *RCM campaign for healthy workplaces delivering high quality care. Caring for you campaign survey results*. London: Royal College of Midwives.

Scamell, M. (2016). The fear factor of risk – clinical governance and midwifery talk and practice in the UK. *Midwifery, 38*, 14–20.

Stacey, M. (1988). *The sociology of health and healing: A textbook*. London: Routledge.

Starhawk. (1990). *Truth or dare: Encounters with power, authority, and mystery*. San Francisco: Harper Collins.

Stapleton, H., Kirkham, M., Curtis, P., & Thomas, G. (2002). Framing information in antenatal care. *British Journal of Midwifery, 10*(4), 197–201.

ten Hoope-Bender, P., de Bernis, L., Campbell, J., Downe, S., Faveau, V., Fogstad, H., et al. (2014). Improvement of maternal and newborn health through midwifery. *The Lancet, 384*(9949), 1226–1235.

Towler, J., & Bramall, J. (1986). *Midwives in history and society*. London: Croom Helm.

Van Lerberghe, W., Matthews, Z., Achadi, E., Ancona, C., Campbell, J., Channon, A., et al. (2014). Country experience with strengthening of health systems and deployment of midwives in countries with high maternal mortality. *The Lancet, 384*, 1215–1225.

Vincent, C. (2010). *Patient safety*. Oxford: Wiley-Blackwell.

Vincent, C., & Amalberti, R. (2016). *Safer healthcare: Strategies for the real world*. New York: Springer.

Wraight, A., Ball, J., Seccombe, I., & Stock, J. (1993). *Mapping team midwifery*. IMS report series 242. Brighton: Institute of Manpower Studies, University of Sussex.

Yoshida, Y., & Sandall, J. (2013). Occupational burnout and work factors in community and hospital midwives: a survey analysis. *Midwifery, 29*, 921–926.

Young, N. (2012). An exploration of clinical decision-making among students and newly qualified midwives. *Midwifery, 28*(6), 824–830.

Young, C. M., Smythe, L., & McAraCouper, J. (2015). Burnout: lessons from the lived experience of case loading midwives. *International Journal of Childbirth, 5*, 154–165.

Further Reading

Edwards, N., Mander, R., & Murphy-Lawless, J. (Eds.). (2018). *Untangling the maternity crisis*. London: Routledge.

This contemporary text contains a compilation of writings from a number of authors and has at its heart to bring about 'best possible experiences of childbearing' for women and those caring for them..

The first part concentrates on the Birth Project Group survey (BPG), the second part addresses the traumatic experiences of women, midwives, families and wider communities and the final part explores practical and political strategies to bring about change within the maternity arena..

Mander, R., & Fleming, V. (2014). *Becoming a midwife* (2nd ed.). Abingdon: Routledge.

This second edition explores what it is to be a midwife, examining the factors that make midwifery such a special profession, alongside some of the challenges. It is suitable for those contemplating a career in midwifery and provides an opportunity for more experienced midwives to reflect on their careers to date. All chapter authors introduce their own theme and recount a vignette that throws light on their understandings of midwifery and reasons for becoming (or not becoming) a midwife and any subsequent career moves. Supported by commentaries and drawing together these insights, the editors demonstrate what it means to be a midwife today..

Mander, R., & Murphy-Lawless, J. (2013). *The politics of maternity*. Abingdon: Routledge.

This book explores the complex issues surrounding contemporary childbirth practices, analysing the current clinical, managerial and policymaking environments. It is designed to help professionals cope with the transition from education to the reality of the system within which they learn and practise in a changing healthcare work environment..

Useful Websites

Association for Improvements in Maternity Services: https://www.aims.org.uk

Caring Midwives: https://studentmidwife.net

International Confederation of Midwives: https://www.internationalmidwives.org/

The *Lancet* midwifery series: http://www.thelancet.com/series/midwifery

Midwife Diaries: https://midwifediaries.com

National Childbirth Trust: https://www.nct.org.uk

Royal College of Midwives: https://www.rcm.org.uk

CHAPTER 2

Standards for Midwifery Education and Professional Regulation

Jayne E. Marshall ▪ Carmel Lloyd

CONTENTS

LEARNING OUTCOMES

By the end of this chapter the reader should be able to:

- understand the rationale for the existence of global standards for midwifery education
- identify the standards and directives governing the design and delivery of pre-registration midwifery education programmes
- recognize the role of the regulator in monitoring midwifery education standards
- appreciate how the midwifery profession is regulated across the world
- recognize the principles of midwifery regulation and what it aims to achieve
- understand the history of midwifery regulation in the United Kingdom
- acknowledge the recent regulatory changes to midwifery regulation in the United Kingdom and their implications for midwives and midwifery practice
- reflect on the limitations of the regulation of individuals and the part that systems regulators play in ensuring the safety of the public.

Overview

This chapter explores the standards for midwifery education and professional regulation of midwives from an international and United Kingdom (UK) perspective. It provides an overview of the standards and directives governing pre-registration midwifery education programmes and identifies the role that the regulator plays in monitoring the standards are being maintained. The history of midwifery regulation in the UK from the Midwives Act of 1902 to the most recent changes in 2017 is discussed, including the introduction of revalidation and the removal of the regulatory framework for the supervision of midwives. The impact of public inquiries into failings within the National Health Service (NHS) that contributed to the need for regulatory reform is also discussed. Within the chapter are activities for readers to undertake to assist them in contextualizing the theory that is presented.

Introduction

Midwifery (and midwives as the primary professional group to provide midwifery care) is considered a vital solution to the challenges of providing high-quality maternal and newborn care for all women and newborns in all countries (Renfrew et al 2014). Several international organizations are involved in the strengthening of the midwifery profession, in particular the International Confederation of Midwives (ICM), the World Health Organization (WHO) and the United Nations Population Fund (UNFPA). With the aim of achieving global goals for sexual, reproductive, maternal and neonatal health, the ICM has identified three pillars for midwifery practice and development as shown in Fig. 2.1. These pillars consist of *education*, to provide a highly competent, qualified workforce; *regulation*, to set the scope of practice, and licensing and relicensing requirements ensuring that midwives provide high-quality midwifery care; and *association*, which

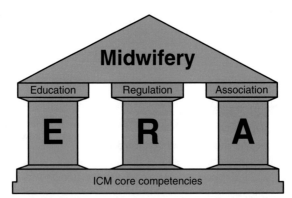

Midwives save lives with cost-effective, quality care. A strong midwifery profession is dependent on three interconnected pillars: Education of competent providers; ongoing supportive Regulation of those providers; and a strong professional Association. The essential Competencies for basic midwifery practice underpin these pillars. ICM Global Standards provide Midwives Associations and governments with frameworks to review and strengthen the supporting structures that create a professional midwifery workforce, responsive to the needs of its country and in line with international standards.

Fig. 2.1   International Confederation of Midwives' pillars: the foundation of a strong midwifery profession.

consists of 'an organised body of persons engaged in a common professional practice, sharing information, career advancement objectives, in-service training, advocacy and other activities' and supports the strengthening of the workforce (UNFPA and ICM 2016).

The ICM *Core Documents* set out the International Definition of the Midwife as shown in Box 2.1 (ICM 2017), the International Code of Ethics for Midwives (ICM 2014a) and the Philosophy and Model of Midwifery Care (ICM 2014b). The ICM has also published *Global Standards for Midwifery Education* (ICM 2013) and *Global Standards for Midwifery Regulation* (ICM 2011). These standards and the ICM founding values and principles provide a professional framework that can be used by midwifery associations, midwifery regulators, midwifery educators and governments to strengthen the midwifery profession and raise the standard of midwifery practice in their jurisdiction. By working within such a professional framework, midwives are supported and enabled to fulfil their role and contribute fully to the delivery of maternal and neonatal care in their country. These standards and founding values and principles will be discussed throughout the chapter.

Standards for Midwifery Education

The unprecedented changes in the health and maternity care landscape continue to prove a challenge to midwifery educationalists in that all pre-registration midwifery education standards continue to be fit for purpose, ensuring the future midwife is appropriately educated and trained to meet the demands of such a dynamic role wherever they practise. In addition, all midwifery education programmes should comply with the standards for pre-registration midwifery education, endorsed by the recognized professional regulatory body of the country in which the programme is undertaken, that are also guided by the *International Definition of the Midwife* (ICM 2017) as detailed in Box 2.1.

In the UK, it is a requirement that midwifery education programmes are developed in accordance with the ICM (2013) *Global Standards for Midwifery Education*, the European Union directive (2013/55/EU) for midwifery education and the Nursing and Midwifery Council (NMC) (2009a) pre-registration standards for midwifery education with the International Definition of the Midwife (ICM 2017) at their core.

BOX 2.1 ■ International Definition of the Midwife

'A midwife is a person who has successfully completed a midwifery education programme that is based on the ICM Essential Competencies for Basic Midwifery Practice and the framework of the ICM Global Standards for Midwifery Education and is recognized in the country where it is located; who has acquired the requisite qualifications to be registered and/or legally licensed to practise midwifery and use the title 'midwife'; and who demonstrates competency in the practice of midwifery.'

Reproduced with permission from International Confederation of Midwives (2017).

THE ICM GLOBAL STANDARDS FOR MIDWIFERY EDUCATION

The ICM global standards for midwifery education (ICM 2013) were developed in 2010 to strengthen midwifery worldwide by preparing fully qualified midwives to provide childbearing women, their babies and their families with high-quality, evidence-based health care. However, these standards represent the *minimum* expected from a quality midwifery programme with emphasis on competency-based education rather than academic degrees; that is, as detailed in *Essential Competencies for Basic Midwifery Practice* (ICM 2018).

All midwifery educationalists have the responsibility to ensure that the curriculum content aligns with but does *not* exceed the regulatory authority for midwifery practice in the specific country where the programme is delivered; however, this may include some knowledge and skills that the ICM would identify as *additional.* This would mean acquiring knowledge and skills that enhance the scope of practice, which might be particularly important depending on the environment in which the individual midwife practises (e.g. *life saving*).

EUROPEAN UNION DIRECTIVE 2013/55/EU

Under European Union law, midwifery and nursing are defined as sectoral professions, and through the *Professional Qualifications Directive (2005/36/EC)* (amended by *Directive 2013/55/EU*) they are part of the automatic recognition regime across European member states. However, with the decision of the UK Parliament in 2016 to withdraw from the European Union, the full effect that this will have on the future mobility of health professionals, and ultimately health care provision within the UK, remains uncertain. These directives specify the training requirements of midwives, including the theoretical and clinical components and the professional activities that each student midwife should undertake during their programme of study.

NMC (2009) PRE-REGISTRATION STANDARDS FOR MIDWIFERY EDUCATION

In the UK, the NMC is undertaking a consultation to review the current pre-registration midwifery education standards (NMC 2009a). It is anticipated the new standards will be fully adopted by 2021 and will establish the competencies required of the future midwife in 2025, being *outcome focused,* accessible to the public and open to objective assessment. They will build on the professional values set out in *The Code* (NMC 2018), be informed by best midwifery practice from the UK and internationally and be unambiguous, transparent and succinct.

THE PHILOSOPHY OF MIDWIFERY EDUCATION

The components of any educational philosophy statement should be twofold: it should look *inward* to the parent discipline (midwifery competencies and practice) and *outward* to educational practice (teaching and learning). The following sections provide details of the fundamental inward and outward components that a midwifery education philosophy should comprise.

All midwifery education programmes should be based on recognizing that individuals are unique and should promote equal rights, regardless of sex, race, religion, age and nationality (WHO 2011). The training should embrace the whole of a woman's life continuum as opposed to focusing on pregnancy, birth and the postnatal and neonatal periods, and should explicitly address the circumstances of the country situation in which the family resides, including the specific public health challenges. Ultimately, it should be woman and family centred to promote safe motherhood, with the student being prepared to deliver health services in a full variety of settings, including the local community, to ensure they have some understanding of the realities of the lives of childbearing women.

The education of the future midwife should focus on meeting the holistic needs (psychological, emotional, physical, social and spiritual) of the woman in a sensitive and competent manner, acting as her advocate and working in partnership with her and her family to promote a safe and satisfying experience of childbirth and motherhood. The programme should aim to prepare individuals who will be quick-thinking and caring midwives, possessing a sound knowledge base and competent clinical skills, by using student-centred learning methods that will develop their

> **BOX 2.2 ■ Quality Assessment of Midwifery Education Programmes**
>
> A variety of forms are used to assess the quality and ensure standards are upheld:
> - institutional review by the Quality Assurance Agency for Higher Education
> - Nursing and Midwifery Council accreditation and monitoring
> - Research Excellence Framework (institutional research activity contributes directly to the student learning experience)
> - Teaching Excellence Framework to recognize and reward excellent learning and teaching: implemented from 2017
> - annual report from external examiners
> - educational audits of clinical placements
> - student feedback (student–staff consultative committees, module evaluations, practice placement evaluations, national student survey, etc.).

critical-thinking, analytical and problem-solving skills. Educational and clinical staff should encourage all students to reflect on their practice and take responsibility for their own learning, so that they develop into lifelong learners who are capable of recognizing their own needs for continuing professional development (CPD).

EVALUATION AND QUALITY ASSURANCE

Midwifery educationalists are required to evaluate the quality and effectiveness of their teaching and of the learning that takes place. Evaluation usually takes place within defined (professional, national and internal) quality assurance frameworks that have common features (Box 2.2). *Quality assurance* refers to the policies, processes and actions through which quality is maintained, developed, monitored and demonstrated (McKimm 2009).

ACTIVITY 2.1 ■

Review your university's philosophy of midwifery education and compare it with the Word Health Organization's (2011) philosophy.
Create a statement that reflects your philosophy of what midwifery education should consist of.
You may wish to consider the following statements and questions:
Look *inward* to the midwifery competencies and practice: How should you practise midwifery?
Look outward to educational practice: How should you facilitate learning with adults?

In the UK, all institutions that wish to offer pre-registration midwifery and nursing education have to first be approved by the NMC to ensure that there are robust processes in place to support the entire student learning experience, acquiring the status of Approved Education Institution (AEI). It is only once AEI status has been achieved that curriculum planning can proceed. The NMC undertakes the approval of all new pre-registration midwifery education programmes in conjunction with the AEI in which they are delivered. This is to ensure that the programmes not only meet the professional regulatory standards but also comply with the academic regulations of the university and the Quality Assurance Agency for Higher Education (2015) *UK Quality Code for Higher Education*. As a consequence, this enables all students who successfully complete the programme to register as a midwife on the NMC's professional register as well as acquire a higher education qualification (minimum being *first* degree level) from the AEI. The maximum length of approval is 5 years, after which time further revalidation of the programme is undertaken by the NMC and AEI.

The role of the Lead Midwife for Education [LME] (Marshall 2015) is crucial for the approval of midwifery education programmes leading to entry to the midwives' part of the professional register. The LME consequently is a vital intermediary between the NMC and the university who forms an essential part of the quality assurance process, demonstrating to the NMC that the standards leading to registration are being maintained. It is usual for the AEI to appoint a suitably qualified academic midwife as an external examiner to independently monitor the assessment process and student achievement of the theoretical and practical components of midwifery programmes, determining that these are comparable with similar programmes at other AEIs.

Box 2.2 shows the various forms by which the quality of midwifery education programmes is assessed and standards are upheld.

Professional Regulation

The aim of regulation is to support midwives to work autonomously within their full scope of practice. By the raising of the status of midwives through regulation, the standard of maternity care and the health of mothers, their babies and their families will be improved. The goal of the ICM (2011) *Global Standards for Midwifery Regulation* is therefore to promote regulatory mechanisms that protect the public (women and families) by ensuring that safe and competent midwives provide high standards of care to every woman and baby. This is achieved through the following six key functions, as shown in Box 2.3.

BOX 2.3 ■ Purpose of Regulation

The safety of the public is achieved through:
1. setting the scope of practice
2. pre-registration education
3. registration
4. relicensing and continuing competence
5. complaints and discipline
6. codes of conduct and ethics.

Modified with permission from International Confederation of Midwives (2011).

The ICM (2011) founding values and principles include recognition that:
- Regulation is a mechanism by which the social contract between the midwifery profession and society is expressed. Society grants the midwifery profession authority and autonomy to regulate itself. In return, society expects the midwifery profession to act responsibly, ensure high standards of midwifery care and maintain the trust of the public.
- Each woman has the right to receive care in childbirth from an educated and competent midwife authorized to practise midwifery.
- Midwives are autonomous practitioners; that is, they practise in their own right and are responsible and accountable for their own clinical decision-making.
- The midwife's scope of practice describes the circumstances in which the midwife may make autonomous clinical decisions and in what circumstances the midwife must practise in collaboration with other health professionals, such as doctors.
- Midwifery is a profession that is autonomous, separate and distinct from nursing and medicine. What sets midwives apart from nurses and doctors is that *only* midwives can exercise the full scope of midwifery practice and provide all the competencies within this scope.

- Wherever a registered/qualified midwife with a midwifery practising certificate works with pregnant women during the childbirth continuum, no matter what the setting, they are practising midwifery. Therefore when a midwife holds dual registration/qualification as a nurse, They *cannot* practise simultaneously as a midwife *and* a nurse. In a maternity setting a registered/qualified midwife *always* practises midwifery.

The ICM (2011) also identifies the following principles of good regulation to provide a benchmark against which regulatory processes can be assessed.

- **Necessity:** Is the regulation necessary? Are current rules and structures that govern this area still valid? Is the legislation purposeful?
- **Effectiveness:** Is the regulation properly targeted? Can it be properly enforced and complied with? Is it flexible and enabling?
- **Flexibility:** Is the legislation sufficiently flexible to be enabling rather than too prescriptive?
- **Proportionality:** Do the advantages outweigh the disadvantages? Can the same goal be achieved better in another way?
- **Transparency:** Is the regulation clear and accessible to all? Have stakeholders been involved in development?
- **Accountability:** Is it clear who is responsible to whom and for what? Is there an effective appeals process?
- **Consistency:** Will the regulation give rise to anomalies and inconsistencies given the other regulations already in place for this area? Are best practice principles being applied?

INTERNATIONAL TRENDS IN THE REGULATION OF MIDWIVES

The ICM (2011) global standards mainly reflect existing midwifery regulatory frameworks in many parts of the developed world, with the exception that regulation should be midwifery specific, with the governance of the regulator having a majority of midwives on their Board. A survey of European midwifery regulators undertaken by the NMC (2009b) identified that midwifery is mostly regulated either within an autonomous nursing and midwifery regulatory body such as in the UK or through a shared responsibility between a ministry and a midwifery or nursing and midwifery regulatory body. France is the only country where midwifery is regulated by an autonomous midwifery regulatory body. In some countries, such as Denmark and Norway, there is a board of health which is the regulatory authority for all health professionals.

The United States of America presents a complicated picture with regard to midwifery regulation. While midwifery is defined and regulated across all 50 states, the legal status, definitions, regulations and scope of practice differ markedly. This creates confusion for policymakers, consumers and insurance companies, and can limit services to women. In 2012, seven US midwifery organizations representing professional associations, education/accreditation and certification, known collectively as the US Midwifery Education, Regulation, and Association (US MERA), began working together to achieve common goals in midwifery that align with the ICM global standards for strengthening midwifery. One of the first projects identified as a priority by the US MERA was building consensus on the legal recognition of all nationally certified midwives.

In Australia and New Zealand there is a consistent framework for regulation across the health professions but individual regulatory bodies. In Australia there is a Nursing and Midwifery Board, which has separate standards and codes of conduct for nurses and midwives. In New Zealand there is a separate Midwifery Council.

Following the publication of the global standards, the African Health Profession Regulatory Collaborative for Nurses and Midwives was set up to convene leaders responsible for regulation from 14 countries in east, central and southern Africa. This regulatory collaborative supports four to five countries per year in implementing locally designed regulation improvement projects, and over time aims to increase the regulatory capacity of health professional organizations and ultimately improve regulation and professional standards within this region of Africa. However, many low- and middle-income countries in Africa and other regions of the world have limited or non-existent regulatory processes as identified in the *State of the World's Midwifery 2014* (UNFPA et al 2014). Although there is evidence of increasing effort to improve midwifery education and strengthen the profession through association, more work needs to be done in the development of legislation for midwifery regulation in these countries (Castro Lopes et al 2016).

THE REGULATION OF MIDWIVES IN THE UK

The statutory regulation of health professionals has existed in the UK for over 500 years (Mc-Givern et al 2015). Historically, this legislation came about not as a consequence of political or public pressure to ensure the quality of care for the public but rather as a result of lobbying by the profession itself. *Professional self-regulation* was developed to recognize specialist skills and ensure that only those individuals meeting such standards set by their peers gained professional status.

The first regulatory body for health professionals in the UK was set up following the Pharmacy Act of 1852, which was followed by the Medical Act of 1858 and then the Midwives Act of 1902. The Midwives Act 1902 created the Central Midwives Board (CMB) as the regulatory body and introduced the state registration of all midwives in England and Wales, with the midwives' register opening in 1905. Further acts introduced the registration of midwives in Scotland in 1915 and Ireland in 1918. The intention of these acts was to protect women from uneducated and unqualified midwives; however, unlike other professional regulatory bodies that were largely constituted of members of the occupation to be regulated, the CMB was dominated by doctors, who had long opposed the regulation of midwives.

The CMB established the statutory functions of:

- maintaining a register of qualified midwives
- framing rules to regulate, supervise and restrict, within due limits, the practice of midwives to keep the public safe
- arranging for the training of midwives and the conduct of examinations
- setting up professional conduct proceedings with power to remove from the register any midwife found guilty of misconduct.

The Midwives Act was followed by the Nurses Registration Act in 1919, which established the General Nursing Council (GNC) for England and Wales, followed by the establishment of councils in Scotland and Ireland. The two professions were regulated separately until the Nurses, Midwives and Health Visitors Act of 1979 established the United Kingdom Central Council for Nursing, Midwifery and Health Visiting (UKCC) in 1983. National boards were established in each of the four UK countries to approve and monitor pre- and post-registration education and training as well as be responsible for the supervision of midwives (see Chapter 10).

Similarly to the CMB and Nursing Councils, the key tasks of the UKCC were to:

- maintain a register of qualified nurses, midwives and health visitors
- set standards of nursing, midwifery and health visiting education, practice and conduct
- provide advice for nurses, midwives and health visitors on professional standards
- consider allegations of misconduct or unfitness to practise due to ill health.

During the passage of the 1979 Nurses, Midwives and Health Visitors Act, there were concerns from the midwifery profession that the UKCC register and Council would be dominated by nurses and that midwives would lose control of their profession. Midwives lobbied for, and succeeded in, establishing a special clause to be inserted into the act and put into legislation the requirement for a *statutory midwifery committee*. The remit of the Midwifery Committee was for it to be consulted on all midwifery matters and to formulate the rules for the practice and supervision of midwives.

Two underlying principles of the Nurses, Midwives and Health Visitors Act of 1979 were the protection of the public and self-regulation by the three professions. This was achieved by most members of the UKCC being elected by the three professions from the four countries of the UK. This dichotomy – between the public interest and professional interest – has been central to the development of the regulation of the professions and has played a key part in recent reforms of midwifery regulation in the UK.

A review of the function of the UKCC undertaken by J.M. Consulting in 1998 concluded that more effective regulation required the balancing of the interests of the professions with those of employers, service users, educators and others. In tandem with the emergence of patient- and women-centred care in the 1990s, *professional self-regulation* gave way to *professional regulation* in the public interest. It was against this background that the Nursing and Midwifery Order 2001 was drafted. The order encompassed the main recommendations made by J.M. Consulting (1998) and strengthened the accountability of the professions to the public in general and, in particular, around fitness to practise. The Nursing and Midwifery Order 2001 created the legal framework for the Nursing and Midwifery Council (NMC), which came into being in 2002. The UKCC and the English National Board (ENB) for Nursing, Midwifery and Health Visiting were abolished, and the regulation, education and quality assurance functions of the ENB were transferred to the NMC. The national boards in Northern Ireland, Scotland and Wales were also abolished, and some of their functions were transferred to other bodies. In Northern Ireland, responsibility for post-registration education and training was transferred to the Northern Ireland Practice and Education Council for Nursing and Midwifery (NIPEC), and in Scotland it was transferred to NHS Education for Scotland (NES). These changes strengthened the sector-wide shift from professional self-regulation to independent regulation.

The NMC is the current independent statutory regulator of nurses and midwives in the UK. Accountable to the UK Parliament, the NMC is required by its governing legislation to:

- establish and maintain a register of all qualified nurses and midwives eligible to practise in the UK
- set standards for their education, practice and conduct
- take action when those standards are called into question.

REGULATORY REFORM

In the late 1990s, public trust in the health professions' abilities and willingness to call those they regulated to account had failed. Two significant inquiries into failings within the NHS, the Bristol Royal Infirmary Inquiry (Kennedy 2001) and the Shipman Inquiry (Smith 2004), identified a *'club culture'* among doctors which caused them to put their own professional loyalties and relationships before the safety of patients. A number of the recommendations from both inquiries concerned the regulation of health care professionals, including their education and training, assessment of competence, registration, CPD and revalidation.

ACTIVITY 2.2 ■

All registered health professionals are regulated in the United Kingdom to protect the public.
For you to understand how different health professionals are regulated, visit the following websites and compare the regulatory processes for each profession, identifying the similarities and differences:

- General Medical Council at https://www.gmc-uk.org
- Health and Care Professions Council at https://www.hcpc-uk.org
- Nursing and Midwifery Council (NMC) at https://www.nmc.org.uk.

You will find that the key concepts from all the regulators are very similar.
Add the NMC website to the *favourites* on your electronic device or record it in another way that will be useful to you and visit it regularly for updates.

Following these inquiries, a new statutory body was established in 2003 to oversee the nine health professions' regulators, namely the Council for Healthcare Regulatory Excellence (CHRE). The CHRE (now known as the Professional Standards Authority for Health and Social Care [PSA]) was given legal powers as an independent body to monitor the performance of the regulators and report to Parliament. The PSA holds the regulatory bodies to account and provides annual reports to the UK Parliament on their performance. The PSA also conducts audits and investigations, and can appeal fitness to practise cases in the courts if it considers that sanctions applied by the regulators are insufficient to protect the public. In addition, it has undertaken three special reviews of the NMC (PSA 2008, 2011, 2012) and has just commenced a fourth review on the handling of complaints and lessons learned (PSA 2017). The PSA has also suggested that the regulation of health professionals needs a radical overhaul and has called for *right-touch* regulation (PSA 2015) and further reform (PSA 2016), including the need for new legislation as recommended by the Law Commission, Scottish Law Commission and Northern Ireland Law Commission (Law Commission et al 2014). Such proposals are primarily focused on enhancing public protection and professional responsibility, supported by more effective, efficient and responsive regulatory processes.

Following the Bristol Royal Infirmary and Shipman inquiries, the government commissioned a further two reviews, and the resulting reports by Donaldson (2006) and the Department of Health (DH; 2006) led to the publication of a white paper – '*Trust, assurance and safety: the regulation of health professionals in the 21st century*' (DH 2007). This resulted in significant reforms to the governance arrangements of all the health profession regulators, moving from elected and professionally dominated boards to appointed boards with equal profession and lay representation. The reforms also modernized and harmonized some of the fitness to practise procedures and sanctions and required all health professions to adopt a form of *periodic revalidation*.

Revalidation

Revalidation is the mechanism that allows professionals to demonstrate that their knowledge and skills remain contemporary and continue to meet the standards of conduct and performance set out by the regulator. Following the passing of the legislation in the Health and Social Care Act 2008, all statutorily regulated professionals, medical and non-medical, are required to have systems in place to demonstrate their continued fitness to practise in the form of *revalidation.*

Taking effect from April 2016, the NMC's (2019) revalidation requirements are designed to enable midwives and nurses to demonstrate that they practise safely and effectively and *live* the standards as set out in *The Code* (NMC 2018). Revalidation replaces the previous post-registration education and practice requirements and necessitates registrants to revalidate every 3 years. In the 3 years before they renew their registration, nurses and midwives are required to undertake and provide proof of:

- 450 hours of practice specific to their area of employment (e.g. clinical, education, management or research), or 900 hours if they are renewing their registration as both a midwife and a nurse
- 35 hours of CPD, of which 20 hours must be *participatory* learning (see Chapter 15)
- five accounts of practice-related feedback
- five written reflective accounts (see Chapter 5)
- a reflective discussion with a fellow NMC registrant
- a health and character declaration
- a professional indemnity arrangement
- confirmation by a registered practitioner.

It is a midwife's responsibility to maintain their professional registration by engaging in lifelong learning and maintaining a portfolio to evidence that their CPD meets the standards required by the regulatory body (i.e. their knowledge and skills are contemporary). The NMC has a microsite on its website that provides detailed explanation and resources to support each midwife and nurse with their revalidation. The Royal College of Midwives (RCM) also provides a number of i-learn modules to support CPD and an electronic portfolio system (i-folio) where midwives can store all their information, documents and learning activity in preparation for when they are required to revalidate.

Changes to Midwifery Regulation in the UK

A wide range of public inquiries, including, most recently, the Mid Staffordshire NHS Foundation Trust Public Inquiry (Francis 2013) and the Morecambe Bay Investigation (Kirkup 2015), identified that the actions, motivation, responsibility and accountability of individual health professionals are important in upholding the standards of the profession and contributing to patient safety culture. However, advocates of patient safety science see all, or most, errors as products of the system or organization of care (Walshe 2003, 2009). This sentiment was also supported by Berwick (2013), who stated that culture will trump rules, standards and control strategies every single time and consequently a safer NHS will depend far more on major cultural change than on a new regulatory regime.

During the Parliamentary and Health Service Ombudsman (PHSO) in England investigation into the failures in maternity care at Morecambe Bay NHS Foundation Trust, an exploration of the additional tier of regulation which applied to midwives – the *statutory supervision of midwives* (see Chapter 10) was also undertaken (PHSO 2013). Concerns were expressed that there was a structural flaw which permitted the local investigation of midwives by midwives, which could lead to potential muddling of the supervisory and regulatory roles of midwives and the possibility of a perceived conflict of interest. The report recommended two principles for the future model of midwifery regulation (PHSO 2013):

- midwifery supervision and regulation should be separated
- the NMC should be in direct control of regulatory activity.

The PSA (2014) also considered the report and added that:

- There was a lack of evidence to suggest that the risks posed by contemporary midwifery practice required an additional tier of regulation.
- The imposition of regulatory sanctions or prohibitions by one midwife on another without lay scrutiny is not in line with good regulatory practice.

In response to these findings, the NMC commissioned an independent review of midwifery regulation by the King's Fund. The scope for the review required the King's Fund to recommend a future model that would be fit for public protection, would be fair and proportionate and would give the NMC sufficient regulatory control to be accountable for its outcomes. The report, published in 2015, recommended that the additional layer of regulation for midwives should end, that the NMC should restrict its role to the core functions of regulation and that the governments of the four UK countries should consider other ways to ensure that the functions of supervision and professional development are provided by other organizations in the health system (Baird et al 2015).

In January 2015, the NMC decided to ask for a change in its legislation to remove the additional tier of regulation applying to midwives, which included the supervision of midwives as a statutory function with a regulatory role. Following the NMC's decision, the Secretary of State for Health announced on 16 July 2015 that the government would change the legislation governing the NMC's regulation of midwives. The main effect of the changes would be to remove the supervision of midwives out of the NMC's statutory legislation.

Gillman and Lloyd (2015) outlined in their paper to the NMC that these changes would be more far-reaching than just the removal of the supervision of midwives from statute; it would include the removal of the *Midwifery* section of the Nursing and Midwifery Order 2001 (Section 60) which provided the legislation for:

- the Midwifery Committee
- rules as to midwifery practice
- local supervision of midwives.

Following consultation and debates in Parliament (House of Lords Hansard 2017), the Nursing and Midwifery (Amendment) Order 2017 was passed. This removed the statutory requirement for the NMC to convene a committee (which advises the NMC at their request. or otherwise, on matters affecting midwifery and who the NMC must consult on the exercise of its functions insofar as they affect midwifery) and removing provisions relating to the local supervision of midwives, including the Midwives Rules (NMC 2012). It also amended Part V of the Nursing and Midwifery Order 2001 in respect of certain fitness to practise functions of the NMC relating to both midwives and nurses.

The NMC (2017) has stated that the changes do not affect:

- the separate registration of midwives
- direct entry to the register as a midwife
- the protected title of a midwife
- the protected function of midwives attending a woman in childbirth
- separate competencies and pre-registration education standards for midwives.

The statutory supervision of midwives has been replaced by an employer-led model of clinical supervision based on the principles set out by the DH (2016), which are discussed further in Chapter 10. However, the PSA and NMC consider that the current regulatory arrangements in the UK still require fundamental reform to make them fit for purpose in a modern health service. Many organizations have argued that less emphasis should be placed on the use of external pressures such as regulation to improve health services. There needs to be improved collective and collaborative responsibility, not only from individual health professionals but also from their employers, as well as service users and policymakers (Bell and Jarvie 2015). Effective regulation requires enhanced integrated approaches to ensuring safety and quality, connecting the systems that regulate the provision of health and maternity care with those that regulate the professions.

To keep up to date with the changes to the regulation of health professionals in the UK, midwives should add the PSA, NMC and RCM websites to their *favourites* on their electronic devices and sign up to the respective newsletters to keep involved in shaping the future of the midwifery profession.

ACTIVITY 2.3 ■

Consider the changes to midwifery regulation arising from the *Nursing and Midwifery (Amendment) Order 2017.*
What effect do they have on the following?

- Midwifery at the Nursing and Midwifery Council (NMC).
- The NMC Midwifery Panel.
- Midwifery education.
- Practising as a midwife in the United Kingdom.
- Midwifery supervision.

Compile a report of what you have learned and add to your portfolio to demonstrate your continued professional development.

Conclusion

This chapter has discussed the standards for midwifery education and professional regulation from a global and UK perspective and has highlighted the value of how a professional framework can serve in strengthening the midwifery profession and raise the standard of midwifery practice worldwide. It is vital that pre-registration midwifery education standards are always fit for purpose so that the future midwife is educated and trained to meet the challenges of contemporary midwifery practice. Furthermore, by working within such a professional framework, midwives are continually supported and enabled to fulfil their role competently and confidently contribute fully to the safe delivery of maternal and neonatal care in their country of registration.

The role that the regulator plays in monitoring the standards in countries outside the UK has been outlined and compared briefly with the function of the NMC. The history of midwifery regulation in the UK, from the Midwives Act of 1902 to the most recent changes in 2017, was discussed, which provides the reader with the context in which to fully appreciate the introduction of the requirement for revalidation in 2016 and the disestablishment of the regulatory framework for the supervision of midwives in 2017. The latter change is evidenced by the gradual move away from the regulatory arrangements that focused on the interests of the professions towards arrangements where the primary purpose is public protection and patient safety, as well as the drive for regulatory reform as a consequence of recent inquiries into failings within the NHS.

More priority needs to be given to supporting staff, learning from mistakes and sharing best practice. To do this, the respective regulatory frameworks need to put in place rules, standards and guidance which are proportionate to the level of risk that enables health professionals to work to their full scope of practice. A philosophy of lifelong learning and access to CPD with support and appropriate supervision is key to protecting the public as well as to improving the quality of health and maternity services.

KEY POINTS

- It is essential to the health and well-being of childbearing women, their babies and their families that all midwives are educated and trained to the ICM Global Standards for Midwifery Education as a *minimum.*
- A strong midwifery profession and the safety of mothers and babies worldwide are dependent on three interconnected pillars – *education, regulation* and *professional association –* that are underpinned by essential competencies for basic midwifery practice.
- Midwifery education programmes should not only meet the professional regulatory standards but should also comply with the academic regulations of the university and the Quality Assurance Agency for Higher Education.
- Evaluation of midwifery education programmes should take place within defined (professional, national and internal) quality assurance frameworks that have common features.
- Regulation, both nationally and internationally, is currently undergoing continuous reform, and midwives need to keep abreast of developments and contribute to ongoing debates and consultations.
- Whilst there is increasing effort to improve midwifery education and strengthen the profession through association, more work needs to be undertaken in developing legislation for midwifery regulation in low- and middle income countries.
- Revalidation is the mechanism in the UK that allows midwives to maintain their registration through demonstrating that their knowledge and skills are contemporary and that they use *The Code* (NMC 2018) in their everyday practice.

References

Baird, B., Murray, R., Seale, B., Foot, C., & Perry, C. (2015). *Midwifery regulation in the United Kingdom.* Available at: https://www.nmc.org.uk/globalassets/sitedocuments/councilpapersanddocuments/council-2015/kings-fund-review.pdf.

Bell, D., & Jarvie, A. (2015). Preventing 'where next'. Patients, professionals and learning from serious failings in care. *Journal of the Royal College of Physicians of Edinburgh, 45*, 4–8.

Berwick, D. (2013). *A promise to learn – a commitment to act: Improving the safety of patients in England.* London: Department of Health.

Castro Lopes, S., Nove, A., ten Hoope-Bender, P., de Burnis, L., Bokosi, M., Moyo, N. T., & Homer, C. S. E. (2016). A descriptive analysis of midwifery education, regulation and association in 73 countries: the baseline for a post-2015 pathway. *Human Resources for Health, 14*, 37.

Department of Health. (2006). *The regulation of the non-medical healthcare professions. A review by the department of health.* Available at: https://www.pmguk.co.uk/data/page_files/publications%20and%20reports/2006/R.RegulationNon-medicalHealthProf.pdf.

Department of Health. (2007). *Trust, assurance and safety: the regulation of health professionals in the 21st century.* London: The Stationery Office.

Department of Health. (2016). *Proposals for changing the system of midwifery supervision in the UK.* Available at: https://www.gov.uk/government/publications/changes-to-midwife-supervision-in-the-uk/proposals-for-changing-the-system-of-midwifery-supervision-in-the-uk.

Donaldson, L. (2006). *Good doctors, safer patients: Proposals to strengthen the system to assure and improve the performance of doctors and to protect the safety of the public.* London: Department of Health.

Francis, R. (2013). *Report of the Mid Staffordshire NHS Foundation Trust Public Inquiry.* London: The Stationery Office.

Gillman, L. J., & Lloyd, C. (2015). *Re-framing midwifery supervision: a discussion paper.* Available at: https://www.rcm.org.uk/sites/default/files/Re-framing%20supervision%20-paper%20for%20discussion%20final%2023%203%202015.pdf.

International Confederation of Midwives. (2011). *Global standards for midwifery regulation.* Available at: https://internationalmidwives.org/assets/uploads/documents/Global%20Standards%20Comptencies%20Tools/English/GLOBAL%20STANDARDS%20FOR%20MIDWIFERY%20REGULATION%20ENG.pdf.

International Confederation of Midwives. (2013). *Global standards for midwifery education.* Available at: http://www.internationalmidwives.org/assets/uploads/documents/CoreDocuments/ICM%20Standards%20Guidelines_ammended2013.pdf.

International Confederation of Midwives. (2014a). *The international code of ethics for midwives.* Available at: http://internationalmidwives.org/assets/uploads/documents/CoreDocuments/CD2008_001%20V2014%20ENG%20International%20Code%20of%20Ethics%20for%20Midwives.pdf.

International Confederation of Midwives. (2014b). *The philosophy and model of midwifery care.* Available at: http://internationalmidwives.org/assets/uploads/documents/CoreDocuments/CD2005_001%20V2014%20ENG%20Philosophy%20and%20model%20of%20midwifery%20care.pdf.

International Confederation of Midwives. (2017). *International definition of the midwife.* Available at: https://internationalmidwives.org/assets/uploads/documents/CoreDocuments/ENG%20Definition_of_the_Midwife%202017.pdf.

International Confederation of Midwives. (2018). *Essential Competencies for midwifery practice.* Available at: https://www.internationalmidwives.org/our-work/policy-and-practice/essential-competencies-for-midwifery-practice.html.

J. M. Consulting. (1998). *The regulation of nurses, midwives and health visitors: Report on a review of the Nurses, Midwives and Health Visitors Act 1997.* Bristol: J.M. Consulting.

Kennedy, I. (2001). *The report of the public inquiry into children's heart surgery at the Bristol Royal Infirmary 1984-1995: Learning from Bristol.* London: The Stationary Office.

Kirkup, B. (2015). *The report of the Morecambe Bay Investigation, Preston, Lancashire.* London: The Stationery Office. Available at: https://www.gov.uk/government/uploads/system/uploads/attachment_data/file/408480/47487_MBI_Accessible_v0.1.pdf.

Law Commission, Scottish Law Commission, & Northern Ireland Law Commission. (2014). *Regulation of health care professionals, regulation of social care professionals in England.* London: HMSO.

Marshall, J. E. (2015). The power of the lead midwife for education (LME): The role, function and challenges. *MIDIRS Midwifery Digest, 25*(1), 11–14.

McGivern, G., Fischer, M., Palaima, T., Spendlove, Z., Thomson, O., & Waring, J. (2015). *Report to the General Osteopathic Council. Appendix 2: A review of literature on professions, health professional regulation, revalidation and continuing fitness to practise. Warwick, Warwick Business School*. Available at: http://www.osteopathy.org.uk/news-and-resources/research-surveys/gosc-research/research-to-promote-effective-regulation/.

McKimm, J. (2009). Quality, standards and enhancement. In Fry, H, Ketteridge, S and Marshall S, (Eds.), *A handbook for teaching and learning in higher education; enhancing academic practice* (3rd ed.). (pp. 186–197). London: Routledge.

Nursing and Midwifery Council. (2009a). *Standards for pre-registration midwifery education*. London: Nursing and Midwifery Council.

Nursing and Midwifery Council. (2009b). *Survey of European midwifery regulators*. London: Nursing and Midwifery Council.

Nursing and Midwifery Council. (2012). *Midwives rules and standards*. London: Nursing and Midwifery Council.

Nursing and Midwifery Council. (2017). *Practising as a midwife in the UK. An overview of midwifery regulation*. London: Nursing and Midwifery Council.

Nursing and Midwifery Council. (2018). *The Code. Professional standards of practice and behaviour for nurses, midwives and nursing associates*. London: Nursing and Midwifery Council.

Nursing and Midwifery Council. (2019). How to revalidate with the NMC. Available at: https://www.nmc.org.uk/globalassets/sitedocuments/revalidation/how-to-revalidate-booklet.pdf.

Parliamentary and Health Service Ombudsman. (2013). *Midwifery supervision and regulation: Recommendations for change*. Available at: https://www.ombudsman.org.uk/sites/default/files/Midwifery%20supervision%20and%20regulation_%20recommendations%20for%20change.pdf.

Professional Standards Authority for Health and Social Care. (2008). *Special report to the Minister of State for Health Services on the Nursing and Midwifery Council*. London: Council for Healthcare Regulatory Excellence. Available at: https://www.nmc.org.uk/globalassets/siteDocuments/CHRE/CHRE-Special-report-NMC-2008.pdf.

Professional Standards Authority for Health and Social Care. (2011). *NMC progress review. A review of the NMC's fitness to practise directorate's progress since 2008*. London: Council for Healthcare Regulatory Excellence.

Professional Standards Authority for Health and Social Care. (2012). *Strategic review of the Nursing and Midwifery Council: Final report*. London: Professional Standards Authority for Health and Social Care.

Professional Standards Authority for Health and Social Care. (2014). *Written evidence for the Public Administration Select Committee follow up session on the Parliamentary and Health Service Ombudsman's report into severe sepsis and midwifery supervision and regulation*. London: Professional Standards Authority for Health and Social Care. Available at: https://www.professionalstandards.org.uk/docs/default-source/publications/consultation-response/others-consultations/2014/pase-evidence-severe-sepsis-and-midwifery-supervision-and-regulation.pdf?sfvrsn=55a47f20_9.

Professional Standards Authority for Health and Social Care. (2015). *Rethinking regulation*. London: Professional Standards Authority for Health and Social Care.

Professional Standards Authority for Health and Social Care. (2016). *Regulation rethought. Proposals for reform*. London: Professional Standards Authority for Health and Social Care.

Professional Standards Authority for Health and Social Care. (2017). *Terms of reference for review of Nursing and Midwifery Council*. Available at: https://www.professionalstandards.org.uk/latest-news/latest-news/detail/2017/06/15/terms-of-reference-for-review-of-nursing-and-midwifery-council-announced.

Quality Assurance Agency for Higher Education. (2015). *UK quality code for higher education: Overview and expectations*. Gloucester, Quality Assurance Agency for Higher Education.

Renfrew, M. J., Homer, C. S. E., Downe, S., McFadden, A., Muir, N., Prentice, T., & ten Hoope-Bender, P. (2014). *Midwifery: An executive summary for the Lancet series*. Available at: http://www.thelancet.com/series/midwifery.

Smith, J. (2004). *The Shipman Inquiry: fifth report, safeguarding patients lessons from the past – proposals for the future*. London: The Stationary Office.

United Nations Population Fund, International Confederation of Midwives & World Health Organization. (2014). *The state of the world's midwifery 2014: A universal pathway. A woman's right to health.* New York: United Nations Population Fund.

United Nations Population Fund & International Confederation of Midwives. (2016). Comprehensive midwifery programme guidance. Available at: http://www.unfpa.org/sites/default/files/resource-pdf/Midwifery%20Programme%20Guidance.pdf.

Walshe, K. (2003). *Inquiries: Learning from failure in the NHS?* London: The Nuffield Trust.

Walshe, K. (2009). Regulating health professionals. In Heal. J, and Dugdale. P, (Eds.), *Patient safety first. Responsive regulation in healthcare* (pp. 144–166). Sydney: Allen and Unwin.

World Health Organization. (2011). A philosophy of midwifery education. In *Strengthening midwifery toolkit: Module 5: Developing a midwifery curriculum for safe motherhood – guidelines for midwifery education programmes* (pp. 6–7). Geneva: World Health Organization.

Statutes, Orders and Directives

Directive 2013 /55/EU (*the 'Modernised' Directive*) of the European Parliament and of the Council of 20 November 2013 amending Directive 2005/36/EC on the recognition of professional qualifications and Regulation EU No 1024/2012 on administrative cooperation through the Internal Market Information System (*'the IMI Regulation'*).

Health and Social Care Act. (2008). London: HMSO.

House of Lords Hansard. (2017). *Nursing and Midwifery (Amendment) Order 28*th *February 2017* (Vol. 779). Available at: https://hansard.parliament.uk/Lords/2017-02-28/debates/1B4AAA1D-1823-4038-B24D-7523943A9F37/NursingAndMidwifery(Amendment)Order2017.

Medical Act. (1858). London: HMSO.

(England and Wales). *Midwives Act.* (1902). London: HMSO.

Midwives (Scotland) Act. (1915). London: HMSO.

Midwives (Ireland) Act. (1918). London: HMSO.

(England and Wales). *Nurses Registration Act.* (1919). London: HMSO.

Nurses, Midwives and Health Visitors Act. (1979). London: HMSO.

Nursing and Midwifery Order. (2001). *Statutory Instruments 2002 No. 253.* London: The Stationery Office.

Nursing and Midwifery (Amendment) Order. (2017). *Statutory Instruments No. 321.* London: The Stationery Office.

Pharmacy Act. (1852). London: HMSO.

Further Reading

The Lancet Series on Midwifery. (2014). Available at: http://www.thelancet.com/series/midwifery.

    The Lancet Series on Midwifery consists of four separate articles that have been developed collaboratively by a multidisciplinary group of clinical, academic, research, policy, advocacy and other experts from around the world. Together, the articles address key issues on the role of midwifery in the world today, and challenge much of the current thinking and attitudes about it among health professionals and decision makers.

Pickett, L. (2017). *Professional regulation in health and social care. House of Commons Library briefing paper number CBP8094.* Available at: https://researchbriefings.parliament.uk/ResearchBriefing/Summary/CBP-8094.

    This briefing paper describes the main functions of professional regulators in the United Kingdom in more detail, along with some of the prominent debates surrounding this area of health policy as well as the case for reform. Regulators differ in their policies, functions and operations, so the focus of this briefing is on the largest regulators: the General Medical Council, the Nursing and Midwifery Council, the Health and Care Professionals Council, the General Dental Council and the General Pharmaceutical Council.

Professional Standards Authority for Health and Social Care. (2017). *Right-touch reform. A new framework for assurance of professions.* Available at: https://www.professionalstandards.org.uk/docs/default-source/publications/thought-paper/right-touch-reform-2017.pdf?sfvrsn=5.

    The report covers in detail four main areas of the regulation of health professionals: the role of regulators in prevention of harm; the future of fitness to practise; professional regulators' role in education and training; and modernising registers. The report also provides a detailed summary and analysis of current arrangements and outlines proposals for regulatory reform and future development and improvement.

Useful Websites

Council for Healthcare Regulatory Excellence (see Professional Standards Authority for Health and Social Care)

General Medical Council: https://www.gmc-uk.org

Health and Care Professions Council: https://www.hcpc-uk.org

International Confederation of Midwives: https://www.internationalmidwives.org

NHS Education for Scotland: https://www.nes.scot.nhs.uk

Northern Ireland Practice and Education Council for Nursing and Midwifery: https://www.nipec.hscni.net

Nursing and Midwifery Board of Australia: https://www.nursingmidwiferyboard.gov.au

Nursing and Midwifery Council: https://www.nmc.org.uk

Professional Standards Authority for Health and Social Care: https://www.professionalstandards.org.uk

Quality Assurance Agency for Higher Education: https://www.qaa.ac.uk

United Nations Population Fund: https://www.unfpa.org

US Midwifery Education, Regulation, and Association: http://www.usmera.org

World Health Organization: https://www.who.int

CHAPTER 3

Communicating Effectively in Midwifery Education and Practice

Leontia Pillay ■ Lyndsey Smith

CONTENTS

LEARNING OUTCOMES

By the end of this chapter the reader should be able to:

- understand theories of communication
- assess personal strengths and challenges relating to communication skills
- understand the value of active listening
- differentiate between social and professional boundaries affecting communication
- identify strategies in providing clear communication for women when English is not their first language
- describe how specific communication tools can be used effectively in midwifery education and practice
- appreciate the impact that advances in digital communication and social networking can have on midwifery education and practice.

Overview

This chapter provides a critical debate around the importance of effective communication relating to individual health care professionals, the environment in which they work and the collective values that reflect the culture of the work undertaken (Moss 2012). A range of communication theories and tools will be explored, providing activities to stimulate learning and embed them in practice. Various factors and recent developments that can influence communication in the 21st century, such as social media, are examined in the context of midwifery education and clinical practice.

Introduction

Communication is central to human interaction, an element of life that is often presumed elementary but in reality is a complex and varied process that can be learned and mastered. For the purpose of this chapter, the focus will be on how midwives communicate at a macro level from a professional perspective by learning the process of sharing information using a set of common rules; involving human feelings and attitudes, and combining elements of more than one culture (Northouse and Northouse 1998; Sully and Dallas 2010). Learning best practice in professional communication can be an overwhelming task because of the sheer volume of models and definitions identified in the literature. As experience develops, health care professionals are expected to reflect on their own practice and communication style (Nursing and Midwifery Council [NMC] 2018) (see also Chapter 5). To work in partnership with women and families to ensure that care is effective, elements of different communication tools may be required. *The Code* (NMC 2018) and the requirements for the revalidation of nurses and midwives (NMC 2019) clearly highlight how fundamental communication is in contemporary midwifery education and practice.

England and Morgan (2012) reaffirm that the Midwives Act of 1902 ensured that the practice of midwifery was closely supervised and that midwives became accountable for both their clinical skills and their behaviour. The midwife has a special role in life that presents itself as a partnership with the woman and her family. It is therefore imperative that the midwife is equally skilled in providing the necessary clinical care as well as the ability to offer advice in an appropriate way. The women in the care of a midwife will all be unique. Each woman will have specific nuances which should be recognized and catered for when communicating in order for the midwife to provide the very best, all-encompassing level of care. It is recognized that student midwives learn their professional behaviour, including developing their communication skills, from the midwives (mentors/practice supervisors, practice assessors) with whom they connect in the clinical setting as well as in the university and wider professional context. When communication fails or is substandard, this has a significant impact at a number of levels. The woman's experience of maternity care could be jeopardized, but also, and more importantly, so could her safety. Communication failure can also be a result of ineffective intra- and interprofessional relationships (e.g. midwife to midwife or midwife to doctor).

If one first examines the relationship between midwife and woman it is clear that the complexity of providing contemporary maternity care and the expectation to provide a continuous service creates a number of competing challenges. Midwives, whilst considered to have the knowledge and skills in the physiological process of birth, may also be caring for women who have complex physical and social needs (Chief Nursing Officers of England, Northern Ireland, Scotland and Wales, 2010). There are many women who live in poverty, as well as an increasing number who can speak, read and write little or no English, who require support in accessing services. Furthermore, the latest National Maternity Review (Department of Health [DH] 2016) highlighted the need for good-quality and consistent communication not only with the woman and her family but also for health care professionals to communicate clearly with each other. Women also reported that they expect digital tools to be used for communication and that such information should be up to date and relevant (DH 2016).

It is therefore imperative for every midwife to demonstrate effective communication skills across a broad spectrum of outlets and in a plethora of different instances. *The Code* (NMC 2018) clearly sets out the professional standards midwives and nurses must uphold. For the midwife to practise effectively, they must communicate clearly, including verbal and non-verbal communication, through her record keeping and any digital communication, including social media and networking sites (NMC 2015).

Social Media

The explosion of social media platforms (Fig. 3.1) over the past decade has arguably had the most dramatic effect on society that has ever been experienced. Developments have surpassed predictions, and the social media landscape continues to evolve such that it is now a fundamental part of life and human interaction, consequently playing a significant role in the way individuals communicate.

The access to and acceptance of information online whether through social media or the Internet means health care professionals must become accustomed to and experts in social technology. In health care alone there are 40,000 medical applications *(apps)*, of which many are for pregnancy (Tripp et al 2014; Wirtanen 2012). Most women accessing midwifery services either have grown up with social media or have an understanding of social media services. Likewise, many midwives entering the profession are social media savvy but tend to engage with the technology only for personal use. In contemporary society, it is imperative that midwifery services develop according to the trend towards social media. Communication is a fundamental aspect of midwifery and therefore must incorporate technology, the Internet and social media to improve dialogue not only between the midwife and the public, but also with fellow midwives and health care professionals

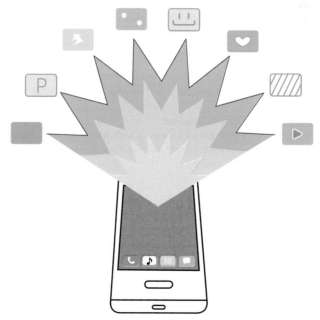

Fig. 3.1   Explosion of social media. (Courtesy Paris Dunlop and Leontia Pillay.)

(Stewart et al 2012). However, whilst there are many advantages to this form of communication, midwives must also be aware of the challenges.

E-professionalism is described as a new construct that accounts for attitudes and behaviours associated with the professional but manifests itself through digital media (Cain and Romanelli 2009). Breaches of confidentiality and indiscretions in professional behaviour can lead to issues related to privacy and safety (Jones and Hayter 2013). The NMC has recognized this and has published guidelines on the use of social media for the professional (NMC 2015).

Many women use the Internet to gain information, and Tripp et al (2014) suggest that this has the potential to be harmful if there is no screening of the information available. Some apps that have been developed can cause a false reassurance or further raise a woman's anxiety, for example *My Baby's Beat* and *Smart Contraction*, which monitor the fetal heart beat and the woman's contraction, respectively, to advise the user of an appropriate time to go into hospital. Whilst both may help reassure the woman, there is also the potential for many things to go wrong. Women may become so dependent on the technology that they lose the ability to recognize the *non-verbal cues* from their own body. As the term *midwife* means *with woman*, every midwife therefore has a responsibility to be the woman's advocate, advising her to be prudent with information found on the Internet (Wylie 2014). At the same time, midwives should embrace this technology and review how and when it can be used to successfully improve communication. Many professional bodies are using different platforms to communicate within the profession. The Royal College of Midwives has a Facebook page and Twitter account. An individual can follow discussion at a conference that they are unable to attend by using the designated hashtag or following other midwives who are tweeting from the event (Wylie 2014). Social media has transformed communication within society, and the challenge for today's midwife is having the ability to combine face-to-face communication with technology to ensure communication is effective and efficient for everyone involved in the woman's care.

England and Morgan (2012) suggest that communication is a learned skill that requires a conscious effort to improve its quality. Theories/models of communication can help midwives in developing a better understanding of the complex nature of communication of one's *self* by supporting reflection and consequential adjustments in their practice as appropriate.

Theories of Communication

The midwife's skill to recognize the context surrounding the communication taking place lies in their ability to appreciate the different parts of their own self. Burnard (1997) describes these markers as:

- the *physical self*, referring to body language
- the *real self*, referring to the character of oneself with which the individual is most familiar but is only apparent to a few other people, such as close friends and family
- the *self for others*, referring to the character that is apparent when one is in the company of others, for example the *social self*, which may be very different to the *professional self*.

The ability to recognize the three forms of markers is prevalent every day for a midwife. Whilst the midwife's role is to be an advocate for the childbearing woman, it is imperative to stay objective and recognize the boundaries in the professional relationship (Kirkham 2010; NMC 2018). Whilst it is recognized that midwives develop effective working relationships with the women they care for, it remains vitally important to acknowledge the situation and not allow the portrayal of the *real* self to emerge by becoming too friendly. Instead the midwife must maintain the *self for others* within a professional working relationship that is commensurate with *The Code* (NMC 2018).

Further success in the art of communication and the practice of midwifery results from the midwife's ability to understand and examine their own interpersonal skills. The greatest influence

TABLE 3.1 ■ **DeVito's (2015) Dimensions of Communication**

The physical dimension	Relates to the actual environment
The temporal dimension	Relates to that moment in time
The social–psychological dimension	Relates to the status and relationship of the participants
The cultural context	Relates to the beliefs and cultures of the individuals communicating

on this develops from the relationship held with the person or people involved in the communication. DeVito (2015) discusses the context in which communication takes place and outlines four dimensions that it can fall into, as shown in Table 3.1:

Undertake Activity 3.1 to help you understand De Vito's (2015) dimensions of communication and use the model as a tool to reflect on your own professional practice.

ACTIVITY 3.1 ■

A midwife meets a family for the first time in the postnatal ward. The baby is dressed in pink and is lying in a cot by the mother's bed. The midwife asks the mother for permission to examine her daughter, and the mother responds 'it's a boy'. The midwife makes a seemingly innocuous remark about the baby being dressed in pink, suggesting that boys wear blue and girls wear pink. The midwife continues with the assessment of the baby, attempting limited interaction with the mother.

- Using DeVito's (2015) four dimensions of communication, consider the scenario above and highlight each dimension.
- Who has the power and the control in this situation?
- How may this affect future communication between the midwife and the mother in this situation?

In all communication each individual goes through an unconscious process. To understand more fully one's ability to communicate and behave during communication, one must first acknowledge this unconscious process. Webb (2011) suggests it helps professionals to have an understanding of their own style of communication and be aware of these processes. *Transactional analysis* is a technique that is used to interpret and analyse the process of communication. Berne (1964), who first described this technique, suggested that each individual personality is made up of three distinct components described as *egos*:

- the *parent*
- the *adult*
- the *child*.

Harris (2004) suggests that the *parent* is a *taught* concept, the *child* is a *felt* concept and the *adult* is a *learned* concept as shown in Fig. 3.2. Each ego state is an entire system of thoughts, feelings and behaviours from which individuals interact with each other and is a consistent pattern of feeling, experience and behaviour.

These egos shape a person's beliefs and behaviours every day, both consciously and subconsciously. Even as an adult one may be strongly influenced by experiences as a child. Take the example of a young girl playing on a beach who stops to look at a woman sunbathing topless and her parent is quick to chastise her for doing so. The young girl is then likely to carry the subconscious feeling that exposing one's breasts in public is 'naughty' and therefore may continue to fear doing so as an adult. Furthermore, this fear may extend to breastfeeding her baby as a new

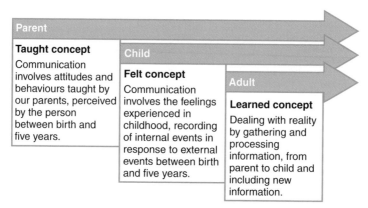

Fig. 3.2   Ego states. (Berne 1964; Harris 2004.)

mother, especially if she has experienced a negative stigma of breastfeeding in public, leading to a preconceived idea that it is '*disgusting*'. This idea may arise from messages learned through her parents as a child, and because of her not having had the chance to change these perceptions in her adult ego, they continue throughout her life.

The adult ego, however, is able take the best experiences from the past and use them appropriately, integrating the positive aspects from the parent and child ego states. If a midwife is aware of this, they are in a better position to help the woman seek information to change her assumptions. This will be most successful when the midwife is able to communicate the information in a way that women understand. In the aforementioned scenario, the midwife should help the new mother to move away from the perception that breastfeeding is disgusting and recognize that breastfeeding is not only a normal physiological event but also has many benefits for both the mother and baby. Education, knowledge and experience are important factors in developing one's self, and an understanding of assertiveness is a vital skill in building successful relationships and outcomes.

Assertiveness

Assertiveness relates to how a person chooses to behave. The principle of *equality* is essential to assertive behaviour and communication. Furthermore, being assertive does not always result in an individual achieving what they want, but sometimes results in the individual realizing a satisfactory compromise (Dickson 2012). The assertive professional is someone who can state clearly what they want and hold firm during a professional disagreement as well as having the confidence to repeat what they have to say (Burnard 1989; Sully and Dallas 2010). Therefore, as well as being aware of one's self and one's environment, assertiveness is a skill required to communicate effectively. An assertive approach to communication will strengthen a midwife's ability to manage the anxiety and stress of a difficult situation and convey the appropriate information to both the childbearing woman and colleagues.

To become appropriately assertive a person must first recognize the difference between assertive behaviour and behaviour which is aggressive, passive or manipulative. The underlying philosophical belief regarding assertive behaviour is based on the concept of *I'm OK you're OK* (Harris 1970). In this concept, four response styles, which Darling (2002) describes as *life positions*, are described to simply demonstrate *aggressive*, *submissive*, *manipulative* and *assertive* communication, as seen in Fig. 3.3. If the assertive life position represents the best form of communication, the other three life positions can be seen as indirect ways of communicating which reflect the imbalance of power between the people communicating. In the perspective of Darling (2002), *I'm OK*

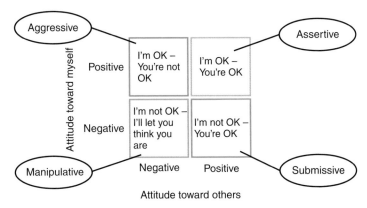

Fig. 3.3 The four life positions. (Courtesy Paris Dunlop and Leontia Pillay. Adapted from Darling 2002.)

you're OK is the *assertive* life position and therefore what people should aspire to. From here it can be seen that *I'm OK you're* not *OK* represents *aggressive* behaviour; *I'm not OK, I'll let you think you are* is *manipulative* or indirectly aggressive *and I'm not OK you're OK* demonstrates *submissive* behaviour. These three life positions are communication types that present when one feels under threat for whatever reason. They are closely related to one's stress response: *fight* (aggressive) or *flight* (passive). It is clear how a combination of self-awareness and assertiveness gives the individual control over their behaviour and communication.

Self-confidence and assertiveness do not come naturally to all people. Even those who are confident in some situations may be less so in others because of the factors previously mentioned. This is especially true for those who are starting a new journey either as a student midwife or as a newly qualified midwife. Self-confidence and assertiveness, however, can be learned and improved by all. Setting small achievable goals which work towards improving self-confidence will go a long way to helping improve one's overall abilities to communicate and therefore perform the role of a midwife, gradually moving towards more challenging activities. It is useful to note that self-esteem tends to be enhanced when an individual chooses to do something which is good for them rather than do something because they feel they ought to.

A midwife must also have strong interpersonal skills to effectively connect with the woman, her partner and family, and colleagues working within the multiprofessional team. The midwife needs to have an understanding of theories underpinning skills required for good communication: techniques such as the appropriate use of verbal and non-verbal communication, questioning and active listening, all of which allow the woman's voice to be heard (DH 2010).

Review the two models of communication as shown in Fig. 3.4 (Darling 2002).

The model in Fig. 3.4A (one-way communication) can be reflected through record keeping where one midwife, the sender, writes *the message* in the notes and the second midwife as *the recipient* reads the notes. No other interaction takes place between the first and the second midwife as it is assumed the recipient fully understands the message and that it is clearly written and with no ambiguity. The second model (two-way communication Fig. 3.4B), however, is considered the more successful model. In this communication the first midwife would be able to amend and enhance the message through feedback to improve the chances of the second midwife fully understanding the scenario.

Verbal Communication

Verbal communication involves the use of the spoken word. The giving and receiving of the message can be influenced by not only the words used but also how they are delivered (e.g. the

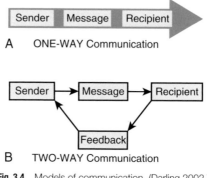

Fig. 3.4   Models of communication. (Darling 2002.)

tone of voice, speed, pitch and language). It is important not to underestimate the intelligence and comprehension of the respondent. As a health professional, the midwife must speak slowly without distorting the natural phrasing and rhythm, speak clearly and distinctly and choose words carefully (e.g. simple common words are better than long and complex ones).

As with Darling's (2002) *four life positions* as described earlier and shown in Fig. 3.3, the words chosen by the midwife can have a subtle but profound effect on how the woman may react to communication. Should the midwife choose to say *'I'm just going to listen to your baby's heart'*, the inclusion of the word *just* can trivialize the procedure, suggesting that the woman should not ask any further questions about the procedure (Simkin et al 2012). Alternatively, the midwife might say *'I'm just going to listen to your baby's heart, okay?'* In this instance the use of *okay?* suggests that consent for the procedure has been obtained when, in fact, the woman may have acknowledged the information but not actively consented to the procedure being undertaken. A further example of a midwife removing power from the woman is demonstrated by the statement *'I just need to take your blood pressure, okay?'* Including the word *need* in this sentence suggests that assessing the blood pressure is extremely important and could be interpreted by the woman that there is no alternative. In addition, midwives must appreciate the importance in recognizing that differences in regional dialect and accent can also create difficulty in understanding what has been said, even when the messenger and recipient speak the same language (Hearnden 2008).

The very best midwives are able to take all of this into account and act accordingly. They will be adept at changing their vernacular to suit and meet the demands of the particular audience. There is an important role for the use of layman's language when communicating with childbearing women to ensure that messages are always fully understood. The midwife is also required to then adapt her language when escalating or sharing clinical information with the multiprofessional team using professional terminology at all times. An example of how a midwife might adapt their professional language to meet the needs of the woman to avoid invoking anxiety is shown below:

> **Professional language:** *'I am going to do an abdominal examination to assess the position of the fetus.'* becomes
> **Layman's language:** *'I am going to feel your tummy to see which way your baby is lying.'*

Midwives must also think beyond the actual spoken word when communicating with women. The role of the midwife entails having to communicate with women in many different situations for a variety of reasons, such as the first formal interview with the woman where the data collected

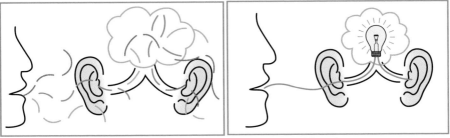

Hearing
- Accidental
- Uncontrolled
- Effortless

Listening
- Concentrated
- Chosen
- Intentional

Fig. 3.5 Hearing and listening. (Courtesy Paris Dunlop and Leontia Pillay.)

are used to inform the subsequent care pathway or an informal liaison in which the midwife has already established a good relationship with the woman and her family. Regardless of the situation, some basic communication skills are required. According to Miller and Webb (2011), these include *active listening*, *attending*, *hearing* and *understanding and remembering*. The environment needs to be appropriate for the interaction, such as a private room to respect confidentiality when the midwife is conducting an interview that also has easy access for a disabled woman, as well as good lighting for the woman who is deaf and wishes to lip read.

Hearing and Listening

The next stage to effective communication is the ability to take information in. To '*hear*', a whole range of aspects of communication must be taken into consideration. The skilled midwife will draw on a range of factors to '*hear*' clearly so as to avoid making assumptions which could result in misunderstandings. Listening is vital to hearing, and there are two types of listening (Miller and Webb 2011):

- *passive listening*, where the recipient shows no signs of hearing the message being related
- *active listening*, where there are clear indications that the message is being both heard and understood by the recipient.

The midwife may use paraphrasing to demonstrate they are listening and understanding (Faulkner 1998; Miller and Webb 2011). Figure 3.5 highlights the subtle differences between hearing and listening in that hearing is an accidental act, relating to the senses, whereas listening requires some effort on the part of the individual.

To actively listen, the midwife must understand that there are three aspects to the conversation. The first is the *spoken word*, known as *linguistic aspects*. For the spoken words to have meaning, an awareness of the subtle nuances of verbal communication is required. These are described as *paralinguistic aspects*, which include the timing, volume and pitch of the spoken word. These aspects begin to add emphasis and significance of meaning to what the person is saying. The volume and pitch of the spoken word may indicate anger/excitement should the individual speak loudly and conversely weakness/fear in a person who is softly spoken. Add to this the non-verbal aspect relating to body language and the midwife has a clearer picture of what the woman or health professional is trying to communicate (Burnard 1997; Miller and Webb 2011). The midwife uses these skills in their everyday work when interviewing women in many different situations. To be successful, an understanding of the interview process is essential.

Interviewing

The structure of the interview will influence its success. The beginning and end of the interview are as important as asking the right type of questions. The midwife's introduction at the beginning of the interview is important to put the woman at ease, informing her of how long the interview is likely to last, the purpose of the interview and that her consent will always be sought should any procedures be required. This will provide a foundation for the midwife to build a professional relationship with the woman based on mutual respect. It is also important to effectively complete the interview. Some women may leave their questions to the end of the interview, but if they are unaware as to when this is likely to be, they are likely to feel frustrated if they have not had the opportunity to articulate their questions (Miller and Webb 2011). A great way to avoid such disappointment is to inform the woman that the interview is nearing an end with a few simple words such as *'I have only a couple of questions left'* or *'I should finish in 5 minutes'* (Miller and Webb 2011). The woman can then ask the midwife questions in the middle of the interview rather than the end.

There are numerous reasons for asking questions; for example, the woman's first contact with the midwife or the first meeting between the midwife mentor/practice supervisor and the student midwife. In these examples the midwife requires a lot of information to be able to determine the most appropriate care pathway for the woman to follow in her pregnancy or to ascertain the learning needs of the student to plan appropriate teaching opportunities during the clinical placement, respectively. Formulating the appropriate type of question will ensure that the midwife is able to gather the information she needs in the most effective way. There are three main types of questions – *open, closed* and *leading* – as shown in Fig. 3.6. The *open question* allows the respondent to answer as they wish and may be helpful in situations where the midwife wishes to ascertain how a woman/student is feeling. The *closed question*, on the other hand, restricts the answer to a simple yes or no response or is aimed at eliciting specific information such as the woman's name and address/stage of training the student is at. The *leading question* implies a preferred answer from the respondent by the way the question is structured; for example, *'Where do you want to give birth to your baby, this hospital or at home?'* or *'How much did you enjoy your learning experience in the birth centre?'*

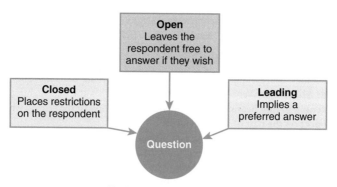

Fig. 3.6 Types of questions.

Undertake Activity 3.2, considering the range of questions the lecturer/academic assessor and midwife mentor/practice assessor may use during a tripartite meeting with a student midwife towards the end of a placement within the birth centre. Decide whether the questions are *open, closed* or *leading,* and consider the advantage and disadvantage of the type of question posed.

ACTIVITY 3.2 ■ **Tripartite Meeting in Birth Centre Between Lecturer/Academic Assessor, Midwife Mentor/Practice Assessor and Student Midwife**

Question From Lecturer/Academic Assessor or Midwife Mentor/Practice Assessor	Type of Question (Open/Closed/Leading)	Advantage	Disadvantage
You enjoyed this placement?			
How do you feel you have settled into working within the birth centre team?			
How many births have you undertaken during this placement?			
You have not had any time off sick during this placement, have you?			
Have you achieved all your learning outcomes that you set with your mentor/practice supervisor at the start of this placement?			
Were there any disappointments from this placement?			
What was the most interesting experience you had during this placement?			
Are you happy with your progress?			
Overall, how do you feel about this placement?			
What will you take forward from this placement to your next placement in the hospital?			

During an interview, not all the information collected is from the spoken word/verbal communication, and so the interviewer must also be aware of the non-verbal cues so as to collect all the relevant information to ensure the interview is successful.

Non-Verbal Communication

Verbal communication and non-verbal communication are closely interrelated (Watzlawick et al 2009). Overall, if verbal and non-verbal messages do not match, it is the non-verbal message that is more likely to be believed. The non-verbal message validates the verbal dimensions of an interaction and therefore the words should always match the body language (Northouse and Northouse 1998).

The midwife has a role in safeguarding vulnerable individuals, be it the childbearing woman, her baby or both, and consequently should attempt to elicit whether the woman has ever experienced any emotional or physical abuse by a family member or close friend so as to be considered at risk. If the woman verbally responds that she has not experienced this but does not make any eye contact with the midwife, speaks quietly with little confidence and appears anxious throughout the interview, these are subliminal messages that the midwife must be aware of that could potentially relate to a case of domestic abuse. Midwives experience incredibly sensitive aspects of people's lives and therefore they must learn to 'read the picture' (Moss 2012) to get as full an insight as possible as to what is being communicated.

In a more practical sense non-verbal communication can be used to effectively inform women about the process of childbirth. When caring for women who are deaf or have learning disabilities, midwives can use visual aids such as pictures or DVDs to assist with communication. For blind women, audio tapes and recordings may be used, with the midwife using models, such as a doll and pelvis, to explain the process of childbirth through encouraging touch.

In addition to reading the non-verbal cues from the woman, the midwife must always be aware of the message she is portraying with her own body language. Gestures can be used to amplify the spoken word. Posture is usually subconscious but can affect who is in control of the situation or can sometimes indicate disinterest. Position and distance can portray messages both positive and negative (England and Morgan 2012).

PROXEMICS

Proxemics is the study of the human use of space: *the personal space* (Toshitaka et al 2011). The relationship between individuals will determine their personal space. At the first interview, for example, if the midwife is positioned too close to the woman, the woman is likely to feel uncomfortable, whereas as the relationship develops, the acceptable personal space between the midwife and the woman is much more likely to change and become closer.

NON-VERBAL CUES BETWEEN MOTHER AND BABY

The relationship between the mother and the baby is enhanced when the woman learns to read the non-verbal cues from her baby. The distance of eye contact between a mother when she is holding her baby is sufficiently close enough for her to elicit the baby's non-verbal cues as well as the baby learning to visualize the mother's facial characteristics. This is particularly important when the midwife is helping the mother to breastfeed her baby. Although it is recognized that breast milk is the best source of nutrition for the human baby, the prevalence of breastfeeding differs across cultures. Where exposure to breastfeeding has been limited, it is important that the midwife educates the woman to watch for early feeding cues, such as the baby rooting, encourage skin to skin contact to calm the baby and follow the baby's lead (UNICEF UK 2012).

Information Transfer and the Value of Record Keeping

In the United Kingdom, communication issues, particularly poor communication between professionals and inadequate communication of risk factors, have been consistently identified in significantly contributing to patient safety incidents resulting in morbidity and mortality (Lewis and Drife 2004; Lewis 2007; Knight et al 2015). Childbearing women have also voiced concern over the interruption to continuity of care and carer nationally and locally (Care Quality Commission 2015). It could be argued that this sentiment reinforces issues that appear in the literature with accounts of information loss and communication failures particularly between shift changes of staff. The King's Fund *Safe Births* recommendations (Kings Fund 2008) and the Healthcare Commission's (2009) review of maternity services have identified areas in need of improvement. These include multidisciplinary team working through joint training and handovers, adequate staffing and clearly defined roles. Underpinning this is the need for good-quality standardized communication. *Towards Better Births* (Healthcare Commission 2008) highlights the importance of good communication for woman-centred care. In addition, multidisciplinary working and communication continue being acknowledged as vital for successful outcomes (DH 2007, 2016).

Most midwifery models of care require the support of the wider maternity team when escalation or referral is required because of a concern or when there is deviation from the normal physiological processes. These characteristics lead to a dependence on a number of means for transferring information, processing this information and ensuring effective coordination of care (Mackintosh et al 2009), all of which can be victim to human error (Brindley and Reynolds 2011).

To facilitate the transfer of relevant maternity patient information between consecutive shifts requires collaboration and two-way communication between teams or individuals which is commonly known as *handover* (Randell et al 2009). The student in the clinical area needs to be able to identify these skills and recognize them in the practitioners they are working with. There is evidence that the quality of handover in maternity care can be poor (Healthcare Commission 2004, 2005; Smith and Dixon 2007; Department of Health Ireland 2014) and thus the key to success is to identify the national and local barriers and facilitators in this process. Although there are limited published studies focused on shift handovers in relation to maternity services (Sabir et al 2006; Beckett and Kipinis 2009), much can be learned from studies in other health care settings, such as the emergency department and ambulance services (Apker et al 2007; Budd et al 2007; Jenkin et al 2007; Yong et al 2008; Horwitz et al 2009) and surgical and medical wards, which rely on communication of information across a multiprofessional platform (Fassett and Bollipo 2006; Broekuis and Veldkamp 2007; Randell et al 2009; Welsh et al 2010).

The quality of handover of care is pivotal in circumstances where health care professionals are required to convey important information and ensure the smooth transition and transfer of responsibility from one professional to another, hence why this is fundamental to ensuring the safety of the childbearing woman and her baby. The use of mnemonics as a standardized approach has received a surge of attention in recent years. A systematic literature review by Risenberg et al (2009) identified 46 articles describing 24 different handover mnemonics. The most frequently cited communication mnemonic was *SBAR: situation, background, assessment,* and *recommendation* (NHS Institute for Innovation and Improvement 2008). The SBAR tool can be used to frame all clinical communication, especially clinical communication that necessitates immediate attention and action, either face to face or by telephone between individual team members or through collaboration at multidisciplinary team meetings.

Use of the SBAR tool may appear simple, but it may take some effort on the part of health professionals to adapt their way of communicating and be assertive, especially with senior colleagues. For the inexperienced midwife/student midwife, making recommendations to more senior colleagues may appear daunting and a challenge, which is an important stage of the SBAR process as it conveys the action the messenger requires. In such situations, a supportive preceptor or lecturer to assist the midwife or student midwife, respectively, in trying out the tool to allay anxiety and build personal confidence is a useful strategy to adopt (NHS Institute for Innovation and Improvement 2008).

The three different situations when SBAR is used are:
- escalation of a situation (e.g. postpartum haemorrhage)
- transfer of care from one area to another (e.g. from the birthing unit to the postnatal area)
- shift handover (e.g. transfer home).

Activity 3.3 provides an opportunity to apply the stages of the SBAR tool to a typical midwifery scenario and provide concise and pertinent information to other members of the multiprofessional team, either face to face or by telephone. It is also worth noting that clear, concise record keeping is essential in documenting the specific management decisions that are made with the woman's and her baby's or the student's interests always at the forefront to ensure the best possible outcome (NMC 2018).

Figure 3.7 demonstrates how SBAR can be used in each of the above situations.

ACTIVITY 3.3 ■

You are working in triage and a healthy primigravida attends at 39 weeks with spontaneous rupture of membranes and contracting every 3 minutes. On examination, you discover there to be significant meconium present. You commence a cardiotocograph, which appears to show features of a suspicious trace. Maternal observations are as follows:
- blood pressure 120/76 mmHg
- pulse 76 beats/minute
- temperature 36.9 °C.

Record your subsequent communication to members of the multiprofessional team in this situation using the SBAR mnemonic:

Situation:
Background:
Assessment:
Recommendation:

Escalation	• **S** Woman in midwife led unit, is having a postpartum haemorrhage (PPH): she gave birth 5 minutes ago. • **B** Low-risk woman, normal progress in labour, physiological third stage of labour. Blood loss 700 mls from ? uterine atony. • **A** All observations are within normal limits • **R** She requires immediate review by the obstetric team.
Transfer of care	• **S** Para 1, Ventouse birth 2 hours ago with episiotomy. Blood loss 400 mls, Baby 3690g. • **B** Low risk antenatally with prolonged rupture of membranes. Rhesus negative. • **A** All maternal and neonatal observations within normal limits. First breastfeed achieved by baby, who has passed meconium. • **R** Routine postnatal care, 24-hour observations of baby: temperature and pulse (sepsis). Review baby's blood group in view of Rhesus-negative mother.
Shift handover	• **S** Para 1, Emergency caesarean section 2 days ago. Been well post-operative. Baby 3320g is reluctant to breastfeed. • **B** Low risk antenatally. • **A** All maternal observations within normal limits. Baby is well hydrated and passing urine. • **R** Provide enhanced support with breastfeeding prior to considering transfer home to community midwife.

Fig. 3.7   Examples of SBAR in different maternity contexts.

Feedback From Women

Deane-Gray (2008) has noted that when women complain about their maternity care, one of the main reasons for dissatisfaction is lack of communication. Use of the second of Darling's (2002) models would allow more feedback between all parties. The situation would remain the same between the midwife and the woman but in this model the woman is able to ask questions and clarify queries, and consequently the midwife is able to develop a better message to convey to colleagues also involved in the woman's care.

The Friends and Family Test (DH 2012) has been implemented to instigate a culture of continuous improvement in the quality of care within the National Health Service (NHS) as well as to provide insight into good practice, including enhancing communication with patients. It is an important feedback tool that enables everyone accessing NHS services to provide feedback on their experiences and whether they would recommend the same services to others. However, it does not replace the NHS complaints procedure. For maternity services, feedback is sought from women at the 36 weeks antenatal appointment, at discharge from the ward/birthing unit/following a home birth and at discharge from the care of the community midwife around the 10th day following the baby's birth.

All letters received from women must be investigated and an answer must be provided. The scenario in Activity 3.4 is based on letters received from childbearing women about the care they received from the midwife. Now undertake Activity 3.4 using the resources contained within this chapter.

ACTIVITY 3.4 ■

Jane Brown has been given a date for induction of labour and asked to arrive at the hospital at 8 a.m. As she is leaving home she receives a message from the midwife to say that there are no beds available at present and to come in at midday. Jane had previously been informed that she needed to have the induction of labour because of placental insufficiency that could lead to the baby becoming distressed. Jane is very anxious that the procedure has been delayed as she is now 42 weeks pregnant.

Consider how this situation may have been avoided using the questions below and how you may respond to Jane and in what form of communication:

■ What were the errors that occurred in this situation?
■ How could they have been avoided?
■ What are the ethical considerations?
■ How could communication be developed to prevent similar incidents from happening in the future?

Conclusion

This chapter has explored the importance of midwives developing effective communication skills to meet the challenges of 21st century midwifery education and practice. The explosion of social media has had a dramatic effect on how individuals communicate, and the platforms are continuing to expand, requiring each health professional to keep abreast of these developments. Having an understanding of communication theory enables both the student midwife and the practising midwife to appreciate the context and the requirement to convey complex information in a way that others will understand. All types of communication are equally important, whether verbal, non-verbal or written: each plays a part in helping to comprehend a much clearer picture.

KEY POINTS

- Effective communication skills are fundamental to midwifery education and practice to develop and maintain good working relationships with students, colleagues and childbearing women.
- Students and practising midwives should be fully conversant with the construct of *e-professionalism* and always use social media appropriately.
- The midwife's skill to recognize the context surrounding the communication taking place lies in their ability to appreciate the different parts of their self/ego.
- Appropriate use of verbal and non-verbal communication, questioning and active listening are essential to achieving effective communication.
- Theories of communication and communication tools can assist students and practising midwives to understand the complex nature of human interaction and develop ways in which to convey messages that can be understood by the recipient.
- A supportive learning and working environment is essential to nurture students and inexperienced health professionals in becoming confident and assertive when interacting with others.

References

Apker, J., Mallak, L. A., & Gibson, S. C. (2007). Communicating in the "gray zone": perceptions about emergency physician hospital list handoffs and patient safety. *Academic Emergency Medicine, 14*, 884–894.

Beckett, C., & Kipinis, G. (2009). Collaborative communication: integrating SBAR to improve quality/patient safety outcomes. *Journal for Healthcare Quality, 31*(5), 19–28.

Berne, E. (1964). *Games people play, the psychology of human relationships*. London: Penguin Books.

Brindley, P. G., & Reynolds, S. F. (2011). Improving verbal communication in critical care medicine. *Journal of Critical Care*, *26*(2), 155–159.

Broekhuis, M., & Veldkamp, C. (2007). The usefulness and feasibility of a reflexivity method to improve clinical handover. *Journal of Evaluation in Clinical Practice*, *13*(1), 109–115.

Budd, H. R., Almond, L. M., & Porter, K. (2007). A survey of trauma alert criteria and handover practice in England and Wales. *Emergency Medicine Journal*, *24*(4), 302–304.

Burnard, P. (1989). *Effective communication skills for health professionals* (2nd ed.). London: Nelson Thorpe.

Burnard, P. (1997). *Know yourself: Self-awareness activities for health care professionals*. London: Whurr.

Cain, J., & Romanelli, F. (2009). E-professionalism: a new paradigm for a digital age. *Currents in Pharmacy Teaching and Learning*, *1*(2), 66–70.

Care Quality Commission. (2015). *Maternity services survey*. Available at: http://www.cqc.org.uk/content/maternity-services-survey-2015.

Chief Nursing Officers of England, Northern Ireland, Scotland and Wales. (2010). *Midwifery 2020: delivering expectations*. London: Department of Health.

Darling, M. (2002). *Managing communication in health care*. Edinburgh: Bailliere Tindall and the Royal College of Nursing.

Deane-Gray, T. (2008). Effective communication. In Peate, I. & Hamilton, C. (Eds.), *Becoming a midwife in the 21st century* (pp. 11–27). Chichester: John Wiley and Sons.

Department of Health. (2007). *Maternity matters: Choice, access and continuity of care in a safe service*. London: Stationery Office.

Department of Health. (2010). *Essence of care 2010. Benchmarks for communication*. Available at: http://www.gov.uk/government/uploads/system/uploads/attachment_data/file/216695/dh_119973.pdf.

Department of Health. (2012). *The NHS Friends and Family Test: Implementation Guide*. London: Department of Health.

Department of Health. (2016). *Better births: Improving outcomes of maternity services in England. A five year forward review for maternity care*. Available at: http://www.england.nhs.uk/wp-content/uploads/2016/02/national-maternity-review-report.pdf.

Department of Health Ireland. (2014). Communication (clinical handover). In *Maternity services national clinical guideline no 5*. Available at: http://health.gov.ie/wp-content/uploads/2015/01/National-Clinical-Guideline-No.-5-Summary-Clinical-Handover-Nov2014.pdf.

De Vito, J. A. (2015). *The interpersonal communication book* (14th ed.). New York: Longman.

Dickson, A. (2012). *A woman in your own right, assertiveness and you (revised 30th anniversary* (ed.). London: Quartet Books.

England, C., & Morgan, R. (2012). *Communication skills for midwives challenges in everyday practice*. Maidenhead: Open University Press.

Fassett, R. G., & Bollipo, S. J. (2006). Morning report: an Australian experience. *Medical Journal of Australia*, *184*(4), 159–161.

Faulkner, A. (1998). *Effective interaction with patients* (2nd ed.). London: Churchill Livingstone.

Harris, T. (1970). *I'm ok – you're ok*. London: Pan Books.

Harris, T. (2004). *I'm ok – you're ok'*. New York: Quill.

Healthcare Commission. (2004). *A summary of the investigation into maternity services provided by the Royal Wolverhampton Hospitals Trust at New Cross Hospital*. London: Healthcare Commission. Available at: https://www.cqc.org.uk/_db/_documents/04011739.pdf.

Healthcare Commission. (2005). *Review of maternity services provided by North West London Hospitals NHS Trust*. London: The Stationary Office.

Healthcare Commission. (2008). *Towards better births*. London: The Stationary Office.

Healthcare Commission. (2009). *Investigations into Mid-Staffordshire NHS Foundation Trust*. London: The Stationary Office.

Hearnden, M. (2008). Coping with differences in culture and communication in health care. *Nursing Standard*, *23*(11), 49–57.

Horwitz, L. I., Meredith, T., Schuur, J. D., Shah, N. R., Kulkarni, R. G., & Jenq, G. Y. (2009). Dropping the baton: a qualitative analysis of failures during the transition from emergency department to inpatient care. *Annals of Emergency Medicine*, *53*(6), 701–710.

Jenkin, A., Abelson-Mitchell, N., & Cooper, S. (2007). Patient handover: time for a change? *Accident and Emergency Nursing*, *15*(3), 141–147.

Jones, C., & Hayter, M. (2013). Social media use by nurses and midwives: a 'recipe for disaster' or a 'force for good'? *Journal of Clinical Nursing, 22*(11–12), 1495–1496.

Kings Fund. (2008). *Safe births: Everybody's business: An independent study into the safety of maternity services in England*. Available at: https://www.kingsfund.org.uk/sites/files/kf/field/field_publication_summary/safe-births-summary-onora-oneill.pdf.

Kirkham, M. J. (2010). *The midwife-mother relationship* (2nd ed.). Basingstoke: Palgrave Macmillan.

Knight, M., Kenyon, S., Brocklehurst, P., Neilson, J., Shakespeare, J., & Kurinszuk, J. J. (Eds.). (2015). *Saving lives, improving mothers' care – lessons learned to inform future maternity care from the UK and Ireland confidential enquiries into maternal deaths and morbidity 2009-2012*. Oxford: National Perinatal Epidemiology Unit. Available at: https://www.npeu.ox.ac.uk/downloads/files/mbrrace-uk/reports/MBRRACE-UK%20Maternal%20Report%202015.pdf.

Lewis, G., & Drife, J. (2004). *Why mothers die 2000 - 2002: the sixth report of the Confidential Enquiries into Maternal Deaths in the United Kingdom*. London: RCOG Press.

Lewis, G. (Ed.). (2007). *The Confidential Enquiry into Maternal and Child Health (CEMACH). Saving mothers' lives: reviewing maternal deaths to make motherhood safer - 2003-2005. The seventh report on Confidential Enquiries into Maternal Deaths in the United Kingdom*. London: Confidential Enquiry into Maternal and Child Health. Available at: http://www.publichealth.hscni.net/sites/default/files/Saving%20Mothers'%20Lives%202003-05%20Midwifery%20Summary.pdf.

Mackintosh, N., Berridge, E.-J., & Freeth, D. (2009). Supporting structures for team situation awareness and decision making: insights from four delivery suites. *Journal of Evaluation in Clinical Practice, 15*(1), 46–54.

Miller, E., & Webb, L. (2011). Active Listening and attending: communication skills and the healthcare environment. In Webb, L. (Ed.), *Communication skills in practice*. Oxford: Oxford University Press.

Moss, B. (2012). *Communication skills in health and social care* (2nd ed.). London: Sage Publications.

NHS Institute for Innovation and Improvement. (2008). *SBAR: Situation, background, assessment and recommendation tool*. Available at: https://improvement.nhs.uk/resources/sbar-communication-tool/.

Northouse, L. L., & Northouse, P. G. (1998). *Health communication strategies for health* (3rd ed.). London: Prentice Hall International.

Nursing and Midwifery Council. (2015). *Guidance on using social media responsibly*. Available at: http://www.nmc.org.uk/standards/guidance/social-media-guidance/.

Nursing and Midwifery Council. (2018). *The code: Professional standards of practice and behaviour for nurses, midwives and nursing associates*. London: Nursing and Midwifery Council. Available at: http://www.nmc.org.uk/standards/code/.

Nursing and Midwifery Council. (2019). *Revalidation: How to revalidate with the NMC*. Available at: https://www.nmc.org.uk/globalassets/sitedocuments/revalidation/how-to-revalidate-booklet.pdf.

Randell, R., Wilson, S., Woodward, P., & Galliers, J. (2009). Beyond handover: supporting awareness for continuous coverage. *Cognition, Technology and Work, 12*(4), 271–283.

Riesenberg, L. A., Leitzsch, J., & Little, B. W. (2009). Systematic review of handoff mnemonics literature. *American College of Medical Quality, 24*(3), 196–204.

Sabir, N., Yentis, S. M., & Holdcroft, A. (2006). A national survey of obstetric anaesthetic handovers. *Anaesthesia, 61*(4), 376–380.

Simkin, P., Stewart, M., Shearer, B., Glance, J. C., Rooks, J., Lyerly, A. D., et al. (2012). The language of birth. *Birth, 39*(2), 156–164.

Smith, A., & Dixon, A. (2007). *The safety of maternity services in England*. London: King's Fund.

Stewart, S., Sidebottom, M., & Davis, D. (2012). International networking: connecting midwives through social media. *International Nursing Review, 59*(3), 431–434.

Sully, P., & Dallas, J. (2010). *Essential communication skills for nursing and midwifery* (2nd ed.). Edinburgh: Mosby.

Toshitaka, A., Hamid, I., Makota, Y., & Masayuki, N. (2011). Personal space-based simulation of non-verbal communication. *Entertainment Computing, 2*(4), 245–261.

Tripp, N., Hainey, K., Liu, A., Poulton, A., Peek, M., Kim, J., et al. (2014). An emerging model of maternity care: smartphone, midwife, doctor? *Women and Birth, 27*, 64–67.

UNICEF, U. K. (2012). *Guide to the Baby Friendly Initiative standard*. Available at: https://www.yumpu.com/en/document/view/27571830/guide-to-the-baby-friendly-initiative-standards-unicef-uk.

Watzlawick, P., Beavin, J. H., & Jackson, D. D. (2009). Principles of human communication. In van Servellen, G. (Ed.), *Communication skills for the health care professional: Concept, practice, and evidence* (2nd ed.) (pp. 23–48). London: Jones and Bartlett Publishers International.

Webb, L. (2011). How to relate to others effectively. In Webb, L. (Ed.), *Nursing: communication skills in practice* (pp. 33–51). Oxford: Oxford University Press.

Welsh, C. A., Flanagan, M. E., & Ebright, P. (2010). Barriers and facilitators to nursing handoffs: recommendations for design. *Nursing Outlook, 58*(3), 148–154.

Wirtanen, M. (2012). Smartphone = Smart Health? Available at: https://www.alliedhealthworld.com/visuals/smartphone-healthcare.html.

Wylie, L. (2014). The social media revolution. *British Journal of Midwifery, 22*(7), 502–506.

Yong, G., Dent, A. W., & Weiland, T. J. (2008). Handover from paramedics: observations and emergency department clinician perceptions. *Emergency Medicine Australasia, 20*, 149–155.

Further Reading

Berne, E. (2015). *Transactional analysis in psychotherapy: A systematic individual and social psychiatry.* Eastford: Martino Fine Books.

This is a reprint of psychiatrist Eric Berne's first book compiled from all his published articles that outlined his theories on transactional analysis, including the parent–adult–child model. The underlying precept is that humans are social creatures and that all individuals are multifaceted beings who change when in contact with another person in their world. It is an ideal book for readers looking to learn more about transactional analysis and its origins.

Kirkham, M. J. (2010). *The midwife-mother relationship* (2nd ed.). Basingstoke: Palgrave Macmillan.

This text examines the relationship between the midwife and the mother from a variety of perspectives that should assist the reader in developing a good working relationship with childbearing women and in so doing enhance the quality of maternity care they provide.

NHS Institute for Innovation and Improvement. (2008). *SBAR: Situation, background, assessment and recommendation tool.* Available at: https://improvement.nhs.uk/resources/sbar-communication-tool/.

This provides an overview of the SBAR tool, including an example of its application in an acute medical situation which demonstrates how it can create a shared expectation between the sender and the recipient of the information being shared.

Useful Websites

Care Quality Commission. (https://www.cqc.org.uk.

ChangingMinds.org (transactional analysis). (https://www.changingminds.org.

King's Fund. (https://www.kingsfund.org.uk.

Nursing and Midwifery Council. (https://www.nmc.org.uk.

Royal College of Midwives. (https://www.rcm.org.uk.

CHAPTER 4

Conceptual and Philosophical Bases of Midwifery

Val Collington ▣ Gina Finnerty

LEARNING OUTCOMES

By the end of this chapter the reader will be:

- cognizant of the language surrounding the philosophical bases that underpin the art of midwifery practice
- able to demonstrate knowledge of key global philosophical principles of midwifery education and practice
- able to identify personal beliefs and values as they relate to midwifery care and practice
- able to devise a personal philosophy of midwifery and appraise it.

Overview

With woman. That is the essence of midwifery. More than a job, more than a profession, midwifery is a philosophy: it is never just a function.

MURPHY 2004: 1

Throughout this chapter the reader is encouraged to examine philosophies that frame their everyday thinking in midwifery education and clinical practice. It explores theories that underpin a midwifery philosophy, midwifery values and beliefs and global perspectives in relation to midwifery ideology. In addition, some of the challenges within midwifery education, practice and research, including a number of case scenarios, are presented to enable the reader to place the theory into context.

Introduction

In the United Kingdom (UK), an inspectorate body, the Care Quality Commission (CQC) exists to improve quality through effective regulation and registration. Robust systems are now in place to improve quality and standards of care following the Francis Inquiry (Mid Staffordshire NHS Trust Public Inquiry 2013) in which substandard levels of care were found in one National Health Service (NHS) Trust in England. Each CQC visit to a maternity unit will inevitably be preceded by a flurry of practical and paper exercises to demonstrate that high-quality care is indeed being delivered. One of these activities may be revisiting the working philosophy of a specific clinical area or department such as a maternity unit.

The Nursing and Midwifery Council (NMC) code (NMC 2018) makes reference to legal and ethical obligations of the midwife and values, whilst *Standards for Pre-registration Midwifery Education* (NMC 2009) emphasizes that midwives must focus on the provision of holistic care for women and their families which respects their individual needs, contexts, cultures and choices. These principles of equity and fairness are deemed fundamental values, which must be addressed in all midwifery education programmes. NMC approval and monitoring of universities explores these elements, and the philosophy underpinning midwifery education programmes is checked to see if they meet professional requirements.

This chapter will have resonances with Chapters 5 and 6. The reader is encouraged to think critically about their inherent values and beliefs about women, birth and being a midwife in challenging practice settings as well as developing their individual philosophy of care in response to this. In addition, they are challenged to consider some relevant theoretical and conceptual models and to use the activities and case scenarios within the chapter as a focus for philosophical discussions with their peers. Some may trigger uncomfortable feelings but it is believed that philosophy should not be an indulgent added *extra* in midwifery curricula and in clinical care, but should be central to the process of making appropriate decisions and judgements in education, clinical practice and research.

Activity 4.1 is a prompt to encourage the reader to reflect honestly on the extent to which a formal, written philosophy has direct relevance to their own practice, whether in clinical practice or as an academic.

ACTIVITY 4.1 ■

- To what extent does the publicly presented philosophy of midwifery guide your interactions with women and their families and, specifically, your daily midwifery care?
- As a midwifery lecturer, how does your philosophy impact on your teaching of students, both in theory and in practice as a link/liaison lecturer or tutor?

So often, a midwifery shift on a busy antenatal ward or day assessment unit means '*getting through the work*' to achieve targets, avoiding blocking NHS beds, rather than providing personalized care to women, their babies and their families. Similarly, pressures on all lecturers to publish in high-impact journals as well as fulfil their teaching commitments can create tension. It is important for midwives to return to their own philosophy on a regular basis so that they remain authentic and true to their belief systems.

Philosophies and Their Relationship to Midwifery

Collins English Dictionary (Knight 2003) defines philosophy as

> *the academic discipline concerned with making explicit the nature and significance of ordinary and scientific beliefs and investigating the intelligibility of concepts by means of rational argument concerning their presuppositions, implications, and interrelationships; in particular, the rational investigation of the nature and structure of reality (metaphysics), the resources and limits of knowledge (epistemology), the principles and import of moral judgement (ethics), and the relationship between language and reality (semantics).*

It is important to consider the extent to which the definition comprises rhetoric or reality within woman-centred midwifery care. The principles underlying an individual's thinking and professional conduct can have a long-lasting impact on women.

The term *philosophy* is also meant to indicate critical examination of practices and assumptions. Dewey (2008) describes philosophy as reflective thinking that lays the context for experience. A philosophy can be viewed as a critical and systematic way of thinking about current beliefs and practice and adds intentionality and deliberation to the work an individual undertakes (Dewey 2008). Considering the fundamental nature of midwifery practice, the knowledge, values, behaviours and actions require critical examination.

Historically, philosophy has been divided into broad categories: *metaphysics, epistemology, value theory* and *logic*. Garvey and Stangroom (2012) suggest that philosophy is actually an activity that uses reasoning and argument to promote human flourishing. The challenge is to embed core ancient arguments into modern midwifery practice and degree programmes. The application of philosophy to midwifery education is central for encouraging students to think critically in applying their belief systems whilst working within the discipline and course philosophy.

Table 4.1 provides an extract from the Philosophy and Model of Midwifery Care of the International Confederation of Midwives (ICM) (2014).

TABLE 4.1 ■ Philosophy of Midwifery Care

1. Pregnancy and childbearing are usually normal physiological processes.
2. Pregnancy and childbearing is a profound experience, which carries significant meaning to the woman, her family, and the community.
3. Midwives are the most appropriate care providers to attend childbearing women.
4. Midwifery care promotes, protects and supports women's human, reproductive and sexual health and rights, and respects ethnic and cultural diversity. It is based on the ethical principles of justice, equity, and respect for human dignity.
5. Midwifery care is holistic and continuous in nature, grounded in an understanding of the social, emotional, cultural, spiritual, psychological and physical experiences of women.
6. Midwifery care is emancipatory as it protects and enhances the health and social status of women, and builds women's self-confidence in their ability to cops with childbirth.
7. Midwifery care takes place in partnership with women, recognising the right to self-determination, and is respectful, personalised, continuous and non-authoritarian.
8. Ethical and competent midwifery care is informed and guided by formal and continuous education, scientific research and application of evidence.

From International Confederation of Midwives (2014: 2).

It is recommended that keywords are identified that resonate with an individual's own philosophy of midwifery. Bearing in mind that midwives play a significant role in orchestration of the maternity care environment (Murphy 2004), the reader is asked to consider the following questions:

- To what extent are you able to practise within this framework so that it becomes a working philosophy?
- In what specific ways is your own midwifery practice emancipatory?
- How do you balance tensions between medicalization and promoting normalcy to demonstrate autonomous practice, holistic care and empowerment of women and their partners?

These issues will be explored throughout the chapter. To answer the above questions, it is first necessary to examine global models of midwifery care in use.

Philosophy of Midwifery Care Within a Global Framework

The *Lancet* series on midwifery care (Renfrew et al 2014) includes four articles with a focus on a new evidence-informed global framework. Central to the framework is the role of the midwife in low-, medium- and high-income countries in the provision of quality maternal and newborn care. Whilst a philosophy of care was not specifically mentioned or addressed, the seminal research drew attention to the need in demonstrating midwives' common beliefs and a solid philosophy of midwifery care in which the safety of women and babies is paramount.

The ICM has an overarching role in providing global guidelines for ethics and philosophy as highlighted in Table 4.1. A model of midwifery care has also been developed as shown in Table 4.2 (ICM 2014).

It is important that, as a community of practitioners, midwives critically examine all statements which have direct implications for provision of care. Considering the ICM (2014) Model of Midwifery Care in Table 4.2:

TABLE 4.2 ■ Model of Midwifery Care

1. Midwives promote and protect women's and newborns' health and rights.
2. Midwives respect and have confidence in women and in their capabilities in childbirth.
3. Midwives promote and advocate for non-intervention in normal childbirth.
4. Midwives provide women with appropriate information and advice in a way that promotes participation and enhances informed decision-making.
5. Midwives offer respectful, anticipatory and flexible care, which encompasses the needs of the woman, her newborn, family and community, and begins with primary attention to the nature of the relationship between the woman seeking midwifery care and the midwife.
6. Midwives empower women to assume responsibility for their health and for the health of their families.
7. Midwives practice in collaboration and consultation with other health professionals to serve the needs of the woman, her newborn, family and community.
8. Midwives maintain their competence and ensure their practice is evidence-based.
9. Midwives use technology appropriately and effect referral in a timely manner when problems arise.
10. Midwives are individually and collectively responsible for the development of midwifery care, educating the new generation of midwives and colleagues in the concept of lifelong learning

From International Confederation of Midwives (2014: 2-3).

- To what extent do you agree with its contents?
- How could the model be enhanced/improved?
- What language do you use to advocate non-intervention when working in a busy materni unit/birthing suite?

The next section explores the theory and ideology underpinning midwifery education and practice.

Theory Related to Midwifery Philosophy

Theory is defined in the *New Oxford Dictionary* as a supposition or a system of ideas intended to explain something, especially one based on general principles independent of the thing to be explained (Pearsall 2001). So, theory can be viewed as a set of statements, principles or ideas by which authority claims are made; for example, about midwifery practice or midwifery education. In other words, a theory is an explanation that helps structure action by identifying key relationships that can be used to explain, predict or change what an lecturer may engage a midwifery student in reflective conversations about, such as decisions regarding care options. Relevant questions might be:

- Why was the decision made?
- What drove the decision?
- Who is responsible for making the decision?

The midwifery lecturer or clinical practitioner may be informed by a particular theory to engage students in reflective thinking to help them make meaning of an educational or practice experience (see Chapter 5). Discussions need to be facilitated by both practitioners and lecturers in which motivated staff confidently role-model their philosophical beliefs. An example of a theoretical model which can be put into practice if it matches an individual's own philosophy is that of Carl Rogers, a humanistic psychologist and educator. Rogers (1961) used humanistic approaches in his practice as a psychoanalyst and teacher to help others reach their full potential. His theory provides one example of how humanistic strategies can be woven into a midwife's philosophy, whether a clinical midwife, a lecturer or a researcher.

In relation to the *essence of midwifery* and the concepts that influence day-to-day practice and care provision, although the effectiveness of midwifery care has been established in many studies, the processes by which midwives accomplish successful outcomes are not well understood. Kennedy et al (2003) conducted a metasynthesis to address this deficit. The themes that emerged relating to the *essence of midwifery* included the midwife as an instrument of care using attributes, such as being non-judgemental, clinically competent and experiencing joy in one's work, to affect the process of care. Another theme related to the woman as a partner in care that is individualized and includes respect and self-determination. In addition, an alliance in midwifery care demonstrated by a relationship with trust, mutual control and shared decision-making was also found. The impact of the environment in the process of midwifery care with emphasis on the midwife protecting normalcy and being present was also noted (Kennedy et al 2003). The essence of care is obviously complex, and the discussion in the following section aims to highlight issues that influence professional practice and care provision.

Midwifery Values and Beliefs

Each professional has their own values, beliefs and attitudes that have developed throughout the course of their lives. Family, friends, community and the experiences an individual has had all contribute to the sense of who they are and how they view the world. If midwives are to provide a service that meets the needs of women and their families and helps them to feel empowered, they need to be aware of their own personal values, beliefs and attitudes and be prepared to adopt the midwifery professional values rather than imposing their own ideas on others.

Values are principles, standards or qualities that an individual or group of people hold in high regard. These values guide the way an individual lives their life and the decisions they make. A value may be defined as something that is held dear: those things/qualities which are considered to be of worth, commonly formed by a particular belief that is related to the worth of an idea or type of behaviour. Values can influence many of the daily judgements that are made as well as have an impact on the support a midwife may give to childbearing women. It is important that midwives do not influence a woman's decisions on the basis of their own values but work from the basis of supporting the woman's values instead.

Beliefs provide context for the experiences an individual has, connecting them to their values and criteria. Beliefs and values are interdependent; that is, they cannot be separated from each other.

In 2012 the NMC and the General Medical Council issued a joint statement (General Medical Council 2012) reinforcing their joint professional values. The statement emphasized the importance of individuals raising concerns when appropriate, in line with ensuring a quality service and public safety. The NHS Constitution for England (Department of Health 2015) has since drawn up a set of NHS values which are highlighted in Table 4.3.

TABLE 4.3 ■ **NHS Values**

Working together for patients	Patients, public and staff have helped develop this expression of values that inspire passion in the National Health Service (NHS) and that should underpin everything it does
Respect and dignity	Every individual who comes into contact with the NHS and organizations providing health services should always be treated with respect and dignity, regardless of whether they are a patient, a carer or a member of staff.
	The NHS aims to foster a spirit of candour and a culture of humility, openness and honesty, where staff communicate clearly and openly with patients, relatives and carers.
Commitment to quality of care	The NHS aspires to the highest standards of excellence and professionalism in the provision of high-quality care that is safe, effective and focused on patient experience.
	The delivery of high-quality care is dependent on feedback.
Compassion	Compassionate care ties closely with respect and dignity in that individual patients, carers and relatives must be treated with sensitivity and kindness.
Improving lives	The core function of the NHS is emphasized in this value – the NHS seeks to improve the health and well-being of patients, communities and its staff through professionalism, innovation and excellence in care.
Everyone counts	Nobody should be discriminated or disadvantaged, and everyone should be treated with equal respect and importance.

From Department of Health (2015).

NHS England has included the treatment of both staff and patients in the drive towards excellence and professionalism across the health service, highlighting that patient safety, experience and outcomes are all improved when staff are valued, empowered and supported (NHS Choices 2015).

ETHICAL CODES AND VALUES

Several national and international associations have determined midwifery ethical codes. In the UK, *The Code* (NMC 2018) sets the professional standards for practice and professional behaviours and incorporates specific ethical and legal obligations. The ethical decisions made in practice are based on an individual's values and their philosophy of midwifery and are explored in more detail in Chapter 6.

Ergin et al (2013) recognized the importance to define and practise ethical rules and codes for professionalization. In Turkey, ethical rules and codes that would facilitate midwifery becoming professionalized are still to be determined, and the study by Ergin et al (2013) was planned to contribute to the professionalization of midwifery by determining national ethical values and codes. A total of 1067 Turkish midwives completed the survey. The preferred professional codes chosen by them were as follows:

- absence of conflicts of interest
- respect for privacy
- avoidance of deception
- reporting of faulty practices
- considerations of mothers and newborns as separate beings
- prevention of harm.

Ergin et al (2013) concluded that cultural values, beliefs and expectations of society cannot be underestimated in their influence on adoption of ethical codes.

In the UK, additional conflicts which may arise in practice include issues around National Institute for Health and Care Excellence (NICE) guidelines conflicting with midwives' individual beliefs based on experiential knowledge. It is pivotal for midwives to use the extensive evidence base in all areas of care. Involvement in quality meetings and multidisciplinary groups to write guidelines and protocols is essential so that midwife practitioners are heard and enabled to work within both the local Trust's philosophy and their personal philosophy.

The following section provides a mini *toolkit* and helpful hints to assist the reader in developing a personal philosophy to use and maintain in their professional portfolio.

Developing a Personal Philosophy

To articulate a personal philosophy, it will be crucial to recall the reason why you entered the midwifery profession and what attracted you to such a demanding role. Remembering specific reasons and the core values and beliefs that led to your applying for and undertaking a challenging preparation programme may be the attraction to be with childbearing women, their babies and their families. It is worth considering whether such reasons, values and beliefs have changed as it is possible that the *norms* which governed clinical settings in previous decades have imperceptibly changed.

Before one embarks on devising or revising a personal philosophy for midwifery education and practice, it may be relevant to consider what comprises *an optimal* birth and what, for the profession, makes a *good* midwife. Kennedy (2000) undertook a Delphi survey to obtain consensus on midwives' views of exemplary practice. Some of the processes midwives highlighted as being exemplary care were:

- supporting the normalcy of pregnancy and birth
- vigilance and attention to detail
- respecting the uniqueness of the woman.

Kennedy (2000) found that the critical difference that emerged was the art of doing nothing well, whereas Smith (2014) reflects on what motivated her to continue to be a midwife. She asserts that

> *The midwife's role is inimitable in mothers' lives, providing care that is centred on their unique needs–ideally ensuring that it is holistic, empowering, proactive and sensitive to the social context and changes in healthcare provision.*

(Smith 2014: 675)

Smith (2014) continues to describe the ongoing challenge of being an advocate for women and working in true partnership with them, stressing the need for midwives to be aware of their own prejudices and unconscious bias so that women's decisional autonomy is not compromised. This is particularly important in settings where the birth culture is dominated by litigation alongside evidence-based care models (Jomeen 2010). A powerful exercise which may help the reader in identifying any prejudices or stereotyping behaviour centres on questioning their *unconscious bias*. This is an essential activity to help maximize equality and to promote fair decision-making. Consider the example in Activity 4.2.

ACTIVITY 4.2 ■

You are driving to work and pass a travelling community camped in a fenced-off disused petrol station. You reflect on the place in society/experience of childbearing women and their young families in that particular culture.

- What does your subconscious tell you about the lives of these childbearing women and the choices they make?
- Do you stereotype these women as being powerless and vulnerable or reckless in their decision to live outside the community?
- How do your values and beliefs about travellers influence your communication with similar families and the care you provide?

It is essential that your personal philosophy is overarching and values *all* women, their babies and their families. Denehy (2001) clearly articulates that the first step in creating a personal philosophical statement is for the individual to identify their core values. As postulated earlier, this will usually emerge from the individual's own culture, family, education, etc. The next step is to delineate their professional values which may stem from the ICM global philosophy of midwifery care (Table 4.1) or perhaps their organization's vision/mission statement.

Box 4.1 presents a '*Statement of Purpose*' from an NHS trust in London. The statement opens with the trust's objectives followed by the corporate objectives.

Whilst the statement of purpose contains an '*overall strategic vision*' and strapline, there needs to also be ownership by all stakeholders and continued support to translate the statement into a

---

BOX 4.1 ■ Statement of Purpose From a National Health Service Trust (Example)

Trust Objectives

'*The overall strategic vision for the Trust is to build on its current position to consistently be a high performing organisation with a sustainable future, to continue to work with patients, the public and stakeholders to enhance its reputation and to provide both acute and community health services to the population of [the NHS Trust] and its surrounding areas. This vision is articulated in the following strap-line:*

"**Delivering excellent integrated care for you and your family, when and where you need it**".'

Corporate Objectives of the Trust

- 'To deliver high quality, integrated patient-centred services
- To ensure staff are able, empowered and responsible for the delivery of effective and compassionate care
- To achieve best practice performance standards
- To secure value for money and ensure the financial sustainability of the Trust
- To work with partners to improve the health and wellbeing of the people of [the NHS Trust]'

realistic philosophy. Each department and team needs encouragement to adapt the objectives (e.g. at annual away days) so they continue to be fit for purpose.

The same principle should, ideally, be applied in universities when a new midwifery curriculum is designed. The mission statement or overarching philosophy can help to guide the teaching. The combined articulation of values and beliefs can be powerful, creative and positive. Whilst creating one's own philosophical statement can seem an enormous challenge, the activities presented in Chapter 5 involving honest reflexivity, in combination with the mission statement from the organization in which the individual works/studies, can provide the platform for a fresh approach.

Figure 4.1 provides a word map to help in formulating a personal philosophy.

The words within the word map have been selected specifically for this chapter, but readers are encouraged to identify their own words that are meaningful to their own area of practice.

Examples of midwives' informal philosophies can be found on websites such as that of *One-to-One Midwives*, a caseload team: http://www.onetoonemidwives.org/. It may help the reader to reflect on the best practice they have observed during their midwifery careers so far: e.g. what is a '*good*' birth and what comprises a '*good*' midwife?

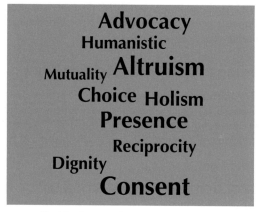

Fig. 4.1 A personal philosophy word map.

Normal Birth Dichotomies

Darra (2009) provides an examination of concepts surrounding the normal birth versus natural birth argument, speculating that the concept of *normal* birth is difficult to define in retrospect, as it is so subjective. Consequently, Darra (2009) suggests that *good-enough* birth is a more appropriate term. This stems from the theory of salutogenesis, which promotes the health of the individual rather than focusing on illness. As Downe (2008) claims, a more in-depth analysis of normality is needed. Kitzinger (2005) purports that there has been a *pathologizing* of the birth experience, leading to tocophobia (fear of birth), with some women's perception of trauma lasting for many years. Talbot (2014) examined what constituted a *good* birth from the women's perspective and found that women were empowered by midwives' provision of respectful care. In addition, Robertson (2016) asserts that the hallmarks of being *with woman* are flexibility and openness. Undertake Activity 4.3.

ACTIVITY 4.3 ■

- With reference to the philosophy of midwifery care of the International Confederation of Midwives (2014) (Table 4.1) that considers the importance of promoting normality, consider other hallmarks that you could add to the definition and essence of midwifery.
- Current debates have a focus on *optimal* birth. How is this reflected in the language used within the birth setting in which you work and/or the higher education settings in which you work or study?

Hatem et al (2008) investigated the benefits of *midwife-led* care versus other models of care for childbearing women. The underpinning philosophy of midwife-led care in this context was described as being *normality, continuity of care* and *being cared for by a known and trusted midwife during labour* (Hatem et al 2008). Findings from this study demonstrated that outcomes were improved for women and babies when the midwife was the lead professional, leading to an increase in models of care such as caseloading.

What appear to be sometimes neglected, however, are the needs of women who have high-risk pregnancies and births. Berg (2005) devised a midwifery model of care for women who had pregnancies considered to be of high risk which demonstrated that mutuality between the midwife and woman was essential to maximize openness, equality and connection within the caring relationship. When the ICM requirements are considered, the expectations of outcomes for women and babies apply in different global contexts and can prove challenging when one is working within different, often conflicting belief systems.

Midwifery Ideology: Different Perspectives

Murphy (2004) articulated that being with woman (*the essence of midwifery*) is also how individuals relate to their families and significant others. It is *being present* to the other, to ourselves, and to the mutuality of the relationship that is created by being *with* someone. The following section explores some of the conflicting ideologies, disparate belief systems and paradoxes in knowledge across the globe.

CONFLICTING IDEOLOGIES (UK AND AUSTRALIA)

Hunter (2004) found there were conflicting ideologies at play for practising midwives through exploring how a range of midwives experienced and managed emotion in their work. Hunter (2004) discovered that community and hospital environments presented midwives with fundamentally different work settings that had diverse values and perspectives. The result was two primary occupational identities and ideologies that were in conflict. Hospital midwifery was dominated by meeting service needs, via a universalistic and medicalized approach to care; the ideology was, by necessity, *with institution*. Community-based midwifery was more able to support an individualized, natural model of childbirth reflecting a *with woman* ideology. According to Hunter (2004), when midwives were able to work according to the *with woman* ideal, they experienced their work as emotionally rewarding. Conversely, when this was not possible, their experience at work was emotionally difficult and required regulation of emotion, (i.e. *emotion work*).

The implications of this for practice is that understanding the dilemmas created by conflicting occupational ideologies is important to improve the quality of midwives' working lives and hence the care they give to women and their families. In the short term, strategies involving education and clinical supervision may be of assistance in enabling midwives to reconcile these conflicting perspectives. However, in the long term, more radical solutions may be required to address the underpinning contradictions. Garratt (2010) asserts that midwives often risk *professional dissociation* when powerlessness is experienced through being more *with institution* than *with woman*. Fenwick et al (2012) found that within a sample of newly qualified midwives, many struggled to provide woman-centred care in cultures which were risk averse. Difficulties appear to be encountered globally if the midwives do not conform to the *cultural norm* of the workplace. Models need to be developed in which women as service users feel empowered.

DISPARATE BELIEF SYSTEMS (NORWAY)

Doing midwifery between different belief systems was the focus of work by Blaaka and Schauer-Eri (2008), who noted that in Norway childbirth had been increasingly concentrated in large centralized hospitals, with a parallel trend towards more birth interventions. These changes had resulted in new ways of framing birth from a woman's physiological life experience to a medical event resulting in intrapartum care being undertaken between two different belief systems: a biomedical system and a phenomenological system. Blaaka and Schauer-Eri (2008) conducted this small study exploring the views of seven skilled midwives to ascertain how they experienced their daily work between a biomedical belief system and a phenomenological belief system within a Norwegian high-technology labour ward. Three themes were identified:

1. sensing where the woman is in labour
2. being available for but not overbearing to the women
3. being in a room of struggle.

The findings were discussed from the perspective of being between these two belief systems, with special focus on what they refer to as wise midwifery judgement as a way of managing the struggle. The themes described here are a reminder of the importance of having a philosophy that guides behaviours and actions in dichotomous situations. Additionally, it relates to the issues raised in Chapter 5 about intuitive decision-making. For example, for Betsch (2008) there appears to be some consensus with the idea that intuition is based on a store of experience which is accessed automatically and without conscious awareness, so the analytical reasoning process is not evident.

DISPUTES ABOUT THE MIDWIFERY PARADIGM AND WHAT IS 'NORMAL' (AUSTRALIA AND UNITED STATES OF AMERICA)

In a similar vein, Reed (2013) examined actions and interactions of a sample of practising midwives in Australia. Through use of a narrative inquiry approach, Reed (2013) concluded that *ritual companionship* should be the recommended model as opposed to use of a *rites of protection* midwifery model for women in labour, the latter being those rites which meet the needs of the institution and promote defensive practice at the expense of providing woman-centred care. Fahy and Parratt (2006) used the term *midwifery guardianship* when developing a theory of birth territory. They concluded that midwives working within the guardianship model created a birth experience which was more positive for women and assisted with both increased satisfaction for women and better adaptation in the immediate postpartum period. It is relevant to analyse the use of language in the Norwegian and Australian studies, questioning to what extent midwives should be *guardians* to women and whether this is at the expense of women feeling truly empowered. It is possible that translations of *protection* and *guardianship* differ across cultures, but critical analysis of the use of language is an important issue for midwives to continually reflect on.

Cragin (2008) examines three theoretical models that were developed in the United States of America to describe the essential components of midwifery practice. The three theories (Lehrman 1988; Thompson et al 1989; Kennedy 2000) demonstrate remarkable consistency in the identification of concepts important to the discipline, which include the following essential characteristics of the midwifery paradigm of care:

1. acknowledgment of connections between the mind and body and the person to the person's life and world

2. assuming the perspective of the woman to investigate meaning and her experience of symptoms or conditions so that a plan of care is developed by the midwife and woman together
3. protection and nurturance of the normal in processes related to women's health, implying a judicious use of technology and intervention.

PARADOXES IN KNOWLEDGE AND EVIDENCE-BASED PRACTICE

In addition, Kennedy and Lowe (2001) postulate that the everyday world of clinical practice is filled with paradigms and paradoxes that stem from the issues of who defines knowledge, how it is generated and how the individual midwife applies it when providing care for women and their families. Kennedy and Lowe (2001) argue that research useful for clinical practice should provide evidence to support scientific approaches (models) or strategies (interventions) in caring for women. In a clinical discipline, the answers to research questions should eventually inform clinical decision-making by providing practical clinical knowledge. Kennedy and Lowe (2001) present the steps for application of research (Stevenson 1990) for the development of clinically applicable knowledge that the midwife can use to analyse and evaluate research findings as a basis for practice decisions. Specific examples of midwifery research are used to illustrate each stage in the process and the circular nature of knowledge development. The challenge is to prepare midwives who can apply research findings skilfully using the best evidence to support clinical practice, as well as to help midwife researchers who will develop systematic programmes of relevant research about midwifery practice and outcomes.

Challenges of Midwifery Education, Practice and Research

The NHS and higher education institutions are suffering severe financial constraints. This has led to reduced resources, limited spaces both for workers and for patients and limited time to complete tasks efficiently whilst simultaneously being woman centred. Problems are compounded by the increased acuity and complexity of women's health problems. The challenges to midwives living out their collective and individual philosophies continue. These include:

- The challenge of consistently providing holistic, woman-centred care in line with the ICM Philosophy of Midwifery Care (ICM 2014). This is often compounded by the risk culture associated with obstetrics and increased complaints from the public.
- The challenge of working together within a multidisciplinary team, providing compassionate care, practising open communication and reducing inequalities, particularly for vulnerable families. These practices need to be in line with the values and principles that guide the NHS (Department of Health 2015). However, issues continually arise because of conflicting medical versus midwifery models.
- One challenge within higher education arises from the disparity which occurs when lecturers facilitate learning using widely differing ideologies. Students need guidance to choose apposition for themselves. Philosophy sessions therefore need to be firmly embedded within the midwifery curriculum.

These examples provide ripe ground for research into midwifery education and practice. A solution to overcoming some of these barriers and challenges could be for midwives to take some time (perhaps once a year) to attend a national or international conference. If funding can be obtained, this provides a perfect opportunity to update, re-energize and gain support for one's role. New information can be taken back to practice or a university to improve services and educational programmes. If the reader is in the position of presenting at a conference, this is the ideal time to articulate their philosophy and invite critique.

Consider the three scenarios in Activity 4.4.

ACTIVITY 4.4 ■

Scenario 1: Breastfeeding

Carly is a 32-year-old woman, who has a 4-day-old baby boy. As Carly is anaemic and exhausted after a caesarean section, a maternity support worker, rostered on a night shift on the hospital postnatal ward, has advised Carly to discontinue breastfeeding. Other senior staff agree with this decision; however, Carly expressed that she wanted to exclusively breastfeed soon after the birth.

- As the named midwife on the day shift (8 a.m. to 4 p.m.), how will you reconcile your deeply set belief that the UNICEF UK Baby Friendly Initiative (2012) standards should be achieved whilst practising within local and national guidelines?

Scenario 2: Mental Illness

Johanna has a history of depression and there is also a history of abuse in her childhood. She is 24 years old and has been admitted to the antenatal ward with hypertension. Several midwives and maternity support workers have seemed brusque in their manner when caring for Johanna and, to you, lack sensitivity in their communication.

- How will you articulate your values, beliefs and underpinning philosophy to persuade the ward staff to work with *The Code* (Nursing and Midwifery Council 2018) and National Institute for Health and Care Excellence (NICE) guidelines?

Scenario 3: Screening

Asha, a midwifery lecturer has been tasked with teaching antenatal screening to a cohort of first-year student midwives. A year ago, Asha experienced a late termination of her second pregnancy for fetal abnormalities (Patau's syndrome).

- What steps should Asha take to objectively share knowledge and what safeguards should be put in place to ensure that students are taught the correct principles of screening?

Conclusion

This chapter has provided opportunities for the reader to address their philosophical beliefs, values and unconscious biases related to women's reproductive health and birth, challenging them to consider what makes a *good* midwife and what comprises an *optimal* birth. A philosophy should be a living one and not just created as a paper exercise. It is therefore essential that a midwife's personal philosophy is overarching and values the diverse group of women, their babies and their families within their care.

The process of revalidation with the NMC provides an excellent opportunity for the reader to visit their personal philosophy (see Chapter 5). Murphy (2004) reminds us that the essence of midwifery is being 'with woman'. The activities woven throughout this chapter will have tested readers' values and beliefs in terms of being able to achieve this. Every interaction an individual has should be grounded in an intentional philosophical perspective and guided by systematically developed theory. Clarity regarding philosophy and theory is critical for the midwifery profession because together they can help clarify what motivates an individual's actions and enhance outcomes, be they be clinical or educational.

KEY POINTS

- Every midwife registrant must work according to the NMC *Code* (2018).
- Midwives need to think critically about their inherent values and beliefs.
- Midwives' underlying principles can have a long-lasting impact on women and their families.
- Philosophical beliefs should be confidently role-modelled in practice and education.
- All midwives need to critically consider and address any unconscious bias in their practice and professional behaviour.
- Devising a philosophy should be not merely a paper exercise but a 'living' tool to guide midwifery practice, teaching and research.

References

Berg, M. (2005). A midwifery model of care for childbearing women at high risk: genuine caring in caring for the genuine. *Journal of Perinatal Education, 14*(1), 9–21.

Betsch, T. (2008). The nature of intuition and its neglect in research on judgement and decision-making. In Plessner, E., Betsch, C., & Betsch, T. (Eds.), *Intuition in judgement and decision-making*. New York: Lawrence Erlbaum Associates.

Blaaka, G., & Schauer-Eri, T. (2008). Doing midwifery between different belief systems. *Midwifery, 24*(3), 344–352.

Cragin, L. (2004). The theoretical basis for nurse-midwifery practice in the United States: a critical analysis of three theories. *Journal of Midwifery and Women's Health, 49*(5), 381–389.

Darra, S. (2009). 'Normal', 'natural', 'good' or 'good-enough' birth: examining the concepts. *Nursing Inquiry, 16*(4), 297–305.

Denehy, J. (2001). Articulating your philosophy of nursing. *The Journal of School Nursing, 17*(1), 1–2.

Department of Health. (2015). *The NHS constitution for England*. London: The Stationary Office. Available at: *https://www.gov.uk/government publications/the-nhs-constitution-for-england/the-nhs-constitution-for-england*.

Dewey, J. (2008). *Democracy and education*. Radford: Wilder Publications.

Downe, S. (2008). *Normal childbirth: evidence and debate*. London: Churchill Livingstone.

Ergin, A., Ozcan, M., Acar, Z., Ersoy, N., & Karahn, N. (2013). Determination of national midwifery ethical values and ethical codes. *Nursing Ethics, 20*(7), 808–818.

Fahy, K. M., & Parratt, J. A. (2006). Birth territory: a theory for midwifery practice. *Women and Birth, 19*(2), 45–50.

Fenwick, J., Hammond, A., Raymond, J., Smith, R., Gray, J., Foureur, M., et al. (2012). Surviving not thriving: a qualitative study of newly qualified midwives' experience of their transition to practice. *Journal of Clinical Nursing, 21*(13), 2054–2063.

Garratt, L. (2010). *Survivors of childhood sexual abuse and midwifery practice*. Abingdon: Radcliffe Publishing.

Garvey, J., & Stangroom, J. (2012). *The story of philosophy: A history of Western thought*. London: Quercus.

General Medical Council. (2012). *Joint statement*. Available at: http://www.gmcuk.org/Professional_values_ joint_statement__August_2012.pdf_49744505.pdf.

Hatem, M., Sandall, J., Devane, D., Soltani, H., & Gates, S. (2008). Midwife-led versus other models of care for childbearing women. *Cochrane Database of Systematic Reviews* (4), CD004667.

Hunter, B. (2004). Conflicting ideologies as a source of emotion work in midwifery. *Midwifery, 20*(3), 261–272.

International Confederation of Midwives. (2014). *The philosophy and model of midwifery care* Core document CD2005_001. Available at: https://www.internationalmidwives.org/assets/files/definitions-files/2018/06/ eng-philosophy-and-model-of-midwifery-care.pdf.

Jomeen, J. (2010). *Choice, control and contemporary childbirth*. Oxford: Radcliffe Publishing.

Kennedy, H. P. (2000). A model of exemplary midwifery practice: results of a Delphi study. *Journal of Midwifery and Women's Health, 45*(1), 4–19.

Kennedy, H. P., & Low, L. K. (2001). Science and midwifery: paradigms and paradoxes. *Journal of Midwifery and Women's Health, 46*(2), 91–97.

Kennedy, H. P., Rousseau, A. L., & Low, L. K. (2003). An exploratory metasynthesis of midwifery practice in the United States. *Midwifery, 19*(3), 203–214.

Kitzinger, S. (2005). *The politics of birth*. London: Elsevier.

Knight, L. S., (Series editor). (2003). *Collins English dictionary (complete and unabridged)*. Glasgow: Harper Collins.

Lehrman, E. J. (1988). *A theoretical framework for nursing-midwifery practice*. Tuscon: University of Arizona.

Mid Staffordshire NHS Foundation Trust Public Inquiry. (2013). *Report of the Mid Staffordshire Foundation Trust Public Inquiry*. London: The Stationery Office.

Murphy, P. A. (2004). Midwifery: a philosophy, not a function. *Journal of Midwifery and Women's Health, 49*(1), 1.

NHS Choices. (2015). *Principles and values that guide the NHS*. Available at: http://www.nhs.uk/nhsengland/ thenhs/about/pages/nhscoreprinciples.aspx.

Nursing and Midwifery Council. (2009). *Standards for pre-registration midwifery education*. London: Nursing and Midwifery Council.

Nursing and Midwifery Council. (2018). *The Code: Professional standards for nurses, midwives and nursing associates*. London: Nursing and Midwifery Council.

Pearsall, J. (Ed.). (2001). *New Oxford Dictionary of English*. Oxford: Oxford University Press.

Reed, R. (2013). *Midwifery practice during birth: rites of passage and rites of protection*. Sippy Downs: University of the Sunshine Coast. PhD thesis.

Renfrew, M., Homer, C., Downe, S., McFadden, A., Muir, R., Prentice, T., et al. (2014). Midwifery. An executive summary for the Lancet's series. Available at: https://www.thelancet.com/series/midwifery.

Robertson, A. (2016). *Are midwives a dying breed?* Available at: https://birthinternational.com/article/birth/are-midwives-a-dying-breed/.

Rogers, C. R. (1961). *On becoming a person: A psychotherapists view of psychotherapy*. Boston: Houghton Mifflin.

Smith, J. (2014). The culture of midwifery and autonomy. *British Journal of Midwifery, 22*(9), 695–696.

Stevenson, J. S. (1990). The development of nursing knowledge; accelerating the pace. In Chaska N., L. (Ed.), *The nursing profession. Turning points*. St. Louis: Mosby.

Talbot, D. (2014). Exploring the 'good' birth: what is it and why does it matter? *British Journal of Midwifery, 22*(12), 854–860.

Thompson, J., Oakley, D., Burke, M., Jay, S., & Conkin, M. (1989). Theory building in nurse midwifery. The care process. *Journal of Nurse-Midwifery, 34*(3), 120–130.

UNICEF UK Baby Friendly Initiative. (2012). *Guide to the Baby Friendly Initiative standards*. London: UNICEF UK Baby Friendly Initiative.

Further Reading

Borrelli, S. E. (2014). What is a good midwife? Insights from the literature. *Midwifery, 30*, 3–10.

> *The author performed a literature review to explore what it is that constitutes a good midwife and also what women most value in a midwife. Important attributes of midwives from the women's perspective included moral and ethical values. This has implications for midwives in practice and for inclusion of philosophy within educational programmes.*

Fahy, K., Foureur, M., & Hastie, C. (Eds.). (2008). *Birth territory and midwifery guardianship*. Edinburgh: Butterworth Heinemann.

> *This multiauthored book provides thought-provoking debates for readers around territory and the sociopolitical factors around birth in the 21st century. There is a useful chapter (Parratt, pp. 39–54, 'Territories of the self and spiritual practices during childbirth') to aid development of the reader's personal philosophy where strategies for coping with change (e.g. using mindfulness) to protect oneself and to enact one's philosophy are presented.*

Gaskin, I. M. (2002). *Spiritual midwifery*. Summertown: Book Publishing Company.

> *This seminal text describes Ina May Gaskin's philosophy of her midwifery work on The Farm in Tennessee in the United States of America in the 1970s. Much of the book is based on stories of home births and celebrates the spiritual elements of birth without intervention.*

Montgomery, E., & Bick, D. (2014). Cultural explorations in midwifery. *Essentially MIDIRS, 5*(9), 7–10.

> *In this article, the authors purport that the impact of culture on midwives' behaviour and attitudes can often be ignored. Because of recent cultural shifts in the National Health Service, the impact on practising midwives has led to burnout. The authors examine models which increase professional autonomy and continuity of care such as caseloading. Development of trusting, empathetic relationships with carers is vital to women, and this means midwives need to embody a robust philosophy of care.*

Useful Websites

Birth Spirit. http://birthspirit.com/about-us/our-philosophy/.

> *This is an American website. Robin Lim suggests that birthing is a profound initiation to spirituality.*

One-to-One Midwives. http://www.onetoonemidwives.org/.

> *This progressive team of midwives has developed a successful caseloading model covering the North West of England and Essex. The website displays the midwives' philosophical values and beliefs and demonstrates their commitment to woman-centred care and empowerment of women.*

CHAPTER 5

Reflection and Intuitive Practice

Val Collington ▓ Jan Fook

LEARNING OUTCOMES

By the end of this chapter the reader should:

- be able to define the concepts of reflection and intuition and the connection between them
- have an understanding of different models of reflection
- be aware of different types of knowledge and ways of knowing
- appreciate how to develop a reflective portfolio
- understand the value of practising reflection and using one's intuition.

Overview

This chapter aims to introduce the reader to the concept of reflection and its link to different ways of knowing, such as *intuition*. The main points covered are: *definitions and understandings of reflection*; *the connection between reflection and intuition*; *different models of reflection*; and *an overview of different types of knowledge and ways of knowing* and practical information on *how to develop a reflective portfolio*. Case studies and activities are included throughout the chapter to illustrate the theories presented.

Introduction

Over the last five decades, reflection and reflective practice have become common ideas in professional practice. Whilst intuition as an idea has been long valued, there has also been a more recent move towards evidence-based practice, which seems to contradict the value of reflection and intuitive ways of knowing (McIntosh 2010). Nevertheless, it is important to recognize their joint value and to integrate the two (Mantzoukas 2007; Brannigan and Moores 2015). To do this, however, it is important to revisit what is meant by *reflection* and *intuition*, and to understand how these concepts contribute to more complex and responsive forms of practice which cannot necessarily be completely evaluated by further scientific evidence. This chapter aims to assist the reader in developing a reflective portfolio by reviewing the basic understandings of reflection and different models for reflecting on practice. By also reviewing different theories of knowledge and ways of knowing, the chapter will show how reflection and intuition are interlinked and can be used successfully in midwifery practice. Activities will help process practice experiences to further illustrate how reflection can be used to improve clinical practice.

The Nature of Reflection

Reflection is a very long-standing concept. Socrates spoke of the *examined life* for ethical and compassionate engagement with the world and its moral dilemmas (Nussbaum 1997), whereas in the 1930s Dewey (1933) declared that reflection was *learning from experience*. Schon (1983), however, is credited with developing the notion of *reflective practice*, based on the idea that professionals are not always aware that they may not be *practising what they preach* as there may often be a considerable gap between theory and practice. Being able to improve professional practice by reflecting on the theories unconsciously embedded in practice, to then align one's thinking more effectively with doing, came to be referred to as *reflective practice* (Schon 1983). The capacity to reflect on practice and to learn directly from the experience of practising is particularly relevant in the current climate and challenges of ongoing change, revised policies and economic cutbacks within the working environment.

There are many different definitions of *reflection* and how to reflect (Fook et al 2006). In this chapter the most basic meanings of *reflection* and *intuition* are outlined to determine how other definitions might fit with these. Taking the ideas from Dewey (1933) and Socrates (Nussbaum 1997) as the starting points, it is important to examine in more detail what *learning from experience* is, and how it might contribute to *the examined life*. Aiming towards *the examined life* for ethical and compassionate engagement with the world and its moral dilemmas directs a person to the clear purpose of reflection, which is to enable them to develop the way they relate to their world and others within it in more ethical and compassionate ways. Dewey (1933) focuses on how this might be achieved: *by learning from personal experience*. Everyone thinks they learn from experience, but this depends on what the person learns, and what is meant by *learning* and *experience*. Furthermore, it could be questioned as to what the exact process is by which people learn.

Put simply, *learning from experience* involves re-examining past personally experienced events to make new meaning of them in the light of later experiences and contexts. Current experience can also be examined in this way. The *learning* should involve turning the thinking involved from that early event into a broader principle or guideline by perceiving patterns or commonalities with other experiences or events. This type of learning should enable more expansive and flexible ways of thinking and acting rather than cause more rigid or restrictive thinking (Fook et al 2017). *Learning* in this context is *changed* or *reshaped thinking* which is more expansive, and the experience being referred to is *personally experienced*. *Expansive learning* denotes learning which enables more options and/or is able to be transferred to other settings. For the learning to be maximized, the experience should be one which somehow does not fit and which Dewey (1933) refers to as the *discrepant experience:* one which seems puzzling or contradictory in terms of perceived patterns to date.

If *reflection* is defined as learning from experience for more ethical and compassionate engagement, then an example of an experience on which a midwife might wish to reflect could be that in Activity 5.1.

ACTIVITY 5.1 ■

As a midwife you relate well to childbearing women and their families as well as your colleagues within the multiprofessional team. On this particular occasion you have clearly explained to a woman during the first stage of labour the rationale for and the procedures involved in undertaking an artificial rupture of the membranes, and she appears to have understood your explanation. However, a newly appointed obstetrician enters the room and interrupts the conversation, leading to the woman becoming unsure about the procedure and appearing more anxious. Usually you are able to assert yourself and support women for whom you are providing care and so you feel annoyed with yourself and uncertain as to how you should challenge the doctor to restore your relationship with this particular woman and regain her trust.

Restrictive learning from experience might simply involve you throwing up your hands and concluding that because you feel disempowered by the obstetrician's interference, considering that they are more powerful than you, there is no point in you trying to communicate directly with the woman, so you will simply leave it up to the doctor to do so instead.

Consider what could be *helpful things* to learn from this experience.

Helpful reflection or learning from this experience in an expansive way might involve some understanding of both *how* and *why* the woman feels more anxious and why you feel more uncertain. You might ask yourself the following questions:

1. What does the whole incident and situation mean to you as a professional and a midwife?
2. Have some of your own fundamental values being contravened?
3. What is important to you in this situation?

Once you have understood these issues better, you will be able to work out what is most important to you and what you might want to prioritize. This will help to establish the most effective ways to deal with such situations. If you believe that it is more important for the woman to feel less anxious, consider asking the obstetrician how the woman can be helped to feel calmer. In this way reflection will help you learn more complex ways of working, which can be modified in different situations.

Processes of Reflection and the Concept of Intuition

Taking into consideration how reflection may be understood from the example in Activity 5.1, the question remains about what processes can be used to put reflection into practice. An easy approach is that provided by Schon's (1983) model of reflective practice. Schon's (1983) approach is based on the notion that all practice has theory embedded in it, referring to these as assumptions on which actions are based. The problem here is that people are not often aware of their assumptions as they are implicit in what a person does. This means that there can be huge contradictions between what a person actually does and what they believe themselves to be acting on. For example:

I always say that I believe in treating people equally, but I am also aware that I often favour the people I like, even if/when I am aware of this and try not to do it.

According to Schon (1983), reflection commences when a person becomes aware of the assumptions (theories) which are implicit or embedded in what they do, and through this awareness exercises a conscious choice about what assumptions (theories) they keep and how they work on this basis. In short, reflective practice is simply being able to align theory and practice and therefore improve the way a person works through reflecting on their actual practice.

With this in mind (pulling together the main aspects discussed so far), the definition of *reflection* outlined above can be expanded by the addition of a description of how it is done, as well as describing what it is and its purpose. As a result, *reflection* can be defined as learning from experience for more compassionate and ethical engagement through a process of examining the embedded assumptions and remaking the meaning of the experience in more expansive ways. This process will be further expanded in a later section in which different models or approaches to reflection are outlined.

It is interesting to explore how *reflection* and *intuition* are related. Intuition is a concept separate from that of reflection, although the two are often discussed together. *Intuition* refers to the often rapid *gut feelings* or *hunches* a person may have about situations without being aware of, or being able to, articulate the concrete or rational reasons for them. For this reason intuition is often contrasted with decision-making based on more scientific methods (Greenhalgh 2002). Because of the inability to account for a clear and deliberative process in intuitive decision-making, there are many different perspectives on how it comes about. Some people feel it bridges a gap between the conscious and unconscious, and refer to a more mystical quality (Betsch 2008). There appears to be some consensus with the idea that intuition is based on a store of experience which is accessed automatically and without conscious awareness (Betsch 2008), so the analytical reasoning process is not evident. That said, it is implied that people without experience are less able to be intuitive (Greenhalgh 2002), and that the basis for intuitive judgements is relatively inaccessible to scrutiny.

There is some similarity here with the concept of reflection, which itself is difficult to pin down and provide hard evidence of its outcomes (Fook et al 2016). Reflection may therefore help unearth the basis of intuition, since it enables the discovery of implicit assumptions of which a person may be unaware. A process of reflection, in this sense, functions as a way of accessing the reasons for an intuitive judgement and may therefore enhance the evidence base for practice. Coupled with reflection, intuition can be a powerful way of providing evidence for professional decisions which may not have been learned through more formalized scientific means. In this way, intuitive decisions, scrutinized through a rigorous process of reflection, may function to humanize and make more holistic professional practice by including learning achieved through experience.

In Activity 5.1, as a midwife you may be very aware of your feelings or instincts and use them as a guide to inform decisions made about undertaking artificial rupture of the membranes. Some of these types of feelings are instinctive and rely on intuition and not facts. Bearing in mind that intuitive decision-making could be based on *experience, curiosity, emotional intelligence, networks, tolerance*, etc. (Matzler et al 2007), consider the issues raised in Activity 5.2.

ACTIVITY 5.2 ■

- Whilst reflecting on your possible reaction to the obstetrician's intervention, do you believe the most important thing is that a person should trust their own feelings and intuition and act accordingly?
- How do you think being intuitive and being reflective fit together?
- How do you perceive your own thinking in practice: is it more intuitive or more reflective, or a mixture of both?
- Are there some situations in which you might be more intuitive and others where you are more reflective, or are both types of thinking integrated for you?

Models of Reflection

There are many different ways of defining *reflection*, and consequently there are a number of different models and processes developed for practising it. In the first part of this chapter the definition of *reflection* that Fook and Gardner (2007) have developed into a complex model for undertaking reflection was introduced. This model incorporates several different theories (*reflective practice, reflexivity, post-structuralism, critical social theories* and *spirituality*) to develop an integrated approach (Kellehear and Fook 2010).

The reflection is organized in two stages:
- Stage 1 focuses on drawing out the hidden assumptions.
- Stage 2 focuses on assisting the person to work out a revised meaning of the experience and its relevance to their future professional practice.

In practice, this approach consists of working in a small group to foster dialogue which enables reflection for each group member. Each person is asked in turn to provide an example of a critical incident (i.e. something that happened to them which they regard as important to their learning). This serves as an example of practice, or the *discrepant experience*, referred to earlier. The group enables each person to learn from that experience by asking questions and engaging in dialogue. This helps the person unearth the hidden or implicit assumptions embedded in the story of their experience, and so reach its deeper meaning. Other questions might include the following:
- Why was this incident critical for you?
- What were you assuming about the other person, or your own responsibility/power?
- What might be other perspectives on the situation?
- What might you have left out or overlooked?

The learning climate of such a group is vital: it is important that a non-judgemental and non-solution-focused climate is set up. The purpose of the group is not to impose judgements on the person reflecting but to create a climate where the person learns to reflect for themselves: to pose their own questions and to search for deeper meaning. The theoretical basis of this approach, and some examples from practitioners who have used it, is detailed elsewhere (Fook et al 2017).

Habermas (1971) has been influential in providing a theoretical framework for reflection, being used extensively in health care, including midwifery settings (Taylor 2006). Habermas (1971) identified three knowledge domains:

1. *the technical:* techniques for controlling/manipulating the environment
2. *the practical:* social interactions and meaning-making
3. *the emancipatory:* self-understanding needed to operate effectively in the social environment.

The last domain is seen as the one concerned most with *critical* reflection, which broadly is reflection that enables a transformation in fundamental thinking. Notably, Johns's (2006) framework for guided reflection that involves a dual focus of both *looking in* at one's own personal psychological and emotional aspects and *looking out* at the external situation is used extensively in the health care context. Johns and Burnie (2013) identified five patterns of knowing: the *aesthetic*, the *personal*, the *ethical*, the *empirical* and the *reflexive* (i.e. the act of self-reference) aspects of the situation.

This model of reflection is designed to be used with another person such as a mentor or supervisor. Another approach to reflection that is used in health care is the framework of Rolfe et al (2011). This is based on the earlier work of Borton (1970) which uses three simple questions to reflect on a situation:
- **What?** *(What...is the problem?...was my role?...happened?...were the consequences?)*
- **So what?** *(So what...was going through my mind?...should I have done?...do I know now about what happened?)*
- **Now what?** *(Now what...do I need to do?...are the broader issues that have been raised?...might happen now?)*

Borton (1970) considers the final question *Now what?* as the one that can make the greatest contribution to practice.

Reflective Practice and Ways of Knowing

Reflective practice is the capacity to reflect on an action so as to engage in a process of continuous learning. According to Bolton (2010), reflective practice involves paying critical attention to the practical values and theories that inform everyday actions by examining practice reflectively and reflexively. A key rationale for reflective practice is that experience alone does not necessarily lead to learning, so deliberate reflection on experience is essential (Loughran 2002).

Reflective practice can be an important tool in practice-based professional learning settings where individuals learn from their own professional experiences rather than from formal learning or knowledge transfer. It may be the most important source of personal professional development and improvement. It is also an important way to bring together theory and practice. Through reflection, an individual is able to observe and label forms of thought and theory within the context of their own work (McBrien 2007). Individuals who reflect throughout their practice are not only looking back on past actions and events but also are taking a conscious look at emotions, experiences, actions and responses, and are using that information to add to their existing knowledge base to reach a higher level of understanding. According to Moon (1999), reflective practice is an active, dynamic action-based and ethical set of skills placed in real time that deals with authentic, complex and difficult situations.

Knight (2015) discusses the process of reflective practice and how it is beneficial to nurses and their practice, claiming there is a growing need for reflective practice in the nursing profession because of the high emotional cost of the work and day-to-day high work pressure. Reflective practice is a structured process that is most effective in facilitated groups and should be tried out in individual teams to gain people's confidence and demonstrate the rewards. The value of group sharing, questioning and learning should be considered within the midwifery and wider health care context. The promotion of reflection in midwifery and nursing education is, according to Taylor (2006), to espouse active adult learning not only from a theoretical perspective but also from that of experiential learning. It is imperative that both midwives and nurses engage in reflective practice to obtain meanings from their experiences to contribute to ongoing professional knowledge and practice development.

Lyons (1999) argues that to continually develop as a discipline, a profession needs to generate a knowledge base that can evolve from education and practice. Reflective midwifery practitioners have the potential to develop clinical expertise directed towards achieving desirable, safe and effective practice. Midwives are *with woman*, providing the family with supportive and helpful relationships as they share the deep and profound experiences of childbirth. To become skilled helpers, students need to develop reflective skills and valid midwifery knowledge grounded in their personal experiences and practice. Midwife educators and practitioners can assist students and enhance their learning by expanding the scope of practice, encouraging self-assessment and the development of reflective and professional skills. In addition, using critical social theory and adult learning principles, Lyons (1999) examines how midwives can assist and thus enhance students' learning through the development of professional and reflective skills in midwifery practice.

The importance of documentary and narrative records in reflection is well established. O'Donovan's (2007) review of the literature clarified the success of reflection as an aid to learning in nursing. Guided reflection according to Johns (2006: 36) is defined as

> *a journey of self-inquiry and transformation for practitioners…to realize desirable practice as a lived reality. The journey is written as a narrative that reveals the transformative drama unfolding. Along the journey, the vision of desirable practice is constantly explored and shifting as new understandings emerge.*

Moreover, reflective practice and guided reflection are both respected and essential as learning and assessment methods in educational and training programmes (Donaghy and Morss 2000; Ash and Clayton 2004). Reflection can also aid the maintenance and achievement of clinical competence, and hence is an important tool in a health professional's repertoire of skills (Matthews 2004). Reflective journals have been used for a number of years in professional education as purported by Collington and Hunt (2006) in the promotion of reflection and learning in midwifery and midwifery education (Lyons 1999) and within postregistration nursing programmes (Chirema 2007).

In the United Kingdom, context-reflective practice has also become an increasingly influential concept in social work education, being acknowledged as key to ensuring that social workers are better equipped to engage in complex decision-making and effective practice (Wilson 2013). However, there remains a lack of clarity about how this concept is defined and operationalized in teaching and learning, with little systematic empirical examination of its utility in facilitating professional development. Wilson (2013) aimed to develop an understanding of social work students' experiences of reflective practice, and discovered agency systems that have become over-reliant on rules and procedures present formidable obstacles to learning both at an individual level and at an organizational level. Wilson (2013) argues that the relationship between how reflective practice is taught and how it is enacted in practice needs to be better understood if such obstacles are to be overcome. This further highlights the challenges that need to be addressed if reflection and critical thinking are to become embedded within education and practice cultures.

Theories of Knowledge and Ways of Knowing

It is reasonable to suggest that practice draws on several different ways of knowing whilst acknowledging the difficulties often faced by practising midwives in defining what they do and hence what it is that constitutes midwifery practice. Drawing on the literature on the origins of knowledge and the sources of midwifery knowledge, the types of knowledge required to enhance practice are discussed in the following section, focusing on the place of reflection in generating knowledge for midwifery.

Schon (1983) identifies that historically the dominant epistemology of practice was based on *technical rationality* which failed to recognize the practical use of professional knowledge, hence the alternative, *reflection-in-action*. Schon (1983) also stated that the knowledge which characterizes the professional in action is *knowledge-in-use*. Besides the formal theoretical knowledge that a midwife is required to use in her day-to-day work, there is also the dynamic form that comes from experience and builds the capacity to think creatively in context to produce effective action. So, when a midwife undertakes an activity, it is in the light of personal understanding, knowledge and theories.

In considering the *domains of professional education*, Barnett (1992) proposed four areas in which students' critical abilities must be exercised: *core knowledge*, *contextual knowledge*, *professional action* and *professional values*. It is the application of core knowledge that women and employers require from midwives in the maternity services and the expectation of competent performance. Eraut (1994) also suggested an organization of knowledge that underpins performance, referring to *immediacy* as although students realize the relevance of scientific knowledge, they tend to remember only that which they regularly use. Eraut (1994) and Barnett (1992) present similar arguments about professional knowledge, competence and expertise, distinguishing between types of knowledge and how they are acquired. Dewey (1933) expressed concern about the skills used to manipulate knowledge (i.e. reprocessing it) to achieve a purpose. Similarly, Habermas (1971) regarded reflection as a tool used to develop particular forms of knowledge, some of which rely on critique or evaluation of thought and enquiry to understand *the self* in the human context. Considering these issues, Activity 5.3 provides examples of reflection from two different students regarding their views of the value of reflection.

ACTIVITY 5.3 ■

Scenario 1: Writing About Professional Learning

'Last week a woman came into the labour ward during the night. I examined her (with my mentor) to assess whether the cervix was fully dilated and the first thing I noticed was the anterior fontanelle to the right.... It was a deflexed head and a brow presentation. I reflected (written) on the situation (e.g. possible problems resulting from brow presentation) and it helped me, not only in that situation, but it helped me in knowing what an anterior fontanelle felt like as it was my first experience. The reflection was not about my feelings but about what I have learnt. It is about hard facts, physiology and how I am going to know in the future, what I should have done about it, did I do the right thing'

student 10996, collington 2005

Scenario 2: Developing Knowledge

'I think the purpose of these reflections is just to learn about practice, to learn about yourself...mid-wifery.... You obviously need the theory as well. If you want to learn something from the reflection you can't speak about your feelings all the time, you have to go into the theory...it gives you another point of view, more knowledge and understanding. Take active management, for example, if that's what I have seen. I can relate to the other point of view from the research...sometimes you know a better way of managing the second stage.... I will try to do it bearing in mind what researchers say is a better outcome for women. Doing reflections on something...going deep into it develops your knowledge'.

student 10999, collington 2005

- Do you think there are different models of reflection being demonstrated in each scenario?
- If so, which ones?
- How do you think reflection combines learning about facts, feelings, theories and knowledge?

It is argued above that reflection can help in the maintenance and achievement of clinical competence, and hence is an important tool in a health professional's development. Furthermore, practice draws on several different ways of knowing, and writing reflections is a popular means of recording thoughts. With this in mind, the following section provides some guidance for developing a reflective portfolio.

Developing a Reflective Portfolio

A reflective portfolio contains writings that summarize the insights and experiences a midwife or student has gained from their learning from both a theoretical and a clinical perspective. It is used to assess the individual's engagement with professional practice and their ability to use theoretical knowledge in an applied setting. The portfolio itself can take many forms, including an extended written piece, a notebook or binder of short writings and documentary evidence, or can be developed electronically (e-portfolio). The contents of a reflective portfolio will vary according to the discipline, but in general it contains short written pieces that summarize and reflect on the experiences of practical work placements. A student's portfolio, for example, can include the following: samples of personal assignments, journal entries, critical incident reports, records of achievement, personal statements, etc.

Since 2016, all nurses and midwives in the United Kingdom regardless of work setting and role (clinical practice, education, management and research, etc.) are required to undergo a process of revalidation to maintain their registration with the Nursing and Midwifery Council (NMC). This involves each registrant writing reflective accounts based on the four themes of *The Code* (NMC 2018) and engaging in reflective discussions with fellow registrants

---

BOX 5.1 ■ Reflective Questions

Choose an event you would like to learn from and consider the following:
- What was the nature of the continuing professional development (CPD) activity and/or practice-related feedback and/or event or experience in your practice?
- What did you learn from the CPD activity and/or feedback and/or event or experience in your practice?
- How did you change or improve your practice as a result?
- How is this relevant to *The Code*? (Nursing and Midwifery Council 2018). Select one or more themes: *'prioritize people'; 'practise effectively'; 'preserve safety'; promote 'professionalism and trust'*.

(NMC 2019). Feedback to the NMC (2019) has already shown that the reflective discussion is thought to be one of the most rewarding elements of revalidation. Box 5.1 lists reflective questions relating to continuing professional development activity taken from the NMC template for revalidation (NMC 2019).

Detail of what the registrant is expected to do with these themes in linking explicitly to the NMC Code (NMC 2018) is provided, and whilst the guidance above might be deemed less structured than some models of reflection referred to in this chapter, it does, however, provide the direction for thinking about performance in practice and the need to consider improvements. Box 5.2 provides guidance to individuals on how to compile a good reflective portfolio.

BOX 5.2 ■ How to Compile a Good Reflective Portfolio

Be critical

Although the content of a portfolio will be more personalized than other assignments, the individual should use the same level of critical analysis as they would in any essay or examination.

Be comprehensive

A good range of experiences that exemplify the individual's work throughout the duration of the assessment period should be included. One or two periods of work may be highlighted, but these should be contextualized within the individual's overall experience.

Do not worry about revealing weaknesses

Writing about personal professional insecurities and weaknesses can show areas for development. It also enables an individual to reflect on theories and methods that might benefit them in the future.

Have a plan for development

The reflective portfolio should testify to the individual's development as a practitioner. However, to write a really strong portfolio, the individual should also include an action plan for future development that articulates the knowledge and skills required to address the professional weaknesses that the reflections have revealed and how it is envisaged these are to be developed.

Adapted from Ivory Research (2015).

Sowter et al (2011) argue that although the use of portfolios is widespread within health care education, agreement on their purpose, content, assessment and value is still debated. The objective of the study of Sowter et al (2011) was to achieve consensus on quality criteria for clinical practice portfolios that would act as guidance for students and lecturers. The Delphi process (Dalkey 1972) used facilitated exchange of ideas amongst panel *'experts'* about the content and evaluation of clinical practice portfolios, with most debate relating to judgement of competence and rewarding originality and creativity. These issues illustrate the tensions between educational values and professional constraints. The process proved to be an effective method for achieving consensus on quality criteria for clinical practice portfolios and enabled the development of validated guidelines.

It is helpful to consider what might be the specific purposes of a reflective portfolio, and what kinds of pieces might be included to support this. Activity 5.4 supports the reader in determining the design of their reflective portfolio.

ACTIVITY 5.4 ■

If you were asked to design a reflective portfolio to assist in your own learning, consider the following questions:

- What specific aspects of your own learning do you think a reflective portfolio would be able to assist with? (Try to name at least three.)
- What pieces of work would you include to help demonstrate learning on each aspect? (By way of starting, think about some of the activities which normally happen in the course of your day-to-day work. Is there a way of recording what happens and perhaps your own reflections on them? You can be creative here, drawing on a range of activities as outlined in the main text, but also perhaps developing others which have not been mentioned (e.g. non-written methods such as peer observation and feedback; a taped journal; a taped reflective discussion).
- How would you present these pieces of work for assessment and what issues do you imagine there might be in assessing them?

Midwives are required to maintain a professional portfolio as part of their statutory requirements, and one alternative way of doing this is via an e-portfolio. Stewart (2013) notes that some midwives are using open social networking tools and processes to develop an e-portfolio. However, confidentiality of patient and client data and professional reputation must be taken into consideration when one is using online public spaces for reflection. There is little evidence about how midwives use social networking tools for ongoing learning, but Stewart (2013) investigates ways in which reflective midwifery practice may be conducted via an e-portfolio in open, social networking platforms using collaborative processes with peers. Stewart (2013) concluded that the e-portfolio using open social networking tools and processes is a viable option for midwives because it facilitates collaborative reflection and shared learning, although what people think and client confidentiality impact on the nature of open reflection and learning outcomes.

Conclusion

Reflection can be used in various ways, and may work differently for people in different situations. The key to effective reflection, however, for everyone, is to find a meaning and a model which personally works well for them. This would indicate that it has to be something not only which they can apply easily in most situations they find themselves but which also challenges them to think in different ways about their practice and to be forever open to new learning, even from recurring experiences, which sometimes means experimenting with different models.

This chapter has sought to develop an understanding of reflection, as well as different models for practising it. Although the idea of reflective practice is most common in professional circles, an attempt has been made to raise awareness of how reflection is crucial to life in general and not only professional practice. The examples provided, however, should assist midwives in applying reflection to different aspects of professional practice. Different ways of knowing have also been outlined, illustrating how reflection and intuition are interrelated. Finally ideas about developing a reflective portfolio have been provided to assist the reader with ongoing professional development, revalidation and career progression.

KEY POINTS

- Reflection has various meanings.
- Thinking about and learning from experiences are fundamental to reflection.
- Reflection and intuition are interrelated.
- Reflection can help make explicit the more hidden reasons for intuitive responses.
- Intuitive decision-making and implicit assumptions contribute to day-to-day professional practice.
- There are many different models for practising reflection and learning in complex situations.
- Applying theories of knowledge and different ways of knowing is important in ongoing professional development.
- A person should be clear about their own understanding of reflection and the model/s which works for them.

References

Ash, S. L., & Clayton, P. H. (2004). The articulated learning: an approach to guided reflection and assessment. *Innovative Higher Education, 29*(2), 137–154.

Barnett, R. (1992). *Improving higher education: Total quality care*. Buckingham: Society for Research in Higher Education and Open University Press.

Betsch, T. (2008). The nature of intuition and its neglect in research on judgment and decision-making. In Plessner, E., Betsch, C., & Betsch, T. (Eds.), *Intuition in judgement and decision-making* (pp. 3–22). New York: Lawrence Erlbaum Associates.

Bolton, G. (2010). *Reflective practice: writing and professional development* (3rd ed.). Los Angeles: Sage Publications.

Borton, T. (1970). *Reach, touch, teach*. London: McGraw-Hill.

Brannigan, K., & Moores, A. (2015). A model of professional thinking: integrating reflective practice and evidence based practice. *Canadian Journal of Occupational Therapy, 76*(5), 342–350.

Chirema, K. (2007). The use of reflective journals in the promotion of reflection and learning in post-registration nursing students. *Nurse Education Today, 27*, 192–202.

Collington, V. (2005). *An investigation into the perceived influence of reflective journal writing in the process of pre-registration midwifery students' experiential learning*. PhD thesis. London: Kingston University.

Collington, V., & Hunt, S. (2006). Reflection in midwifery education and practice: an exploratory analysis. *Evidence-Based Midwifery, 4*(3), 76–82.

Dalkey, N. C. (1972). The Delphi method: an experimental study of group opinion. In Dalkey, N. C., Rourke, D. L., Lewis, R., & Snyder, D. (Eds.), *Studies in the quality of life: Delphi and decision-making* (pp. 13–54). Lexington: Lexington Books.

Dewey, J. (1933). *How we think: a restatement of the relation of reflective thinking to the education process*. New York: D.C. Heath and Company.

Donaghy, M., & Morss, K. (2000). Guided reflection: a framework to facilitate and assess reflective practice within the discipline of Physiotherapy. *Journal of Physiotherapy, 16*(1), 3–14.

Eraut, M. (1994). *Developing professional knowledge and competence*. London: Falmer Press.

Fook, J., White, S., & Gardner, F. (2006). Critical reflection: a review of contemporary literature and understandings. In White, S., Fook, J., & Gardner, F. (Eds.), *Critical reflection in health and social care* (pp. 3–20). Maidenhead: Open University Press.

Fook, J., & Gardner, F. (2007). *Practising critical reflection: A resource handbook*. Maidenhead: Open University Press.

Fook, J., Collington, V., Ross, F., Ruch, G., & West, L. (Eds.). (2016). *Researching critical reflection: multidisciplinary perspectives*. London: Routledge.

Fook, J., Royes, J, & White, A. (2017). Critical Reflection. In Chambers, M., (Ed.). *Psychiatric and mental health nursing: the craft of caring* (3rd ed.), (pp.117–126). Abingdon: Routledge.

Greenhalgh, T. (2002). Intuition and evidence: uneasy bedfellows? *British Journal of General Practice, 52*(478), 395–400.

Habermas, J. (1971). *Knowledge and human interests*. London: Heinemann.

Ivory Research. (2015). *How to write a good reflective portfolio.* https://www.ivoryresearch.com/library/other-articles/reflective-portfolio-how-to-write-1st-class-reflective-portfolio/.

Johns, C. (2006). *Engaging reflection in practice: A narrative approach.* Oxford: Blackwell.

Johns, C., & Burnie, S. (2013). *Becoming a reflective practitioner* (4th ed.). Chichester: Wiley-Blackwell.

Kellehear, A., & Fook, J. (2010). Using critical reflection to support health promotion goals in palliative care. *Journal of Palliative Care, 26*(3), 295–302.

Knight, S. (2015). Realising the benefits of reflective practice. *Nursing Times, 111*(23–24), 17–19.

Loughran, J. J. (2002). Effective reflective practice: in search of meaning in learning about teaching. *Journal of Teacher Education, 53*(1), 33–43.

Lyons, J. (1999). Reflective education for professional practice: discovering knowledge from experience. *Nurse Education Today, 19*(1), 29–34.

Mantzoukas, S. (2007). A review of evidence-based practice, nursing research and reflection: levelling the hierarchy. *Journal of Clinical Nursing, 17*(2), 214–223.

Matthews, E. (2004). Concordance with pain medication: reflection on an adverse incident. *British Journal of Nursing, 13*(9), 551–555.

Matzler, K., Bailom, F., & Mooradian, T. A. (2007). Intuitive decision-making. *MIT Sloan Management Review, 47*(1).

McBrien, B. (2007). Learning from practice: reflections on a critical incident. *Accident and Emergency Nursing, 15*(3), 128–133.

McIntosh, P. (2010). *Action research and reflective practice.* Abingdon: Routledge.

Moon, J. (1999). *Reflection in learning and professional development: theory and practice.* London: Kogan Page.

Nursing and Midwifery Council. (2018). *The code: Professional standards of practice and behaviour for nurses, midwives and nursing associates.* London: Nursing and Midwifery Council.

Nursing and Midwifery Council. (2019). *How to revalidate with the NMC.* Available at: https://www.nmc.org.uk/globalassets/sitedocuments/revalidation/how-to-revalidate-booklet.pdf.

Nussbaum, M. (1997). *Cultivating humanity: A class defense of liberal reform in education.* Cambridge: Harvard University Press.

O' Donovan, M. (2007). Implementing reflection: insights from the pre-registration mental health students. *Nurse Education Today, 27*(6), 610–616.

Rolfe, G., Jasper, M., & Freshwater, D. (2011). *Critical reflection in practice* (2nd ed.). Basingstoke: Palgrave Macmillan.

Schon, D. (1983). *The reflective practitioner: how professionals think in action.* New York: Basic Books.

Sowter, J., Cortis, J., & Clarke, D. J. (2011). The development of evidence based guidelines for clinical practice portfolios. *Nurse Education Today, 31*, 872–876.

Stewart, S. (2013). Making practice transparent through e-portfolio. *Women and Birth, 26*(4), e117–e121.

Taylor, B. J. (2006). *Reflective practice: A guide for nurses and midwives* (2nd ed.). Maidenhead: Open University Press.

Wilson, G. (2013). Evidencing reflective practice in social work education: theoretical uncertainties and practical challenges. *British Journal of Social Work, 43*(1), 154–172.

Further Reading

Collington, V., & Hunt, S. (2006). Reflection in midwifery education and practice: an exploratory analysis. *Evidence-Based Midwifery, 4*(3), 76–82.
> *This article outlines the strategies that can enable student midwives to reflect on practice experiences.*

Fook, J., & Gardner, F. (Eds.). (2013). *Critical reflection in context: Applications in health and social care.* Abingdon: Routledge.
> *This text includes international case studies of how reflection and critical reflection can be used in different settings and for different purposes: in education, in practice or in research.*

Fook, J., White, S., & Gardner, F. (2006). Critical reflection: a review of contemporary literature and understandings. In White, S., Fook, J., & Gardner, F. (Eds.), *Critical reflection in health and social care* (pp. 3–20). Maidenhead: Open University Press.
> *This is a useful chapter to gain an overview of the different terms and definitions related to critical reflection.*

Greenhalgh, T. (2002). Intuition and evidence: uneasy bedfellows? *British Journal of General Practice, 52*(478), 395–400.
> *This article defines intuition and debates the arguments for and against its use alongside existing evidence.*

Knight, S. (2013). Realising the benefits of reflective practice. *Nursing Times, 111*(23–24), 17–19.
   This article explores the use of reflective practice as a structured process that is most effective in facilitated groups that also seek to gain people's confidence and show the rewards.
Nagel, J. (2014). Intuition, reflection, and the command of knowledge. *Aristotelian Society Supplementary, Vol. 88*(1), 219–241.
   This article argues that action is not always guided by conscious deliberation; in many circumstances, individuals act intuitively rather than reflectively.
Perry, M. A. (2000). Reflections on intuition and expertise. *Journal of Clinical Nursing, 9*(1), 137–145.
   This article describes an experience drawn from clinical practice and education in French-speaking Switzerland, followed by explicit reflection grounded in questions generated by Johns's model for structured reflection.
Wilson, G. (2013). Evidencing reflective practice in social work education: theoretical uncertainties and practical challenges. *British Journal of Social Work, 43*(1), 154–172.
   This article provides a sophisticated coverage of the issues surrounding reflective practice and its use in providing evidence.

Useful Websites

Ivory Research. (2015). *How to Write a Good Reflective Portfolio.* Available at: https://www.ivoryresearch.com/library/other-articles/reflective-portfolio-how-to-write-1st-class-reflective-portfolio/.
   This focuses on what a reflective portfolio should contain and guides the reader on how to construct a good one.
Meadows, C. (2006). *How Do Healthcare Providers Use Intuition?* Available at: https://www.takingcharge.csh.umn.edu/explore-healing-practices/intuition-healthcare/how-do-healthcare-providers-use-intuition.
   This article notes that few research studies have been undertaken on health care professionals' use of intuition or their patients' attitudes toward its use. In general, most health care professionals are reluctant to discuss intuition in practice because of others' perception that it is not a legitimate part of evaluation and decision-making procedures.

CHAPTER 6

Ethical Decision-Making in Midwifery Education and Practice

Sima Hay ▪ Jayne E. Marshall

CONTENTS

LEARNING OUTCOMES

By the end of this chapter the reader should be able to:

- appreciate the importance of how ethics and morals shape personal and professional decisions
- understand how ethical theories, ethical principles and personal values influence decision-making in midwifery education and practice
- reflect on how professional codes of conduct guide a midwife's practice in a range of contexts
- discuss the role of the midwife as an advocate in midwifery practice
- understand the value of using an ethical decision-making framework when faced with ethical dilemmas in education and practice.

Overview

This chapter explores the ethical theories that underpin the decisions and subsequent actions an individual may take from both a personal and a professional perspective, especially in the context of midwifery practice. The four ethical principles approach within the context of health care is discussed. Making an ethical decision requires not only a trained sensitivity to ethical issues but also a practised method for exploring the ethical aspects of a decision and weighing up the consequences that could impact on the choice of a course of action. Use of a framework to inform an ethical decision is absolutely essential and an important aspect of midwifery education that will ultimately impact on the development of a midwife's individual philosophy and future practice. Case studies and activities are included throughout the chapter to illustrate the theories presented.

Introduction

There are three types of ethics:
1. *metaethics*, which focuses on universal truths and where and how ethical principles are developed
2. *normative ethics*, which focus on the moral standards that regulate behaviours
3. *applied ethics*, which focus on specific difficult issues such as euthanasia/end-of-life care, termination of pregnancy and health inequalities.

In the midwifery profession, frequent ethical issues arise simply because of the nature of midwifery practice. Throughout their education and practice, midwives must exercise sound judgement when making decisions, and having a better understanding of ethical theories and decision-making frameworks will help them in managing complex situations as and when they arise more effectively.

Defining Terms

VALUES

Values are attitudes, beliefs or ideals that an individual or group holds and what they use to guide their behaviour and actions (Thompson 2004). Values are usually expressed in terms of right and wrong, hierarchies of importance or how an individual should behave. Beliefs and values are very personal, are freely chosen and are shaped by a range of things, such as a person's background, the type of society they have been brought up in, including the impact of their schooling and media, and the principles and concepts learned since childhood, such as veracity and honesty. It is important to recognize that in a community or culture many of these beliefs and values will be the same, but there may also be different perspectives. Whilst the interpretation of moral codes may be different, an individual will usually be judged by societal codes or what is accepted in civil law. Thompson (2004) refers to a *values lens* that forms one's initial view on how individuals should treat others in society.

Health Education England (2016) developed a national values-based recruitment framework following the publication of the Mid Staffordshire NHS Foundation Trust Public Inquiry report (Francis 2013), which identified substandard care and failings by many staff in exhibiting core values such as care and compassion. This framework not only encourages health and social care employers to complement their existing recruitment processes with values-based recruitment but also encourages higher education institutions to do the same, ensuring that successful candidates to health care programmes, such as preregistration midwifery education programmes, have the appropriate values as well as the intellectual capacity to become compassionate midwives (Department of Health and Social Care 2015).

MORALS

Morals, on the other hand, are established rules of conduct to be used in situations where a decision about right and wrong must be made. Morals therefore provide standards of behaviour that guide the actions of an individual or social group, such as *it is wrong to steal*. Morals are learned over time and tend to be influenced by life experiences and culture.

ETHICS

Ethics is the branch of philosophy that explores the nature of moral virtue and evaluates or reflects on human actions that may be *codified* as in the ethical code of a profession (Mepham 2008). Ethics is concerned with the fundamental principles of right and wrong and what people ought to do, and consequently informs the judgements and values that determine the course of action taken (Bennett 2015). The word "ethics is derived from the Greek "*ethos*," which means "*custom* or "*habit*" and denotes the theory of right action and the greater good. It is not limited to specific acts and defined moral codes, but encompasses the whole of moral ideals and behaviours (Bennett 2015).

Jones (2000: 8) defines ethics as *'the application of the processes and theories of moral philosophy to a real situation'*.

BIOETHICS

The application of ethical theories and principles to moral issues or problems in health care is known as *bioethics*. In the 1970s, as health care providers began to embrace a holistic view of the patient and the rights of the individual, in addition to treating and curing disease, bioethics or *biomedical ethics* came into existence as an area of ethical enquiry

However, the terms *ethics* and *morals* are often used interchangeably despite there being subtle differences between them, and how they may influence others can present in different ways. Put simply, morals are seen as *personal and internally driven*, guiding the individual into doing what they believe to be right and avoiding what is thought to be wrong, whereas ethical theories and principles are *externally driven* from a societal perspective, providing professionals with guidance or rules on their conduct. Clarke (2015) states that this can be applied to midwifery in the way midwives behave, support and conduct the care of women in childbirth; e.g. following an ethical principle because society expects this of the midwife, but also morally, from a personal belief that is internally driven. Midwives need to fully understand the strengths and limitations of the individual values they hold and, wherever they practise, it is essential that they reflect and examine their *value lens* for discriminatory behaviours based on gender, culture, family or societal norms.

It is worth noting that in some situations an ethical and moral decision may also be informed by legal aspects; however, the law is entirely separate at opposite ends of the spectrum (see Chapter 7). Nevertheless, as the concept of the law is to protect the public from harm, and failing to do so would result in an individual facing prosecution, it is argued that protecting life is rooted within an ethical principle. Furthermore, such a decision is likely to also be supported by a personal moral belief that in failing to follow the law and ethics harm could be done. It is therefore vital that midwives reflect on their own perspective and further develop their understanding of ethical theory and accompanying frameworks so as to support their decision-making in a non-judgemental way.

Ethical Theories

Ethical theory has been debated since ancient times by philosophers who have tried to explore and define how things are and should be. There are different ethical theories, and these can be

---

BOX 6.1 ■ Major Ethical Theories

Utilitarianism: consequentialism/teleological theory
Deontology: duty-based ethics
Virtue ethics
Feminist bioethics
Principles

---

applied to different situations to inform an individual's thinking and support their personal and professional decision-making (Clarke 2015). There are five major ethical theories that attempt to specify and justify moral rules and principles as shown in Box 6.1, and each will be explored in the following sections.

UTILITARIANISM (CONSEQUENTIALISM/TELEOLOGICAL THEORY)

The utilitarian approach argues that actions have no intrinsic ethical character but acquire their moral position from the consequences that follow them. It originates from the Greek *telos* meaning *end* or *purpose* and is sometimes known as *teleological theory*. This theory is described as doing the greatest good/having the greatest benefit for the greatest number of people. It is therefore attractive in that this approach can aid decision-making for the masses in that an action is good if it provides benefit for the majority. Utilitarianism originates from the thinking of Jeremy Bentham and John Stuart Mill in the 18th and 19th centuries based on hedonistic values in relation to happiness and pleasure. However, the use of the term *happiness* has been criticized as for some individuals the consequences of an action may not always result in happiness, and subsequently this has led to changes in the interpretation of the theory (Devlin and Magill 2006).

Utilitarianism is one of the most powerful and persuasive approaches to ethics in the history of philosophy. It is generally accepted that the morally right action is the action that produces the best outcome (Mepham 2008). Utilitarian principles tend to be the basis for many aspects of health and maternity care, such as health promotion and screening programmes. However, health care professionals should be aware that for some individuals making a decision to take part in any health care activity, such as antenatal screening, may evoke anxiety and fear and consequently result in a degree of unhappiness.

There are two types of this theory: *act utilitarianism* and *rule utilitarianism*. Act utilitarianism is the purer form, and expects every potential action to be assessed according to its predicted outcomes in terms of benefit. Rule utilitarianism, on the other hand, considers moral rules that are intended to ensure the greatest benefit such that each act is assessed as to what extent it conforms to the rules.

DEONTOLOGY: DUTY-BASED ETHICS

In contrast, deontological ethics is an approach to ethics that focuses on the rightness or wrongness of the specific actions rather than whether their consequences are right or wrong. This approach derives from the Greek *deon* meaning *obligation*, *duty* or *rule* and is focused on making decisions based on one's duties and other's rights, and is often referred to as *duty-based ethics* (Mepham 2008)

The 18th century German philosopher Immanuel Kant is considered the most influential thinker of deontological or duty-based ethics. Kant judged morality by examining the nature of actions and the will of the person rather than the resulting outcomes. To act morally is concerned with truth telling and respect for duty, regardless of the circumstances. The interpretation of duty may vary according to an individual's personal situation, their values and their beliefs, which can be based on natural laws and religion (e.g. *traditional deontology*). The actions of an individual should always be rational and stem from goodwill; namely the *categorical imperative* that is defined as follows:

- *Act only according to that maxim by which you can also will that it will become a universal law.*
- *Act in such a way that you always treat humanity, whether in your own person or any other, never simply as a means, but always at the same time as an end.*

According to the deontological approach, an action can be moral only if it can be applied to everyone universally: if everyone were to act in the same way. Kant believed that everyone is autonomous and rational and should be treated with respect rather than as a means to an end or for personal gain. Whilst it has been argued that the concept of health care provision is essentially utilitarian, health professionals adopt a more deontological approach to the delivery of care. The *duty of care* that all health professionals are familiar with is defined within *The Code* (Nursing and Midwifery Council [NMC] 2018). However, in some instances, there may be conflicting duties that create a dilemma in determining the best course of action, and in maternity care it is essential that midwives respect women as individuals with their own experiences to inform the decision-making process.

VIRTUE ETHICS THEORY

In the late 1950s the Anglo-American philosopher Anscombe expressed an increasing dissatisfaction with the existing forms of deontology and utilitarianism and proposed an alternative view, that of *virtue ethics*, which can be traced to Socrates, Plato and Aristotle (Anscombe 1958). This theory affirms that morality/virtue ascends from the identity and/or character of the individual rather than being a reflection of the actions of the individual (or consequences thereof). Living an ethical life, or acting rightly, requires development and demonstration of the virtues of courage, compassion, wisdom and temperance (McCammon and Brody 2012)

The Aristotelian approach places value on moral character or virtues of the individual above all else, rather than acts or outcomes. It assumes people can learn to act in a virtuous manner through training until they acquire the habit of virtue. In addition, behaving virtuously entails choosing the best approach to create happiness, or acting by deliberating on general principles until the best decision is reached. Virtue ethics rejects the reliance on rules for resolving moral problems, for which it has been heavily criticized (Beauchamp and Childress 2013). Consequently, the position taken is *'we know because we are virtuous'*. A further criticism of virtue ethics is that there is no defined set of approved virtues, so it is never certain when one is behaving virtuously or not (Mepham, 2008)

FEMINIST BIOETHICS

A number of 18th and 19th century philosophers, including Mary Wollstonecraft, John Stuart Mill, Catherine Beecher, Charlotte Perkins Gilman and Elizabeth Cady Stanton, championed the feminist approach to ethics as an attempt to rethink traditional ethics to the extent it depreciates or devalues women's moral experience (Jagger 1992). Consequently, feminist theory aims to eliminate the oppression of any group of people, but most particularly women. Feminist theory requires examination of how an action affects the person in order to come to a moral conclusion (Jagger 1992). The main reasoning of feminist ethics is to make a well-informed ethical decision that is not gender biased and appeals to important core values. It is by nature particularistic, and in this respect it is similar to many virtue ethical approaches. From a feminist perspective the advances in maternal medicine and an awareness of women's health, cultural and social issues are of great importance to midwives, such as termination of pregnancy, reproductive medicine, justice and care, genetic diagnosis, exploitation and abuse of women, female genital circumcision, contraception human immunodeficiency virus, and equal access to (and quality of) health care and health care resources.

In the early 1970s, feminist *bioethics* emerged, initially focusing on medical ethics (Holmes and Purdy 1992; Tong 1997; Warren 2000). Feminist bioethics is concerned with the correct understanding of autonomy as relational autonomy (Mackenzie and Stoljar 2000; Donchin 2001), a strong focus on care and the claim for an equal and just treatment of women that excludes any discrimination within health care provision, including among health care professionals and on many different levels of the organization. Jaggar (1992), however, is critical of traditional ethics for letting women down in several ways, arguing that less concern for women's issues and interests is shown than for men's issues and interests. It is considered that ethics tends to favour *male* ways of moral reasoning, which emphasize rules, rights, universality and impartiality over *female* ways of moral reasoning, which emphasize relationships, responsibilities and partiality (Jaggar 1992).

Ethical Principles

Ethical principles rather than theories have usually provided the foundation to analyse and act on ethical dilemmas in health and maternity care. Midwives appear more conversant with ethical principles than with ethical theories, and consequently, in practice, decisions tend to be made with use of a combination of principles.

PRINCIPLISM: THE FOUR PRINCIPLES APPROACH

The four principles approach within (bio)medical ethics draws on common morality; that is, a set of norms that are shared by all persons committed to promoting goodness/morality (Beauchamp and Childress 2013). This is one of the most widely used approaches, providing a general guide, intended to be an aid in balancing judgement usually in health care settings. The four principles approach, often referred to as *principlism*, consists of four universal prima facie ethical principles – *respect for autonomy*, *beneficence*, *non-maleficence*, and *justice* – as shown in Box 6.2.

These four principles are not ranked in hierarchal order, although in midwifery practice respect for maternal autonomy has assumed a greater significance in the context of maternal choice, underpinned by the requirement to provide the woman with sufficient information to put her in a position to choose.

Professional Codes of Practice

Codes of practice provide advice and guidance to practitioners, setting out clear standards of professional conduct and *best* practice for them to use in their everyday work and are in effect a framework. *The International Code of Ethics for Midwives* (International Confederation of Midwives [ICM] 2014) is part of the ICM *core documents*, which provide a professional framework for international use by midwifery associations, midwifery regulators, midwifery educators and governments to strengthen the midwifery profession and raise the standard of midwifery practice in their jurisdiction. By working within such a professional framework, midwives are supported and enabled to fulfil their role and contribute fully to the delivery of maternal and neonatal care in their respective country.

When a midwife registers with the NMC, they are committed to uphold the standards of *The Code* (NMC 2018), which are underpinned by ethical principles that put the interests of service users first to promote public trust through professionalism. This applies to *all* midwives, whether they provide direct care to individuals, groups or communities or bring their professional knowledge to bear in other roles, such as leadership, education or research. If midwives fail to uphold

> **BOX 6.2 ■ The Four Ethical Principles (Principlism)**
>
> - *Respect for autonomy* values the decision-making capacities of an individual, enabling them to make informed choices. To respect autonomy means that an individual has the right to choose to either accept or decline information or a course of action/treatment. Placing women at the centre of maternity care, empowering them make their own health care decisions, is an essential component of the notion of autonomy.
> - *Beneficence* is compassion and taking positive action to do good or balance the benefits or risks in a given situation, and refers to actions performed that contribute to the welfare of others. There are two principles of beneficence: *positive beneficence*, which requires the provision of benefits, and *utility*, which requires benefits and drawbacks be balanced. The midwife should always act in a way that benefits the childbearing woman, her baby and her family; however, this principle can cause a dilemma when a woman chooses a course of action that may not be in her and her fetus's/baby's best interests.
> - *Non-maleficence* (*primum non nocere*) is the principle of avoiding causing harm or hurt to another. Most treatments involve some harm, even if minimal, but the harm should not be disproportionate to the benefits of the treatment. Non-maleficence asserts an obligation to not inflict harm intentionally, and forms the framework for the standard of *duty of care* that is expected of *all* health professionals.
> - *Justice* refers to treating everyone fairly and equally, in light of what is due or owed to an individual. In addition, *respect for justice* involves a fair distribution and access to resources, such as health and maternity services, including a range of places for giving birth.

The Code, the NMC can take action that may include removing them from the professional register. This also includes the responsible use of social networking in that conduct online should be judged in the same way as conduct in the real world. The consequences of improper postings that cause harm to others could put a midwife's registration at risk or could jeopardize a student midwife's eligibility to join the professional register (see Chapter 3). The NMC (2015) has issued guidance on the use of social media that can be applied to other forms of online communication, such as personal websites and blogs, discussion boards and general content shared online, including text, photographs, images, and video and audio files. Educators can use *The Code* to assist student midwives understand what it means to be a professional and how using *The Code* in practice helps to achieve this. The four standards of *The Code* (NMC 2018) are summarized in Box 6.3.

THE RULES OF FIDELITY AND VERACITY

In addition, midwives must be conversant with the ethical rules of *fidelity* (faithfulness) and *veracity* (truth telling). Being faithful or loyal means honouring one's commitments or promises to another person, and thus creates the trust that is key to any relationship. Burkhardt and Nathaniel (2013) argue, however, that there is no absolute duty to keep promises, but in every situation the harmful consequences of the promised action must be balanced against the benefits of promise keeping.

Through entry into the midwifery profession, every registered practising midwife should always uphold the professional code of practice according to the country in which they are licensed to practise, practise within the scope of midwifery practice and keep their knowledge and skills up to date, including knowledge of national and local policies. Fidelity requires the midwife to meet all reasonable expectations in these areas, and is a fundamental part of the midwife–woman relationship. When midwives are assigned to care for childbearing women, their babies and their families, whether it be on a day-by-day basis or through case-holding throughout the childbirth continuum, there is an expectation they will fulfil such a commitment. Failure to

---

BOX 6.3 ■ The Four Standards of *The Code*

■ *Prioritize people.*
■ You put the interests of people using or needing midwifery services first. You make their care and safety your main concern and make sure that their dignity is preserved and their needs are recognized, assessed and responded to. You make sure that those receiving care are treated with respect, that their rights are upheld and that any discriminatory attitudes and behaviours towards those receiving care are challenged.
■ *Practise effectively.*
■ You assess need and deliver or advise on treatment, or give help (including preventative or rehabilitative care) without too much delay and to the best of your abilities, on the basis of the best available evidence. You communicate effectively, keeping clear and accurate records and sharing skills, knowledge and experience where appropriate. You reflect and act on any feedback you receive to improve your practice.
■ *Preserve safety.*
■ You make sure that service users and public safety are protected. You work within the limits of your competence, exercising your *duty of candour* and raising concerns immediately whenever you come across situations that put service users or public safety at risk. You take necessary action to deal with any concerns where appropriate.
■ *Promote professionalism and trust.*
■ You uphold the reputation of your profession at all times. You should display a personal commitment to the standards of practice and behaviour set out in *The Code.* You should be a model of integrity and leadership for others to aspire to. This should lead to trust and confidence in the profession from service users, other health and care professionals and the public.

Adapted from Nursing and Midwifery Council (2018)

---

provide midwifery care or carry out prescribed care is unethical, providing the prescribed care is safe and consistent with good practice, and may constitute *abandonment* or *neglect* on the part of the midwife, with the consequential formal investigation into their practice.

Veracity is the act of telling the truth or not lying/deceiving others and is vital to the development and continuance of trust between people. Codes of medical ethics surprisingly have ignored obligations and virtues of veracity, when, by contrast, virtues of candour, honesty and truthfulness are among the most widely praised traits of health professionals and researchers in contemporary biomedical ethics (Beauchamp and Childress 2013). Veracity is prima facie binding, not absolute. *Veracity* in health and maternity care refers to comprehensive, accurate and objective transmission of information as well as the way the professional fosters the individual's understanding. The obligation of veracity is based on respect owed to others, in that respect for autonomy forms the basis for rules of disclosure and consent.

When a childbearing woman enters a relationship with a midwife, they gain the right to the truth regarding their care options, procedures and any results, just as the midwife gains the right to truthful disclosures from the woman. The relationship between midwives and childbearing women ultimately depends on trust, and adherence to rules of veracity is essential to foster trust. It is therefore difficult to accept that deception is ever justified if both the midwife and the woman are respectful of each other as individuals. However, two exceptions exist. The first is where an individual requests *not* to be told the truth. In this case the midwife can under the ethical principles of beneficence and non-maleficence withhold the truth. This does not mean that the midwife must lie, but means that they are released from their obligation to report to the woman what they may know. The second exception, which is less common in midwifery, is where an individual is mentally incompetent and as a result autonomy and the capacity for self-determination are diminished, thereby justifying the withholding of health care information. Furthermore, in some instances midwives may feel constrained by organizational pressures and have limited time to spend with women and fully inform them of their maternity options.

This can create an ethical dilemma for those midwives who believe it is unethical to withhold information especially when the woman asks for specific information about their condition or results.

Now undertake Activity 6.1.

ACTIVITY 6.1 ■

Grace is a student midwife in the first year of a 3-year degree programme.

Grace has been very anxious as her Practice Assessment Document (PAD) is due to be submitted for an end-of-year summative assessment. Whilst she has completed all her summative proficiencies, on the day of submission, she notices that her nominated practice assessor, Megan, has omitted signing one of the proficiencies.

Megan is currently off sick, and in a panic Grace copies Megan's signature onto the page with the outstanding proficiency as she believes that she may fail if she does not submit her PAD on time. During the marking process, Grace's personal midwifery tutor notices the signature is different and queries this. She subsequently emails Grace to come in to the university to see her.

With reference to ethical theories:

- What may have led Grace to choose this course of action?
- What alternatives could Grace have considered?
- How should Grace's personal tutor respond?

Ethical Decision-Making

Making good ethical decisions requires a trained sensitivity to ethical issues and a practised method for exploring the ethical aspects of a decision and weighing the considerations that should impact on the choice of a course of action. Having a method for ethical decision-making is essential (Mason 2006). The more difficult the ethical choice, the more is the need to rely on discussion and dialogue with others about the dilemma. Only by careful exploration of the problem, aided by the insights and different perspectives of others, can good ethical choices be made.

Mason (2006: 3) argues that the concept of

> ethics is not that of a single rule'. Rather, 'ethics consists of a number of principles, all of which are designed to the same end – that is, to find the most acceptable answer to a given philosophical problem.

It is highlighted that a decision based on an ethical principle may not be the 'right' decision in everyone's eyes and that although two decisions may be different, each may be 'right' insofar as they have been based on differing ethical principles (Mason 2006).

Ethical dilemmas are encountered at all levels in the health and maternity care setting and affect all practitioners involved in clinical practice. Having a strategy that supports ethical decision-making when faced with dilemmas can enable midwives to formulate appropriate courses of action that have the recipient's (woman's/baby's/family's) interests at heart.

CASUISTRY

Casuistry, or case-based reasoning, focuses not on rules and theories but rather on practical decision-making in particular cases based on precedent. The features of a case are first identified and then a comparison is made with similar cases and prior experiences, attempting to determine not only the similarities but also the differences. An example is whether or not it would be ethical for a midwife to breach their duty of confidence, such as the health risks to others, if information were not disclosed. A comparison is then made with similar cases, identifying the relative risks of non-disclosure. Casuistry, however, should not be divorced from consequentialism, deontology, or virtue ethics but should complement them.

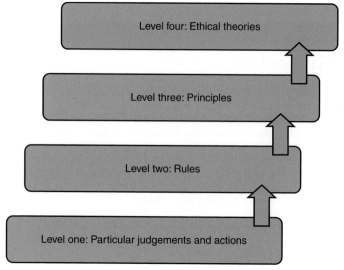

Fig. 6.1   Four-level approach to ethical decision-making.

FOUR-LEVEL APPROACH TO ETHICAL DECISION-MAKING

One ethical decision-making framework is outlined in the work of Beauchamp and Childress (2013), who articulate four levels within a framework, detailed in Fig. 6.1:

- *Level one: judgements and actions.* When midwives are faced with an ethical dilemma, they usually use their intuition, reflecting on their own experiences or those of their colleagues to make a particular judgement and decide on a certain course of action.
- *Level two: rules.* The rules defined within the framework are the rules of veracity (truth telling), privacy, confidentiality and fidelity (promise keeping). Midwives should be familiar with these rules as they are embodied within *The Code* (NMC 2018).
- *Level three: principles.* The four main ethical principles which are usually applied within health care and midwifery practice were discussed earlier and are specifically *respect for autonomy, beneficence, non-maleficence* and *justice* (see Box 6.1).
- *Level four: ethical theories.* These are *utilitarianism* and *deontology.*

When one is using this approach, the use of intuition (*level one*) is a significant starting point in terms of decision-making. *Level two* and *level three* (rules and principles) will further challenge the midwife's decision. However, *level four* (ethical theories) is more challenging, and it may not be possible for the midwife to come to a decision based on one theory alone. One criticism of this approach is the lack of specific reference to *The Code* (NMC 2018), to which the midwife should always refer when contemplating an ethical dilemma.

SEEDHOUSE'S ETHICAL GRID

Seedhouse's (2008) framework for ethical decision-making as shown in Fig. 6.2 was created to support health professionals in their day-to-day work and presents an overview of the elements required for thorough ethical reasoning. The grid is depicted by different layers: from the inner layer at the centre to the second layer, third layer and outer layer. Each layer is described as follows:

- The inner layer: the principles behind health care practice.

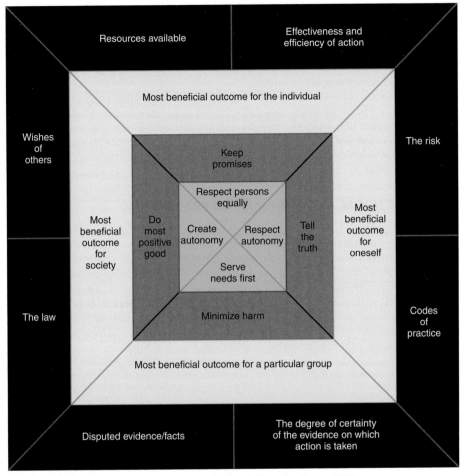

Fig. 6.2 Seedhouse's ethical grid. (From Seedhouse 2008)

- The second layer: the duties a health care worker has.
- The third layer: the nature of the outcomes to be achieved.
- The outer layer: the relevant practical issues.

As can be seen, each layer is formed by a number of boxes that should be considered during the decision-making process. The midwife may make use of some or all of the boxes within one or all of the layers, which offers a degree of autonomy. Seedhouse provides the following suggestions as to how to use the grid:

- *Arrive at an initial intuitive response.* Consider the ethical issue/dilemma intuitively without reference to the grid and try to understand the ramifications of the possible action(s). Clarify the ethical issue/dilemma by key aspects and attempt to list basic pros and cons of the various options for action.
- *Consider the grid.* Consider the *first layer*, which is felt to be the most significant. In most cases this will be the central inner layer (shaded green) as this layer contains the rationale for health care. Ignoring every box in the central inner layer (green) would be unusual for any genuine health care professional.

- *Consider the levels in the rest of the grid.* Select those boxes which offer the most appropriate solution after weighing up and balancing alternatives. The most appropriate solution should be the one that produces the highest degree of morality.
- *Arrange the boxes 'over' the dilemma.* Apply the boxes to the mental picture of the proposed intervention so that the course of action will have been decided and the means to justify it in ethical/moral terms will be available.

As stated previously, two midwives may arrive at different decisions following their analysis of an ethical dilemma. The use of Seedhouse's grid enhances deliberation, throwing light into unseen corners and suggests new avenues of thought, enabling midwives to gain additional support for their decisions in terms of the highest degree of morality. It is good practice for midwives to refer to the grid when an ethical dilemma arises, either from the outset or after the event, so as to reflect on the decision that was made.

SIX-STEP ETHICAL DECISION-MAKING FRAMEWORK

Enck (2014) explores how ethical decision-making in the clinical setting is often overwhelming for clinicians and suggests the use of a framework for ethical decision-making which would offer a process for clinicians to enable them to manage an ethical issue. There is much literature that provides ethical approaches towards resolving an issue, but there are few resources available offering a framework which is practical. This framework is very structured with practical information, consideration and options. It provides a solid decision-making strategy applicable to real-world practice. It also includes the ethical analysis of a health care situation to determine how to make appropriate decisions that are in the best interest of the individual: *a good decision.* Figure 6.3 outlines the six steps of the framework.

Now undertake Activity 6.2.

ACTIVITY 6.2 ■

Rebecca and Simon are in their early 40s and are unable to have children. Rebecca's younger sister Rachel, who has already given birth to three healthy babies, has offered to be a surrogate mother and have a baby for the couple. Rachel used her own eggs, which were artificially inseminated with Simon's sperm, and embryos were subsequently transferred, resulting in Rachel becoming pregnant with twins.

The Couples' Dilemmas

The commissioning parents Rebecca and Simon wish to be present at the birth, but the birth mother, Rachel, wants her own partner to be present instead.

Rachel wishes to give birth according to her own wishes, while the adoptive parents are keen for the quickest and safest birth option for both babies.

The Midwife's Competing Dilemma

The commissioning couple, Rebecca and Simon, wish the midwife to involve them in the arrival of the twins, and yet the relationship between them and the birth mother, Rachel, appears strained. Use Seedhouse's ethical grid as a guide to explore the ethical issues:

- Which of the layers and boxes would inform the rationale for how you would address the dilemma?
- What would your decision be to resolve this dilemma?

Now use another ethical decision-making framework:

- What is the outcome of the dilemma when you use this framework?

Reflect on the use of different ethical decision-making frameworks in resolving the same dilemma and the significance this has on practice.

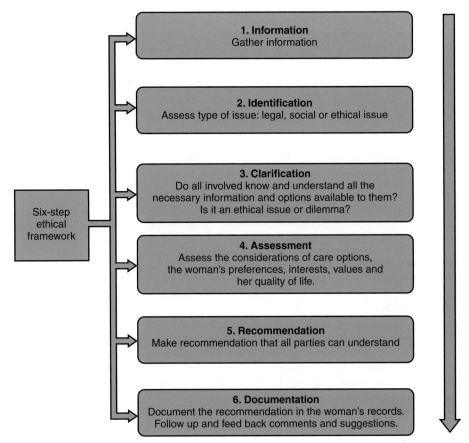

Fig. 6.3 The six-step ethical decision-making framework. (Adapted from Enck 2014)

Being an Advocate

The word *advocate* derives from the Latin *advocare*, which means *to call to one's aid*. The ICM plays a critical role in advocating the provision of the highest quality of care to women, their babies and their families on a global scale. The ICM has defined three pillars of a strong profession – namely *education, regulation* and *association* – as a framework to realize its vision and goals to improve women's health globally and secure their rights and access to midwifery care throughout the childbirth continuum (see Chapter 2). The latter pillar, that of *association*, comprises an organized body of persons engaged in a common professional practice, sharing information, career advancement objectives, in-service training, *advocacy* and other activities which ultimately support the strengthening of the workforce (United Nations Population Fund and ICM 2016).

Being an advocate for childbearing women is an important role of the midwife, standing up for their rights and their best interests at all times. Rules and regulations within a complex health and maternity care setting can often get in the way of the care and treatment the public receives, and an impersonal service can often infringe on a person's rights. This may occur when the environment is stretched and the workload is high, an individual's wishes have not been followed or the care plan requires reviewing and referral to others. Although it is assumed that healthy childbearing women are in a better position to articulate their own wishes, unlike ill patients, it still remains every midwife's responsibility to act as an advocate for women/call to their aid in situations when they are unable to do so for themselves. Such situations may include antenatal screening, choice of place of birth, mode of birth, perineal trauma/female genital mutilation and choices relating to neonatal screening, etc. However, a midwife must also value the woman's self-determination: the right to autonomy and consequential independence in decision-making.

Now undertake Activity 6.3.

ACTIVITY 6.3 ■

Consider situations where you have acted as a woman's advocate in the following:
- Antenatal care
- Intrapartum care and childbirth
- Postnatal care
- Neonatal care

Reflecting on the contents within this chapter:
- Outline the key issues of the situation that required you to become the woman's advocate.
- How did you discuss the situation and options available with the woman?
- From whom and from what did you seek support and guidance?
- How did you feel about supporting a woman's decision that you may not necessarily agree with?
- As a result of undertaking this activity, what are you likely to do in similar situations in the future?

Conclusion

Knowledge of ethics is essential to every midwife. Childbirth can be complex, and ethical dilemmas regularly occur within midwifery education and practice, and it is therefore imperative that student midwives appreciate how ethical theories, rules, principles and judgements can inform the most challenging of decisions made and support their future practice as registered midwives. These concepts are also embedded in *The Code* (NMC 2018) and the ICM (2014) *International Code of Ethics for Midwives* and are fundamental to the practice of every midwife worldwide and the role they play as advocates for childbearing women. Use of any of the ethical decision-making frameworks presented in this chapter can guide the midwife into making appropriate decisions with the interests of women, their babies and their families at heart. The value of *intuition* cannot be underestimated as usually the first gut instinct can often be the most appropriate course of action to take. Use of any of the frameworks can further endorse the rationale for choosing it. The use of activities within this chapter has provided opportunities for the reader to apply the ethical concepts to real-life scenarios to further develop their knowledge and decision-making skills.

KEY POINTS

- An understanding of ethical theories is essential to midwifery practice.
- It is essential that midwives reflect on and examine their *value lens* for discriminatory behaviours based on gender, culture, family or societal norms and their consequential impact on interactions with childbearing women.
- Respect for maternal autonomy has assumed a greater significance in the context of maternal choice and is fundamental to good midwifery practice.
- Dilemmas can occur as a result of conflicts between personal value systems, childbearing women, their families, health care professionals, organizations and society as well as student midwives and their lecturers within the university setting.
- *The Code* (NMC 2018) is underpinned by ethical principles and guides the standards of practice and behaviour for midwives (nurses and nursing associates).
- When acting as a woman's advocate, the midwife attempts to identify the woman's unmet needs and tries to help to address these needs, ultimately referring her to appropriately trained colleagues as and when indicated to minimize any harm.
- An ethical decision-making framework can assist the midwife when the midwife is faced with ethical dilemmas in education and practice.

References

Anscombe, G. E. M. (1958). Modern moral philosophy 1. *Philosophy*, *33*(124), 1–19.

Beauchamp, T. L., & Childress, J. F. (2013). *Principles of biomedical ethics* (7th ed.). Oxford: Oxford University Press.

Bennett, C. (2015). *What is this thing called ethics?* (2nd ed.). Abingdon: Routledge.

Burkhardt, M. A., & Nathaniel, A. (2013). *Ethics and issues in contemporary nursing* (4th ed.). Stamford: Cenage Learning.

Clarke, E. J. (2015). *Law and ethics for midwifery*. Abingdon: Routledge.

Department of Health and Social Care. (2015). *2010 to 2015 government policy: Compassionate care in the NHS*. London: HMSO. Available at: https://www.gov.uk/government/publications/2010-to-2015-government-policy-compassionate-care-in-the-nhs/2010-to-2015-government-policy-compassionate-care-in-the-nhs.

Devlin, B., & Magill, G. (2006). The process of ethical decision making. *Best Practice & Research: Clinical Anaesthesiology*, *20*(4), 493–506.

Donchin, A. (2001). Understanding autonomy relationally: toward a reconfiguration of bioethical principles. *The Journal of Medicine and Philosophy*, *26*(4), 365.

Enck, G. (2014). Six-step framework for ethical decision making. *Journal of Health Services Research and Policy*, *19*(1), 62–64.

Francis, R. (2013). *Report of the Mid Staffordshire NHS Foundation Trust Public Inquiry*. London: The Stationery Office. Available at: https://www.gov.uk/government/publications/report-of-the-mid-staffordshire-nhs-foundation-trust-public-inquiry.

Health Education England. (2016). *Values Based Recruitment Framework*. Available at: https://www.hee.nhs.uk/sites/default/files/documents/VBR_Framework%20March%202016.pdf.

Holmes, H., & Purdy, L. (1992). *Feminist perspectives in medical ethics*. Bloomington: Indiana University Press.

International Confederation of Midwives. (2014). *The international code of ethics for midwives*. Available at: http://internationalmidwives.org/assets/uploads/documents/CoreDocuments/CD2008_001%20V2014%20ENG%20International%20Code%20of%20Ethics%20for%20Midwives.pdf.

Jaggar, A. (1992). Feminist ethics. In Becke., L., & Becker, C. (Eds.), *Encyclopedia of ethics* (pp. 363–364). New York: Garland Press.

Jones, S. R. (2000). *Ethics in midwifery* (2nd ed.). Edinburgh: Mosby.

Mackenzie, C., & Stoljar, N. (Eds.). (2000). *Relational autonomy: feminist perspectives on autonomy, agency and the social self*. New York: Oxford University Press.

Mason, J. K. (2006). Ethical principles and ethical practice. *Clinical Ethics*, *1*(1), 3–6.

McCammon, S., & Brody, D. (2012). How virtue ethics informs medical professionalism. *HEC Forum*, *24*(4), 257–272.

Mepham, T. B. (2008). *Bioethics: an introduction for the biosciences* (2nd ed.). Oxford: Oxford University Press.

Nursing and Midwifery Council. (2015). *Guidance on using social media responsibly*. London: Nursing and Midwifery Council.

Nursing and Midwifery Council. (2018). *The code: Professional standards of practice and behaviour for nurses, midwives and nursing associates*. London: Nursing and Midwifery Council.

Seedhouse, D. (2008). *Ethics: the heart of health care* (3rd ed.). Chichester: John Wiley and Sons.

Thompson, J. B. (2004). A human rights framework for midwifery care. *Journal of Midwifery and Women's Health*, *49*(3), 175–181.

Tong, R. (1997). *Feminist approaches to bioethics: theoretical reflections and practical applications*. Boulder: Westview Press.

United Nations Population Fund & International Confederation of Midwives. (2016). *Comprehensive midwifery programme guidance*. Available at: http://www.unfpa.org/sites/default/files/resource-pdf/Midwifery%20Programme%20Guidance.pdf.

Warren, K. J. (2000). *Ecofeminist philosophy: A Western perspective on what it is and why it matters*. Lanham: Rowman and Littlefield.

Further Reading

Beauchamp, T. L., & Childress, J. F. (2013). *Principles of biomedical ethics* (7th ed.). Oxford: Oxford University Press.
    This popular text provides the reader with a good insight into ethics and morality in health care. Contemporary research and real-life case studies and scenarios assist in placing the theory into context when one is faced with ethical dilemmas and decision-making.

Ekland-Olson, S. (2015). *Who lives, who dies, who decides? Abortion, neonatal care, assisted dying and capital punishment* (2nd ed.). Oxford: Routledge.

This useful text addresses some very difficult ethical dilemmas and poses challenging questions for the reader to contemplate and apply to their practice. It is written in a style that is easy to read and helpful to the reader in clarifying their personal perspectives.

Seedhouse, D. (2008). *Ethics: The heart of health care* (3rd ed.). Chichester: John Wiley and Sons.

This classic ethics text in medical, health and nursing studies is recommended around the world for its user-friendly introduction to ethical analysis. The author ably demonstrates tangibly and graphically how ethics and health care are inextricably bound together, and creates a firm theoretical basis for practical decision-making. The use of the acclaimed ethical grid teaches an essential practical skill which can be productively applied in day-to-day health care. The text includes comprehensive and contemporary examples and case studies, with the addition of an extensive FAQ section.

Walker, M. (2007). *Moral understandings: A feminist study in ethics* (2nd ed.). New York: Oxford University Press.

As a feminist, Walker explores a view of morality and an approach to ethical theory which uses the critical insights of feminism and race theory to rethink the epistemological and moral position of the ethical theorist, and how moral theory is shaped by culture and history.

Useful Websites

Birthrights. http://www.birthrights.org.uk.
Ethics & Compliance Initiative. https://www.ethics.org/.
International Confederation of Midwives. https://www.internationalmidwives.org.
Nursing and Midwifery Council. https://www.nmc.org.uk.
UK Clinical Ethics Network. http://www.ukcen.net.
United Nations Population Fund. https://www.unfpa.org.

CHAPTER 7

Legal Issues Relating to Midwifery Education and Practice

Lindsay J. Gillman ■ Petra Petrocnik

CONTENTS

LEARNING OUTCOMES

By the end of this chapter the reader should have an understanding of:

- the legal framework that governs contemporary midwifery education and practice
- how legal systems and laws relate to midwifery practice
- the importance of treating individuals as equals and respecting their human rights
- legal torts specific to midwifery practices
- the legislation relating to health and safety at work.

Overview

This chapter provides an introduction to a selection of legal issues in relation to childbearing, and explores some of the key areas that affect midwifery education and practice. Case studies and examples are used to illustrate how the law has been applied in a variety of contexts. The legislation relating to the regulation of midwifery practice is explored in more detail in Chapter 2.

Introduction

The midwife's scope of practice is contained within the internationally agreed definition of the midwife produced by the International Confederation of Midwives (2017). However, the freedom to practise midwifery within that scope is determined by the regulation and legislative requirements of the country in which the midwife practises. It is therefore important that every midwife understands the legal framework of the country in which they practise, including their legal accountability, to be effective practitioners. For example, the United Kingdom (UK) Nursing and Midwifery Council (NMC) *The Code* (2018: 18) states in the professional standards of practice and behaviour that midwives and nurses must

> *uphold the reputation of your profession at all times. To achieve this, you must:...keep to the laws of the country in which you are practising.*

In addition to *The Code* (NMC 2018), each midwife must meet Standard 17 in *Standards for Pre-registration Midwifery Education* (NMC 2009), which specifies the competencies and essential skills clusters required of all midwives, which also comply with Article 42 of the European directive on professional qualifications (2005/36/EC). The role and sphere of the midwife's practice is further explored in Chapter 9.

The Law

The law is a system of rules usually made by a government so as to maintain social order, uphold justice and prevent harm to individuals and property. The law can be viewed as a collection of imposed rules that are binding on a population or community. There are usually consequences and sanctions as a result of a failure to follow the rules (Wheeler 2012). Laws are often based on ethical or religious principles and are enforced by the police and criminal justice systems.

THE UK LEGAL SYSTEM

The four principle sources of law in the UK are currently legislation (statute), common law, European Union law and the European Convention on Human Rights (ECHR). *Legislation* is law that is created by a legislature. The most important pieces of legislation are acts of Parliament. The Parliament at Westminster is the only body that has the power to pass laws that apply in all the four UK countries. Parliament is made up of both the House of Commons and the House of Lords. The Scottish Parliament, Northern Ireland Assembly and National Assembly for Wales have powers to pass laws on devolved issues and these laws apply only in the country in which they were passed. England and Wales have a legal system known as *common law*, in which decisions made in the Court of Appeal and the Supreme Court become precedents that must be followed to ensure that similar cases are treated in an equitable way. *European law* has also been a source of UK law, and whilst the UK remains a member state of the European Union (EU), EU law takes precedence over UK law. Equally the UK, as a signatory to the ECHR, requires all courts in the UK to protect the rights of individuals as identified in the ECHR through the Human Rights Act 1998.

The legal system in the UK is complex because it has evolved over centuries rather than being intentionally designed. Magistrates' courts, for example, became an official legal body as far back as 1285, when '*good and lawful men*' were commissioned to keep the King's peace. Since that time Justices of the Peace (magistrates) have undertaken most of the judicial work carried out in England and Wales. Although the UK legal system is complicated and can seem confusing and sometimes contradictory, it is still widely regarded as one of the best and most independent judiciary systems in the world (Courts and Tribunals Judiciary 2016).

THE LAW AND MIDWIFERY ACCOUNTABILITY

The regulation of midwifery practice and the legal system of the country in which the midwife practises are usually intrinsically linked. This system is designed to protect the safety of mothers and babies and to ensure that there is a process by which compensation can occur if this safety is compromised. The law in relation to professional practice enables the identification of the rights of women and the responsibilities of the midwife through a legal relationship. In the UK, there are four areas in which the midwife is accountable: *to society, to mothers and babies, to the professional statutory and regulatory body* and *to the employer* (Griffith et al 2010).

The midwife is accountable to *society* through public (criminal) law and can be called to account if a crime has been committed. Almost all criminal cases will start with a hearing in a magistrates' court, with very serious cases sent to the Crown Court, either for sentencing after the defendant has been found guilty or for a full trial with a judge and jury.

Midwives are accountable to *mothers and babies* by providing safe care. If the duty of care is breached and an individual is harmed as a result of carelessness, a case for negligence can be brought through tort or civil law. Civil cases will be heard initially in a county court, which has the ability to award compensation if harm has been caused through negligence. *The Code* (NMC 2018) states that nurses and midwives must have an indemnity arrangement in place relevant to their scope of practice, in case of a decision to award compensation in case of a decision to award compensation where a claim is successful. This is usually provided through vicarious liability through the contract of employment. The concept of negligence is explored in more detail later in this chapter.

The *professional statutory and regulatory body*, such as the NMC in the UK, will also hold midwives to account for their professional practice. The legislation that governs this public protection role of the NMC is the Nursing and Midwifery Order 2001. The midwife must adhere to the professional standards and codes of practice set out by the regulatory body. If there are concerns over the midwife's practice, or a breach of *The Code* (NMC 2018) has occurred, a fitness-to-practise hearing may be called.

The final sphere of a midwife's accountability is to *the employer* through a contract of employment, which will include the conditions for vicarious liability. A midwife who breaches their contract of employment can be held to account by their employer even though this behaviour may not amount to a crime, civil wrong or professional misconduct, and could face suspension from work, with consequential termination of employment.

Equality and Human Rights

EQUALITY

In the UK, the Equality Act 2010 consolidated the law in relation to forms of discrimination such as race, disability and gender discrimination by simplifying and strengthening the existing anti-discrimination legislation. The Equality Act 2010 provides clear guidance about individual rights and responsibilities through the identification of nine protected characteristics as shown in Box 7.1. Discrimination, harassment and victimization in relation to any of these characteristics within

---

BOX 7.1 ■ Equality Duty

In terms of the provision of health care services, service providers cannot discriminate against individuals or groups and must consider the three facets of equality duty in relation to:

- age
- disability
- gender reassignment
- marriage or civil partnership
- pregnancy and maternity
- race
- religion, faith or belief
- sex
- sexual orientation.

Adapted from the Equality Act 2010 (section 149).

BOX 7.2 ■ Positive Action

An example of *positive action* through the Equality Act 2010 might be the provision of specialist services for an especially vulnerable group, such as pregnant women who are refugees or asylum seekers. These women often have poorer outcomes for a variety of reasons. They may not access services because of language barriers and a lack of appropriate interpreting services, a previous poor experience of maternity services or a fear of being charged high costs for accessing maternity services (Haith-Cooper and McCarthy 2015). This may result in women:

- attending initial antenatal care later than recommended
- not accessing antenatal screening services
- attending fewer antenatal care appointments
- not accessing preparation for parenthood classes (Carolan and Cassar 2010; Phillimore 2016).

Creating bespoke services to meet the needs of this particular group would meet the aims of *positive action* through the provision of favourable treatment to ensure equality outcomes.

---

employment, education and the provision of public services are unlawful. Part of the Equality Act 2010 relates to *equality duty*. This applies to public sector organizations, all of which are required to embed *due regard* within their decision-making processes to eliminate unlawful discrimination, victimization and harassment, promote equality of opportunity and facilitate good relations between groups of individuals. Consideration is required for how employers act, design and deliver services and how they develop policy to ensure the aims of *equality duty* are met (Equality and Human Rights Commission 2016).

The Equality Act 2010 also has provision to assist people who share a protected characteristic and experience disadvantages, or suffer as a result of past or present discrimination. Section 158 of the Equality Act 2010 enables service providers to take *positive action* to ensure that there are better equality outcomes. Positive action can involve the favourable treatment of members of a group who share a protected characteristic. The action taken will not amount to discrimination under this particular Act as long as it meets the conditions of the Act and the test of proportionality. Positive action is lawful and will not amount to discrimination if the disadvantages of a particular group are recognized and enable or encourage persons who share the protected characteristic to overcome or minimize that disadvantage (Equality Act 2010: Section 158.1; Law Society 2012). An example of positive action is shown in Box 7.2.

BOX 7.3 ■ Articles Under the Human Rights Act 1998

The Human Rights Act 1988 sets out the fundamental rights and freedoms that individuals have access to:
Article 2: The right to life
Article 3. Freedom from torture and inhuman or degrading treatment
Article 4. Freedom from slavery and forced labour
Article 5. The right to liberty and security
Article 6. The right to a fair trial
Article 7. No punishment without law
Article 8. Respect for your private and family life, home and correspondence
Article 9. Freedom of thought, belief and religion
Article 10. Freedom of expression
Article 11. Freedom of assembly and association
Article 12. The right to marry and start a family
Article 14. Protection from discrimination in respect of these rights and freedoms
Article 16. The right to participate in free elections

HUMAN RIGHTS

The Human Rights Act (HRA) 1998 came into effect in the UK in October 2000. The HRA incorporates the principles of the ECHR into UK law. The ECHR was created by the Council of Europe following the atrocities of the Second World War with the intention of limiting the interference of the state with the rights of the person. All public organizations and other bodies carrying out public functions have to comply with the ECHR. The specific fundamental rights and freedoms that individuals have access to under the HRA are listed in Box 7.3.

Human rights are a set of universal principles that are based on the acknowledgement that all humans are equally worthy of respect. The principles of *autonomy*, *dignity*, *equality* and *respect* reflect the belief that a person must be treated as *an ends* and not *a means*. The principles of human rights are particularly important in maternity care, when there is the potential for the woman to be viewed as simply a means for carrying an unborn baby. Professionals who care for women during pregnancy and childbirth must ensure that care provision recognizes individuality and autonomy, assuming that women are capable of making autonomous decisions about themselves and their baby (Prochaska 2015).

In the case of *Ternovszky v Hungary* (European Court of Human Rights 2010), the European Court of Human Rights found that the circumstances of giving birth incontestably form part of a person's private life. The court ruled that the Hungarian government had violated Article 8 through its refusal to regulate home birth and failure to enable midwives to attend women giving birth at home.

The court also found that the failure to obtain a woman's consent for the presence of medical students during labour constituted a violation of Article 8 (*Konovalova v Russia*; European Court of Human Rights 2014). The court reiterated the importance of upholding the principles of human rights and for health care professionals to always gain informed consent from an individual requiring health care or treatment regardless of how insignificant the procedure may seem. The legal duties under the HRA require three types of action, which are to *respect*, *protect* and *fulfil* a person's human rights. These actions are explained in Box 7.4.

Confidentiality

All health care professionals must be committed to the principle of upholding the confidentiality of any person in their care. Women who seek maternity care will share private, often sensitive

---

BOX 7.4 ■ Human Rights Duties

- *Respect*
  This action refers to respecting a person's human rights, and avoiding interfering with their rights unless it is absolutely necessary and proportionate to do so.
- *Protect*
  This action means that the necessary steps must be taken to protect a person's human rights.
- *Fulfil*
  This action refers to the steps public authorities must take to ensure that a person's human rights are recognized and realized, and a system must be in place to investigate human rights abuses.

  Examples that relate to childbirth and midwifery care, and a toolkit for practitioners can be found in a guide written by The British Institute of Human Rights (2016) in partnership with Birthrights and the Royal College of Midwives.

  From The British Institute of Human Rights (2016).

---

information with their midwife, who must act in a manner that will protect that information (International Confederation of Midwives 2014; NMC 2018). To build relationships of trust, the midwife should inform women that their details will not be shared and explain any possible limitations of confidentiality, such as those relating to safeguarding. There is much legislation relating to confidentiality and information disclosure that the midwife should be aware of, including the *common law* duty of confidentiality, the Human Rights Act 1998 (Article 8), the Data Protection Act 2018, the Crime and Disorder Act 1998 and the Mental Capacity Act 2005.

INFORMATION DISCLOSURE

There are few exceptions to the principle of confidentiality, and everyone who uses health services should feel confident that information about them and their health is treated with confidentiality. An independent review of information governance in the National Health Service (NHS) was commissioned and undertaken by Dame Fiona Caldicott (Department of Health [DH] 1997) following concerns over patient confidentiality and the ease of access to hospital records. The report recommended a number of principles, known as the *Caldicott principles*, that should be followed to ensure that patient confidentiality and information security is maintained. Implementing these principles became mandatory for the NHS in 1998 and for social care services in 2000. A Caldicott Guardian must also be appointed in each organization to ensure that the Caldicott principles are adhered to and to advise on the ethical and legal aspects of information processing. The Information Governance Review *Information: To Share or Not to Share?* (DH 2013) was undertaken following reports that information sharing had not occurred in some cases where it would have been in the patient's best interest to have done so. When information is shared, the following conditions must be met: sharing must be *necessary, proportionate, relevant, adequate, accurate, timely* and *secure* (Her Majesty's [HM] Government 2015).

There have been a number of occasions when patient confidentiality has been breached within the NHS or social care system. Midwives must ensure that the safeguarding of patient information is prioritized, and must never access medical records unless the information relates to an individual within their care. Midwives and student midwives must also ensure that any woman and her family as well as colleagues and clinical staff referred to in academic writing or reports are not identifiable. Guidance should be available from academic institutions regarding the reporting of case studies, portfolios and the recording of clinical experience, which must be closely followed. Midwives and student midwives must also respect the privacy of others in all forms of spoken and written communication, including digital content, social media and networking sites (NMC 2018, 2015).

SOCIAL MEDIA

The modern era of information technology and social media provides new advantages and threats for individual confidentiality. Social media is a phenomenon that is rapidly growing in popularity and presents new and challenging issues regarding the safety and privacy of personal information. Midwives and student midwives need to exercise extra care when using social media, blogs and other online platforms. The NMC has issued specific guidance for the responsible use of social media in line with *The Code* (NMC 2018) that sets out the principles for professional behaviour and public protection (NMC 2015). Midwives may put their registration at risk if they act in an unlawful or unprofessional manner through social media or other information-sharing websites or applications. It is important to remember that sharing particular characteristics of, locations of or details about an individual may mean that they are identifiable even if they are not specifically named.

SAFEGUARDING

In situations where vulnerable individuals may be at risk of harm, the principle of confidentiality is important in building relationships of trust and enabling concerns and fears to be shared. However, the right to confidentiality in these situations is not absolute. Information sharing is vital to safeguard and promote the welfare of children, young people and vulnerable adults. Sharing appropriate information with the *right people* at the *right time* is central to good safeguarding practice. One of the factors identified in many of the safeguarding serious case reviews is the failure of professionals to record, share and understand the significance of pieces of information that may have prevented serious harm to or death of a vulnerable individual (HM Government 2015). The principles of sharing information according to HM Government (2015) can be seen in Box 7.5.

FEMALE GENITAL MUTILATION

Female genital mutilation (FGM) is illegal in the UK under the Female Genital Mutilation Act 2003 (England, Wales and Northern Ireland) and the Prohibition of Female Genital Mutilation (Scotland) Act 2005. The Serious Crime Act 2015 has strengthened the legislative framework with the aim of reducing the incidences of FGM, and midwives now have a mandatory responsibility for safeguarding children (under the age of 18 years) who have had FGM or are at risk of being subjected to it. If FGM is identified in an adult woman, consideration should be given to the risk of further violence, in addition to the risk of genital mutilation of her unborn baby should the baby be female. There could also be a risk to other children within her care, or to her extended family, and consequently they may need protection. The established safeguarding policy for children should be followed when such cases are identified. Once safeguarding requirements have been considered, women should be offered appropriate culturally sensitive support. The decision to share information, with regard to an adult who has been subjected to FGM, should be based on the principles shown in Box 7.5.

Consent to Treatment and Trespass to the Person

A number of legal and ethical principles underpin the concept of consent; particularly the principle of personal autonomy, which is the individual's right to make their own decisions regarding their care and treatment. The principle of *respect for autonomy* protected under the common law of England and Wales and by Article 8 of the ECHR, is one of the four pillars of medical ethics, the others being those of *beneficence*, *non-maleficence* and *justice* (Beauchamp and Childress 2013), which are discussed further in Chapter 6. UK case law has determined that touching a person

---

BOX 7.5 ■ The Seven Golden Rules to Sharing Information in Health and Social Care Settings

1. *Remember that the General Data Protection Regulation (GDPR), Data Protection Act 2018 and human rights law are not barriers to justified information sharing*, but provide a framework to ensure that personal information about living individuals is shared appropriately.
2. *Be open and honest with the individual* (and/or their family where appropriate) from the outset about why, what, how and with whom information will or could be shared, and seek their agreement, unless it is unsafe or inappropriate to do so.
3. *Seek advice* from other practitioners or your information governance lead, if you are in any doubt if there is any doubt about sharing the information concerned, without disclosing the identity of the individual where possible.
4. Where possible, share information with consent and, where possible, respect the wishes of those who do not consent to having their information shared. Under the GDPR and Data Protection Act 2018 you may share information without consent if, in your judgment, there is a lawful basis to do so, such as where safety may be at risk. You will need to base your judgement on the facts of the case. When you are sharing or requesting personal information from someone, be clear of the basis upon which you are doing so. Where you do not have consent, be mindful that an individual might not expect information to be shared.
5. *Consider safety and well-being*: base your information sharing decisions on considerations of the safety and well-being of the individual and others who may be affected by their actions.
6. *Necessary, proportionate, relevant, adequate, accurate, timely and secure*: ensure that the information you share is necessary for the purpose for which you are sharing it, is shared only with those individuals who need to have it, is accurate and up to date, is shared in a timely fashion, and is shared securely.
7. *Keep a record of your decision and the reasons for it* – whether it is to share information or not. If you decide to share, then record what you have shared, with whom and for what purpose.

From Her Majesty's Government (2018).

---

without valid consent may constitute a civil offence of *assault*, or a criminal offence of *battery*. Therefore to undertake any procedure or treatment against the wishes of a mentally competent adult is a civil wrong, and is considered *trespass against the person*. In some situations, this may even be considered a criminal act. Midwives and all other health care practitioners must therefore always gain the valid consent of any woman for whom they are providing care.

Providing meaningful information is integral to ensuring that any decisions leading to consent are fully informed, and therefore valid. For consent to be valid, defence for an action of trespass against the person, it must have been given freely by a mentally competent person and without duress or fraud (Dimond 2013; Vučemilo et al 2015). The FIGO Committee for the Study of Ethical Aspects of Human Reproduction and Women's Health (2012: 14) defined informed consent as

consent obtained freely, without threats or improper inducements, after appropriate disclosure to the patient of adequate and understandable information in a form and language understood by the patient.

The Code (NMC 2018: statements 2.5 and 4.2) also states that nurses, midwives and nursing associates must ensure that they obtain properly informed consent before carrying out any action, and that they respect, support and document a person's right to accept or decline care and treatment. It must be recognized that pregnant women have a legal right to make informed and autonomous decisions throughout the childbirth continuum, even if such decisions appear to be unwise to health care professionals. Midwives have a legal duty to respect, protect and fulfil such rights of the pregnant woman (see Box 7.4).

TYPES OF CONSENT

There are a number of types of consent that need to be understood in the context of health care provision. Consent may be *expressed* (explicit), confirmed verbally or in writing, or it may be *implied* (implicit) by behaviour such as holding out an arm for blood pressure recording. Implied consent may be unreliable as the person could argue that their actions were misunderstood and consent to touch or treatment was not given. For example, a pregnant woman may hold out her arm expecting her blood pressure to be assessed, but the midwife may assume that implied consent was given for venepuncture or cannulation. Written consent therefore provides the strongest form of evidence of consent. Verbal consent, although valid under English law (Wheeler 2012), is clearly more difficult to evidence unless there is a witness to the conversation. Timely and accurate record keeping is an essential aspect of midwifery practice; therefore when verbal consent is given, this should be documented.

The provision of information and good communication (see Chapter 3) are key components in the process of gaining valid informed consent, to enable the person to make a decision to accept or decline treatment. Information should include the risks and benefits, possible side effects, potential complications, costs of the procedure and the risk in relation to failure of the procedure (Black 2014; Våga et al 2014). The FIGO Committee for the Study of Ethical Aspects of Human Reproduction and Women's Health (2012) highlighted that informed consent is much more complex than simply gaining a woman's signature on a consent form. The importance of gaining informed and valid consent cannot be underestimated, particularly in the unique circumstances of pregnancy and birth when decisions about treatment or procedures may have implications for both the woman and her unborn baby.

CONSENT AND MENTAL CAPACITY

The Mental Capacity Act 2005 is based on the principle that a person must be assumed to have the capacity to make decisions for themselves unless it is established that they lack the ability to do so. This Act also clearly states that a person must not be treated as unable to make a decision merely because the decisions they take may be deemed unwise. Situations in which women decline treatment or refuse to consent to procedures can be emotive particularly if it is considered that the well-being of the woman or the fetus is at risk. Practitioners may feel that there are difficult moral and ethical dilemmas to be resolved; however, it is important to keep the principle of personal autonomy and decision-making capacity as the central focus of care.

The Mental Capacity Act 2005 makes provision for the determination of capacity and for determining *best interest* decisions if a lack of capacity is confirmed. A number of legal safeguards must be applied to determine capacity and to ensure that any decisions fully represent the person's *best interest*. According to Dimond (2013), defining *best interests* includes taking into account an individual's present and past wishes, beliefs and values. Applications can be made to the Court of Protection to get an urgent or emergency court order in situations where it is considered that the life or welfare of someone who lacks capacity is at risk. Court orders will be granted only in situations where a decision has to be made without delay. The controversial case presented in Box 7.6 occurred before the Mental Capacity Act 2005 came into force and demonstrates a situation in which *best interests* were *not* considered.

The DH (2009) highlights that lacking the capacity to consent to a procedure is very different from having the capacity to make an unwise or irrational decision. A person is entitled to make any decision they wish as long as they have the capacity to do so. In a debate about a person's right to make decisions about end-of-life care in the House of Lords (Joffe 2013), Lord Joffe presented the issue of personal autonomy in the context of previous legal judgements:

The patient's right of choice exists whether the reasons for making that choice are rational, irrational, unknown or even non-existent….The right to determine what shall be done with one's own body is a fundamental right in our society. The concepts inherent in this right are the bedrock upon which the principles of self-determination and individual autonomy are based.

BOX 7.6 ■ St George's Healthcare NHS Trust v S (Supreme Court, Court of Appeal (Civil Division) 1998)

S was diagnosed with pre-eclampsia and required admission to hospital for induction of labour. She refused admission for treatment as she did not agree with medical intervention in pregnancy. S was competent and had the capacity to make her own decisions; however, she was detained for assessment under the Mental Health Act 1983*. The obstetric team referred the case to the courts stating that it was a '*life and death*' situation, which resulted in the judge making a declaration overriding the need for S to give consent to treatment. A caesarean section without the consent of S was subsequently carried out.

The Appeal Court later agreed that S's right to autonomy had been violated and that her detention and treatment had been unlawful. The judicial authority for the caesarean section was based on false information, which was that S had gone into labour and the surgery was required urgently, both of which were untrue.

This case highlights the legal position that a *competent* pregnant woman can refuse treatment even if that refusal may result in harm to herself or her unborn child.

*Since the case of S in 1998, the Mental Health Act 1983 has been superseded by the Mental Capacity Act 2005.

THE BOLAM PRINCIPLE

The law relating to informed consent and how to establish whether this duty is properly fulfilled has historically been based on the *Bolam principle*, which has also been used to assess appropriate standards of care in negligence cases. In *Bolam v Friern Barnet Management Committee* (England and Wales High Court 1957), the claimant (Bolam) sustained some serious injuries, including fractures of the acetabula, when undergoing electroconvulsive therapy and argued that the hospital was negligent for not issuing muscle relaxants, not restraining him and not warning him about the risks involved in the procedure. The judge ruled that the doctor was not negligent if he provided treatment in a manner that would be considered appropriate by a *responsible body of medical opinion* held by practitioners skilled in the field in question (DH 2009). However, following the case of *Montgomery v Lanarkshire Health Board* (Supreme Court 2015), the law on informed consent has changed. This change moves away from considering the actions of the *reasonable doctor* and towards that of the *reasonable patient*, highlighting the importance of self-determination and personal autonomy in the consideration of the risks of treatment and consent to treatment as detailed in Box 7.7.

GAINING CONSENT IN OTHER CIRCUMSTANCES

The guidance provided by the DH that doctors could provide contraceptive advice and treatment to girls younger than 16 years without parental consent or knowledge was challenged by Victoria Gillick in the case of *Gillick v West Norfolk and Wisbech Area Health Authority* (House of Lords 1986). This case led to the creation of the term *Gillick competence*, which refers to the legal position of a person younger than 16 years with the capacity to make any relevant decision about themselves. The House of Lords held that a doctor could give contraceptive advice and treatment to a person younger than 16 years if they had sufficient maturity and intelligence to understand the nature and implications of the proposed treatment and that the advice or treatment was in their best interest.

> ### BOX 7.7 ■ *Montgomery v Lanarkshire Health Board* (Supreme Court 2015)
>
> Elizabeth Montgomery had diabetes and was not informed by her obstetrician of the increased risk of shoulder dystocia during childbirth. The obstetrician stated that she routinely chose not to explain this risk to diabetic women as she felt that if she explained all of the risks every woman would ask for a caesarean section.
>
> The risk of shoulder dystocia and subsequent related sequelae is significant for diabetic women, as stated by the Royal College of Obstetricians and Gynaecologists (2012) to be a twofold to fourfold increase in incidences compared with non-diabetic women giving birth to babies of a similar weight. The obstetrician in this case, however, did not consider that these risks were worth explaining to women.
>
> Following this case, the court made it clear that all health care professionals have a clear duty to take *reasonable care* to ensure that patients are aware of all material risks so as to be able to make fully informed choices (Supreme Court 2015).
>
> The Supreme Court judge in this case, Lady Justice Hale, consequently stated:
>
> *An adult person of sound mind is entitled to decide which, if any, of the available forms of treatment to undergo, and her consent must be obtained before treatment interfering with her bodily integrity is undertaken. Gone are the days when it was thought that, on becoming pregnant, a woman lost, not only her capacity, but also her right to act as a genuinely autonomous human being.*

> ### BOX 7.8 ■ Global Issues
>
> The paternalistic model of hierarchy has been the most common model in modern health care systems (Roter and Hall 2006), and unfortunately this can still be seen in some eastern European countries, such as Croatia (Vučemilo et al 2015).
>
> A study in Greece reviewed the level of informed consent in antenatal screening for Down's syndrome. The study findings revealed that 56% of the respondents made an *uninformed* choice before the consenting to antenatal screening procedures (Gourounti and Sandall 2011).
>
> Informed consent in Nigeria is still a problematic issue in midwifery practice, with some procedures such as vaginal examinations often not being discussed with women, or consent not being obtained before the procedure is undertaken (Oyetunde and Nkwonta 2014).
>
> Midwives in the United Kingdom have highlighted that they had inadequate time to facilitate informed decision-making in relation to antenatal screening. Concerns were also raised that informed consent was problematic to obtain in non-English-speaking women (Ahmed et al 2013).

In situations where health care professionals need to make a decision in an emergency with an unconscious individual, Lord Donaldson in the *case Re T* (England Court of Appeal (Civil Division) 1992) clearly stated that decisions must always be made in the best interest of the individual with consideration to any choices that they may have indicated before the emergency. If possible, treatment should be postponed until their consent has been obtained. Consent or refusal to consent cannot be delegated to other family members or the next of kin, as they do not have any legal right to do so.

Recent cases in the UK and Europe that relate to human rights, informed consent and capacity to make decisions have set precedents that can inform midwives and other health care professionals when they are considering how best to respond to complex situations. Box 7.8 highlights some cases in which obtaining informed valid consent during childbirth remains problematic globally.

Negligence and Liability

If a woman or baby is harmed during pregnancy or childbirth through clinical negligence, a claim for personal injury compensation may be made. In England, NHS Resolution (the operating name for the NHS Litigation Authority [NHSLA] since 2017) manages negligence claims against care provided through the NHS. A claim of negligence is one of the most frequent civil actions (torts) brought to obtain compensation. Compensation payments are made to meet the expenses occurred as a result of injury, including loss of earnings, and in recognition of the pain and suffering experienced by the individual. Claims for compensation during pregnancy and childbirth represent 10% of all clinical negligence claims, yet have the highest value of claims reported to NHS Resolution (2018). In the most recent report from 2017/18, maternity claims represented 1067 (10%) of clinical claims by number, but accounted for 48% (albeit a small reduction from 50% in the previous year) of the total value of new claims reported at £2,166.3 billion. However, the number of claims represents a very small percentage of total births, which indicates that the vast majority of births do not result in a clinical negligence claim.

For a claim of negligence to be determined, a three-stage test must be satisfied. This test was introduced following the English tort law case of *Caparo Industries v Dickman* (House of Lords 1990). The three elements of the test are:

- that a person is owed a duty of care
- that a breach of that duty of care has occurred
- that legally recognized harm has occurred as a result of the breach of duty of care.

DUTY OF CARE

The definition of *duty of care* was established in the case of *Donoghue v Stevenson* (House of Lords 1932), which explored if a manufacturer had a duty of care to the consumer regardless of whether they had paid for a product. The statement by Lord Atkin established liability on the basis that a duty of care existed through the *neighbour principle* depicted in Box 7.9. When a duty of care has been established and is subsequently breached, liability for negligence may result, with consequential compensation awarded.

A duty of care exists between the midwife and any woman or baby who is the recipient of their care, as they are classed as the midwife's neighbours according to Lord Atkin's judgement (House of Lords 1932). It has been argued that any woman the midwife comes across in the professional environment is also owed a duty of care (Bryden and Storey 2011). This duty of care includes treatment and care provision, the giving of information, record keeping, supervision and delegation of other staff and management of the clinical situation. All the professional activities of the midwife as identified by the European Parliament would be considered to be part of the midwife's duty of care (European Parliament and the Council of the European Union 2005; Dimond 2013).

BOX 7.9 ■ The Neighbour Principle in *Donoghue v Stevenson* (House of Lords 1932)

You must take reasonable care to avoid acts or omissions which you can reasonably foresee would be likely to injure your neighbour. Who, then, in law, is my neighbour? The answer seems to be – persons who are so closely and directly affected by my act that I ought reasonably to have them in contemplation as being so affected when I am directing my mind to the acts or omissions that are called in question.

STANDARD OF CARE AND BREACH OF DUTY OF CARE

Once a duty of care has been established, a breach occurs where the care provided by the professional has failed to meet the appropriate standard. The standard of care deemed *reasonable* was set by the case of *Bolam v Friern Barnet Management Committee* (England and Wales High Court 1957), which was discussed earlier in this chapter. At the time of the alleged incident, opinion was divided as to whether muscle relaxants should be administered during electroconvulsive therapy as it was not universal practice. It was therefore determined that for negligence to have occurred, it must be established that no reasonable doctor acting in the same circumstances would have acted in the same way.

Therefore breaches of duty of care can be established in circumstances where the individual has not acted with a level of care that would be expected from a reasonably competent professional of similar experience. For newly qualified midwives and student midwives, this is of particular relevance, as the comparison would be made with the standard of care expected of a practitioner at the same grade and level of experience, and not with an expert. The increasing availability of evidence-based clinical guidelines will enable the courts to determine whether a substantial deviation from standard practice has occurred, and to determine whether an appropriate standard of care was given. If a midwife makes a decision to deviate from guidelines, clear documentation of all such decisions is vital so as to be able to support and fully justify such actions, and to defend any claims of negligence. Although maternity claims for negligence are not widespread, they are often prolonged and contentious, which can lead to detrimental effects on the professionals involved (Robertson and Thomson 2015). Through the practice of woman-centred care within a rights-based framework and an understanding of duty within the law, the fear of litigation, which drives defensive practice, should be reduced.

WILFUL NEGLECT

Following a recommendation from the National Advisory Group on the Safety of Patients in England (Berwick 2013), in response to the Francis report into poor standards of care (Mid Staffordshire NHS Foundation Trust Public Inquiry 2013) and the Andrews report in Wales (Andrews and Butler 2014), the Criminal Justice and Courts Act 2015 was enacted for England and Wales in April 2015. This act makes it a criminal offence for a care worker to ill-treat or to wilfully neglect any individual in their care. A care worker is defined as anyone who is paid to provide health or social care, and this therefore includes midwives. The criminalization of ill-treatment and wilful neglect for all patient groups means that poor care in any health or care setting can now lead to prosecution. The numbers of prosecutions for ill-treatment and wilful neglect by nurses and other care workers has risen considerably (Griffith 2015) since the Francis report in England (Mid Staffordshire NHS Foundation Trust Public Inquiry 2013) and the Andrews report in Wales (Andrews and Butler 2014).

Health and Safety at Work

The primary piece of legislation that governs health and safety practice in the workplace in the UK is the Health and Safety at Work Act 1974; in addition, there are a number of pieces of secondary legislation that contribute to the legal framework relating to the working environment. These laws exist to protect the employer, employees and members of the public from harm in the workplace. A full review of health and safety law was undertaken by Lord Young in 2010 (HM Government 2010) following concerns that the law was overly complicated and a compensation culture had developed. The recommendations of the review suggest that a rational, proportionate and common sense approach should be taken to risk management so as to promote health and safety at work.

RISK ASSESSMENT

Employers are required to control the health and safety risks in the workplace by taking reasonable steps to prevent harm through undertaking the process of risk assessment. The steps for undertaking a risk assessment are outlined in Box 7.10. The law does not expect all risks to be

> **BOX 7.10 ■ Five Steps to Risk Assessment**
>
> **1.** Identify the hazards.
> **2.** Decide who might be harmed and how.
> **3.** Evaluate the risks and decide on precautions.
> **4.** Record the findings from activities 1–3 and implement the precautions.
> **5.** Review risk assessment and update if necessary.
>
> ---
>
> From Health and Safety Executive (2014).

removed or that unforeseeable risks are considered, but does expect that reasonable steps have been put in place to protect people from foreseeable harm (Health and Safety Executive 2014). The foreseeable risk of harm in the workplace for midwives tends to be in relation to exposure to hazardous substances and clinical waste, or equipment and environmental factors, including the risk of injury through physical violence.

SUBSTANCES HAZARDOUS TO HEALTH

The regulation for the prevention and control of occupational exposure to biological agents in the health care setting is governed by the Control of Substances Hazardous to Health Regulations 2002 (updated by Health and Safety Executive 2013a). The regulations require action by both the employer and the employee through the use of personal protective equipment (PPE), control procedures and by ensuring that appropriate behaviour occurs to control and prevent exposure to hazardous substances. Employers have a responsibility to provide adequate PPE, and midwives have a responsibility to know why and when PPE such as gloves, aprons and eye protection is required, and should comply with employment policy regarding its use.

SHARPS INJURIES

Injuries from medical needles and scalpel blades (collectively known as *sharps*) are a well-known occupational risk in the health and social care sector. Sharps contaminated with blood from an individual who has a blood-borne infection, such as hepatitis B, hepatitis C or human immunodeficiency virus , can transmit the infection to anyone who becomes injured by them. Because of this transmission risk, these types of injuries can cause considerable concern and stress to the many health professionals who receive them; therefore all employers are required under existing health and safety law to ensure that risks from sharps injuries are properly assessed and the appropriate steps are in place to reduce the risk of occurrence. The Health and Safety (Sharp Instruments in Healthcare) Regulations 2013 (Health and Safety Executive 2013b) provide specific advice and guidance relating to reducing the risk of injury from sharps (Box 7.11).

WORKPLACE VIOLENCE

Midwives may be at risk of being subjected to workplace violence from childbearing women or visitors because they are in contact with a wide range of people who may be experiencing difficult circumstances. There are a number of factors that can lead to acts of violence and aggression when people are receiving health care, such as anxiety, frustration (due to boredom or lack of

> ### BOX 7.11 ■ Key Points From the Health and Safety (Sharp Instruments in Healthcare) Regulations 2013
>
> The employer should ensure that the unnecessary use of sharps is avoided (Regulation 5(1)(a)).
>
> Where it is not reasonably practicable to avoid the use of medical sharps, the Sharps Regulations require employers to:
>
> - use safer sharps (incorporating protection mechanisms) (Regulation 5(1)(b))
> - prevent the recapping of needles (Regulation 5(1)(c))
> - place secure containers and instructions for safe disposal of medical sharps close to the work area (Regulation 5(1)(d)).
>
> Employees must receive adequate training relating to safe use and disposal of sharps (Regulation 6(4)).
>
> Injured employees have a duty to notify their employer of a sharps injury (Regulation 8).
>
> A sharps injury must be recorded and reported (Regulation 7(1)).
>
> ---
>
> Adapted from Health and Safety Executive (2013b).

information), impatience (due to waiting), resentment (due to lack of rights), the effects of drugs or alcohol and any inherent aggression or mental health issues (Health and Safety Executive 2013c). The main risk is that of verbal abuse or physical assault, and employers should work with employees to identify strategies to reduce the risk of workplace violence, including training in conflict resolution to de-escalate threatening situations. There should also be a clear message of zero tolerance of aggressive behaviour within the workplace. The risk of violence and aggression may be increased for midwives who are in situations where they are working alone, and specific risk assessments should be carried out for lone workers to devise and implement preventative and protective measures.

MUSCULOSKELETAL INJURIES

Manual handling injuries account for a significant proportion of all injuries in health care, with absence from work due to musculoskeletal injury or disorder accounting for approximately 40% of all absences within the NHS. This type of injury is also one of the main causes of ill-health retirement (NHS Employers 2014). Midwives, student midwives and maternity support workers are at risk of musculoskeletal injuries as a result of working in clinical environments that may require elements of manual handling in addition to working in prolonged awkward, twisting positions. These positions are more likely to occur when they are supporting women to give birth, especially in water, or during breastfeeding (Long et al 2013).

Several pieces of legislation relate to musculoskeletal injury prevention in the workplace, with responsibilities outlined for both employers and employees. The main legal responsibility for employers is to protect the health and safety of their employees through the Health and Safety at Work Act 1974. The Manual Handling Operations Regulations 1992, as amended by the Health and Safety Executive (2002), require an employer to complete risk assessments on all manual handling tasks that pose a risk and to avoid manual handling for employees as far as reasonably practicable. Identical duties are placed on self-employed individuals, which is an important consideration for midwives who practise independently. There is strong evidence that musculoskeletal injuries can be reduced by a number of modifiable factors, such as ergonomic considerations, equipment or task redesign and training that is tailored for the specific task and environment. Training should also focus on changing attitudes and behaviours, promoting risk awareness and a culture of where risks are continuously assessed and issues reported (Health and Safety Executive 2002).

Conclusion

This chapter has presented some of the main legal issues that midwives and student midwives may encounter during their education and training, particularly in the practice setting. It is important to remember that ignorance is no legal defence and that as professionals, midwives should always ensure that they are aware of the details of all relevant legislation so that they are able to operate within the legal framework of the country in which they practise. The inclusion of examples from practice throughout the chapter should have aided the reader in reflecting on their knowledge of the legal and statutory frameworks and how these can be effectively applied in contemporary midwifery education and practice.

KEY POINTS

- An awareness and understanding of legal accountability is important for midwives to operate within the legal framework of the country in which they practise.
- The principles of *autonomy*, *dignity*, *equality* and *respect* must always be upheld, and care must be provided in accordance with the Human Rights Act 1998.
- Personal autonomy to make decisions, even if those decisions appear to be unwise to health care professionals, is a fundamental human right.
- When considering whether to share information, ensure that this is *necessary*, *proportionate*, *relevant*, *adequate*, *accurate*, *timely* and *secure* to maintain appropriate client confidentiality.
- Midwives may put their registration at risk if they act in an unlawful or unprofessional manner through social media or other information-sharing websites or applications.
- For a claim of negligence to be determined, the person must be owed a duty of care, a breach of that duty must have occurred and harm must have occurred as a result of that breach.

References

Ahmed, S., Bryant, L. D., & Cole, P. (2013). Midwives' perceptions of their role as facilitators of informed choice in antenatal screening. *Midwifery, 29*(7), 745–750.

Andrews, J., & Butler, M. (2014). *Trusted to care: An independent review of the Princess of Wales Hospital and Neath Port Talbot Hospital at Abertawe Bro Morgannwg University Health Board.* Available at: http://gov.wales/docs/dhss/publications/140512trustedtocareen.pdf.

Beauchamp, T. L., & Childress, J. F. (2013). *Principles of biomedical ethics* (7th ed.). Oxford: Oxford University Press.

Berwick, D. (2013). *A promise to learn – a commitment to act. Improving the safety of patients in England.* London: National Advisory Group on the Safety of Patients in England. Available at: https://www.gov.uk/government/uploads/system/uploads/attachment_data/file/226703/Berwick_Report.pdf.

Black, B. P. (2014). *Professional nursing: concepts and challenges* (7th ed.). St. Louis: Saunders.

Bryden, D., & Storey, I. (2011). Duty of care and medical negligence. *Continuing Education in Anaesthesia, Critical Care and Pain, 11*(4), 124–127.

Carolan, M., & Cassar, L. (2010). Antenatal care perceptions of pregnant African women attending maternity services in Melbourne, Australia. *Midwifery, 26*(2), 189–201.

Control of Substances Hazardous to Health Regulations 2002. Available at: http://www.legislation.gov.uk/uksi/2002/2677/pdfs/uksi_20022677_en.pdf.

Courts and Tribunals Judiciary. (2016). *History of the judiciary.* Available at: https://www.judiciary.gov.uk/about-the-judiciary/history-of-the-judiciary/.

Crime and Disorder Act 1998. Available at: http://www.legislation.gov.uk/ukpga/1998/37/pdfs/ukpga_19980037_en.pdf.

Criminal Justice and Courts Act 2015. Available at: http://www.legislation.gov.uk/ukpga/2015/2/pdfs/ukpga_20150002_en.pdf.

Data Protection Act 2018. Available at: http://www.legislation.gov.uk/ukpga/2018/12/contents/enacted.

Department of Health. (1997). *The Caldicott Committee report on the review of patient-identifiable information.* London: Department of Health.

Department of Health. (2009). *Reference guide to consent for examination or treatment* (2nd ed.). London: Department of Health.

Department of Health. (2013). *Information: To share or not to share? The Information Governance Review.* London: Department of Health.

Dimond, D. (2013). *Legal aspects of midwifery.* London: Quay Books.

England Court of Appeal (Civil Division). (1992). *Re T (Adult: Refusal of Medical Treatment) 30 July.*

England and Wales High Court. (1957). *Bolam v Friern Hospital Management Committee [1957] 1WLR 583.*

Equality Act 2010, C.15. Available at: http://www.legislation.gov.uk/ukpga/2010/15/pdfs/ukpga_20100015_en.pdf.

Equality and Human Rights Commission. (2016). *Equality Act guidance.* Available at: https://www.equality-humanrights.com/en/advice-and-guidance/equality-act-guidance#h1.

European Court of Human Rights. (2010). *Ternovszky v Hungary [2010], 14 December.*

European Court of Human Rights. (2014). *Konovalova v Russia [2014], 9 October.*

European Parliament and the Council of the European Union. (2005). Directive 2005/36/EC of the European Parliament and of the Council of 7 September 2005 on the recognition of professional qualifications. *Official Journal of the European Union L.* 255/45. Available at: http://eur-lex.europa.eu/LEXUriServ/LexUriServ.do?uri=OJ:L:2005:255:0022:0142:EN:PDF.

Female Genital Mutilation Act 2003, C. 31. Available at: http://www.legislation.gov.uk/ukpga/2003/31/pdfs/ukpga_20030031_en.pdf.

FIGO Committee for the Study of Ethical Aspects of Human Reproduction and Women's Health. (2012). *Ethical Issues in Obstetrics and Gynecology.* London: FIGO House.

Gourounti, K., & Sandall, J. (2011). The validation and translation of multidimensional measure of informed choice in Greek. *Midwifery, 27*(2), 170–173.

Griffith, R., Tengnah, C., & Patel, C. (2010). *Law and professional issues in midwifery.* Exeter: Learning Matters.

Griffith, R. (2015). Patient protection: ill-treatment and wilful neglect. *British Journal of Nursing, 24*(11), 600–601.

Haith-Cooper, M., & McCarthy, R. (2015). Striving for excellence in maternity care: the Maternity Stream of the city of Sanctuary. *British Journal of Midwifery, 23*(9), 648–652.

Health and Safety at Work Act 1974. Available at: http://www.legislation.gov.uk/ukpga/1974/37/pdfs/ukpga_19740037_en.pdf.

Health and Safety Executive. (2002). *Manual Handling Operations Regulations 1992, as amended by the Health and Safety (Miscellaneous Amendments) Regulations 2002.* London: Health and Safety Executive. Available at: http://www.hse.gov.uk/foi/internalops/ocs/300-399/313_5.htm.

Health and Safety Executive. (2013a). *Control of substances hazardous to health: The Control of Substances Hazardous to Health Regulations (as amended): Approved code of practice and guidance.* London: Health and Safety Executive. Available at: http://www.hse.gov.uk/pubns/priced/l5.pdf.

Health and Safety Executive. (2013b). *The Health and Safety (Sharp Instruments in Healthcare) Regulations.* Available at: http://www.legislation.gov.uk/uksi/2013/645/pdfs/uksi_20130645_en.pdf.

Health and Safety Executive. (2013c). *Violence in health and social care.* Available at: http://www.hse.gov.uk/healthservices/violence/do.htm.

Health and Safety Executive. (2014). *Risk assessment: A brief guide to controlling risks in the workplace.* Available at: http://www.hse.gov.uk/pubns/indg163.pdf.

Her Majesty's Government. (2010). *Common sense common safety; A report by Lord Young of Graffham to the Prime Minister following a Whitehall-wide review of the operation of health and safety laws and the growth of the compensation culture.* London: Cabinet Office.

Her Majesty's Government. (2015). *Information sharing advice for practitioners providing safeguarding services to children, young people, parents and carers.* Available at: https://www.gov.uk/government/uploads/system/uploads/attachment_data/file/419628/Information_sharing_advice_safeguarding_practitioners.pdf.

House of Lords. (1932). *Donoghue v Stevenson AC, 562.*

House of Lords. (1986). *Gillick v West Norfolk and Wisbech Area Health Authority, 17 October.*

House of Lords. (1990). *Caparo Industries plc v Dickman AC 605.*

Human Rights Act 1998, C.42. Available at: http://www.legislation.gov.uk/ukpga/1998/42/pdfs/ukpga_19980042_en.pdf.

International Confederation of Midwives. (2014). *International code of ethics for midwives.* The Hague: International Confederation of Midwives. Available at: https://www.internationalmidwives.org/assets/files/definitions-files/2018/06/eng-international-code-of-ethics-for-midwives.pdf.

International Confederation of Midwives. (2017). *Definition of the midwife.* The Hague: International Confederation of Midwives. Available at: https://www.internationalmidwives.org/assets/files/definitions-files/2018/06/eng-definition_of_the_midwife-2017.pdf

Joffe, J. G. (2013). *Health: end of life motion.* Hansard,12 Dec 2013: Column 922–923. Available at: http://www.publications.parliament.uk/pa/ld201314/ldhansrd/text/131212-0001.htm.

Law Society. (2012). *Equality Act 2010 practice notes.* Available at: http://www.lawsociety.org.uk/support-services/advice/practice-notes/equality-act-2010/.

Long, M. H., Johnston, V., & Bogossian, F. E. (2013). Helping women but hurting ourselves? Neck and upper back musculoskeletal symptoms in a cohort of Australian midwives. *Midwifery, 29,* 359–367.

Mental Health Act 1983. Available at: http://www.legislation.gov.uk/ukpga/1983/20/pdfs/ukpga_19830020_en.pdf.

Mental Capacity Act 2005. Available at: http://www.legislation.gov.uk/ukpga/2005/9/pdfs/ukpga_20050009_en.pdf.

Mid Staffordshire NHS Foundation Trust Public Inquiry. (2013). *Report of the Mid Staffordshire NHS Foundation Trust Public Inquiry.* London: The Stationary Office.

NHS Resolution. (2018). *Annual report and accounts 2017/18.* London: The Stationery Office.

NHS Employers. (2014). *Back in work: Introduction and key messages.* Available at: http://www.nhsemployers.org/case-studies-and-resources/2015/10/back-in-work-back-pack.

Nursing and Midwifery Council. (2009). *Standards for pre-registration midwifery education.* London: Nursing and Midwifery Council. Available at: https://www.nmc.org.uk/globalassets/sitedocuments/standards/nmc-standards-for-preregistration-midwifery-education.pdf.

Nursing and Midwifery Council. (2018). *The code: Professional standards of practice and behaviour for nurses, midwives and nursing associates.* London: Nursing and Midwifery Council. Available at: https://www.nmc.org.uk/globalassets/sitedocuments/nmc-publications/nmc-code.pdf.

Nursing and Midwifery Council. (2015). *Guidance on using social media responsibly.* London: Nursing and Midwifery Council. Available at: https://www.nmc.org.uk/globalassets/sitedocuments/nmc-publications/social-media-guidance.pdf.

Oyetunde, M. O., & Nkwonta, C. A. (2014). Quality issues in midwifery: a critical analysis of midwifery in Nigeria within the context of the International Confederation of Midwives (ICM) global standards. *International Journal of Nursing and Midwifery, 6*(3), 40–48.

Phillimore, J. (2016). Migrant maternity in an era of superdiversity: new migrants' access to, and experience of, antenatal care in the West Midlands, UK. *Social Science and Medicine, 148,* 152–159.

Prochaska, E. (2015). Human rights in maternity care. *Midwifery, 31,* 1015–1016.

Prohibition of Female Genital Mutilation (Scotland) Act 2005. Available at: http://www.legislation.gov.uk/asp/2005/8/pdfs/asp_20050008_en.pdf.

Robertson, J. H., & Thomson, A. M. (2015). An exploration of the effects of clinical negligence litigation on the practice of midwives in England: a phenomenological study. *Midwifery, 33,* 55–63.

Roter, D. L., & Hall, J. A. (2006). *Doctors talking with patients/patients talking with doctors.* Westport: Praeger.

Royal College of Obstetricians and Gynaecologists. (2012). *Shoulder dystocia. Green-top guideline no. 42* (2nd ed.). London: Royal College of Obstetricians and Gynaecologists.

Serious Crime Act 2015, C.9. Available at: http://www.legislation.gov.uk/ukpga/2015/9/pdfs/ukpga_20150009_en.pdf.

Supreme Court, Court of Appeal (Civil Division). (1998). *St. George's Healthcare NHS Trust v S, 30 July.*

Supreme Court. (2015). *Montgomery v Lanarkshire Health Board, 11 March.*

The British Institute of Human Rights. (2016). *Midwifery and Human Rights: A practitioner's guide.* Available at: http://www.birthrights.org.uk/wordpress/wp-content/uploads/2016/09/Midwifery_Web_Version-2.pdf.

The Nursing and Midwifery Order 2001. Available at: http://www.legislation.gov.uk/uksi/2002/253/pdfs/uksi_20020253_en.pdf.

Våga, B. B., Moland, K. M., Evjen-Olsen, B., & Blystad, A. (2014). Reflections on informed choice in resource-poor settings: the case of infant feeding counselling in PMTCT programmes in Tanzania. *Social Science and Medicine, 105*, 22–29.

Vučemilo, L., Milošević, M., Dodig, D., Grabušic, B., Đapić, B., & Borovečki, A. (2015). The quality of informed consent in Croatia – a cross-sectional study and instrument development. *Patient Education and Counselling, 99*, 436–442.

Wheeler, H. (2012). *Law, ethics and professional issues for nursing.* London: Routledge.

Further Reading

NHS Employers. (2013). *Workplace health and safety standards.* Available at: http://www.nhsemployers.org/~/media/Employers/Publications/workplace-health-safety-standards.pdf.

> This is useful document about workplace health and safety standards which provides links to the relevant Health and Safety at Work Act 1974 guidance, and can be used to develop improvement programmes, self-audit or self-assessment of risk in the workplace.

National Health Service (NHS) England. (2014). *Information sharing policy – personal information.* Available at:https://www.england.nhs.uk/wp-content/uploads/2014/08/info-shar.pdf.

> This policy provides a framework for sharing information to deliver better care and considers the controls needed for information sharing. Guidance is given for information sharing to ensure that legal compliance and best practice are followed.

Nursing and Midwifery Council. (2015). *Guidance on using social media responsibly.* Available at: https://www.nmc.org.uk/globalassets/sitedocuments/nmc-publications/social-media-guidance.pdf.

> This document provides principles and guidance for nurses and midwives on how to use social media and social networking sites responsibly, and in line with the requirements of the Nursing and Midwifery Council code (2018). The guidance can also be applied to other online communication applications.

Royal College of Nursing. (2015). *Female genital mutilation: A RCN resource for nursing and midwifery practice* (2nd ed.). Available at: https://www2.rcn.org.uk/_data/assets/pdf_file/0010/608914/RCNguidance_FGM_WEB2.pdf.

> This resource provides information about female genital mutilation; what it is, why it happens and the related legal issues. There are illustrations of good practice, in addition to guidance in working effectively with other agencies and with women and families affected by female genital mutilation.

The British Institute of Human Rights. (2016). *Midwifery and human rights: A practitioner's guide.* Available at: http://www.birthrights.org.uk/wordpress/wp-content/uploads/2016/09/Midwifery_Web_Version-2.pdf.

> This guide and toolkit has been produced in partnership with the Royal College of Midwives and the charity Birthrights to support midwives in providing maternity services that respect human rights. The guide includes decision-making flowcharts and templates.

Useful Websites

Birthrights: http://www.birthrights.org.uk/advice/healthcare-professionals/

> Birthrights is the United Kingdom's only organization dedicated to improving women's experience of pregnancy and childbirth by promoting respect for human rights. The website provides information, factsheets, details of current human rights issues and an email advice service.

Courts and Tribunals Judiciary: https://www.judiciary.gov.uk/about-the-judiciary/history-of-the-judiciary/

> This website gives an overview of the legal system in the United Kingdom and explains the history and traditions of the courts.

Court of Protection: https://www.gov.uk/courts-tribunals/court-of-protection

> The Court of Protection makes decisions on financial or welfare matters for people who are deemed to lack mental capacity at the time important decisions need to be made about themselves. The website provides information and application advice.

Health and Safety Executive: http://www.hse.gov.uk/healthservices/index.htm

> The Health and Safety Executive website provides information about managing the risks in health and social care that can affect employees and users of services. The website provides useful information, e-tools and factsheets for a variety of health and safety issues.

NHS Digital Information Governance: http://systems.digital.nhs.uk/infogov

This website offers guidance on applying the principles of good information governance. The information is designed to help health and care organizations meet the standards required to handle care information appropriately and lawfully.

The Equality and Human Rights Commission: https://www.equalityhumanrights.com/en

The Equality and Human Rights Commission provides accessible information in relation to the Human Rights Act 1998 and the Equality Act 2010. The frequently asked questions sections are useful for understanding and applying the principles of human rights and equality.

CHAPTER 8

Scope of Professional Practice

Jayne E. Marshall ▪ Michelle Butler

LEARNING OUTCOMES

By the end of this chapter the reader should be able to:
- understand the fundamental scope of midwifery practice
- compare and contrast the midwife's scope of practice on a global scale
- recognize the limits of their scope of practice.
- use a framework of responsibility to explore expanding and extending their scope of
  practice
- appreciate the appropriateness of delegating midwifery tasks to others.

Overview

This chapter discusses the role and responsibilities of the midwife in terms of the scope of their professional practice and the controversies of developing and extending their role beyond initial registration to meet the continuing demands of providers and users of the maternity services. Whilst it is recognized that some midwives have developed their skills to fill the void in obstetric and paediatric cover, it is vital that they do not lose sight of the fundamental role of the midwife that is embedded in normal physiological processes. A *framework of responsibility* (Marshall 2010) is presented to support midwives in reflecting on their scope of practice and professional responsibilities when further developing their role and advancing their clinical skills. At the forefront should be comprehensive education and training programmes to ensure not only that the midwives' continuing professional development needs are met but also that the health and well-being of the childbearing woman, her baby and her family remain paramount. To assist the reader in contextualizing the theory that is presented, examples of the more common developments of the midwife's scope of practice are discussed and activities to undertake are provided, including formulating a development plan as part of their ongoing continuing professional development in acquisition of knowledge and skills.

Introduction

The *scope of midwifery practice* refers to the boundaries that are considered appropriate for midwives to practice within and the extent to which a midwife exercises their role in the provision of care for childbearing women, their babies and their families. The International Confederation of Midwives (ICM) core documents include the *International Definition of the Midwife* (ICM 2017), which clearly defines the midwife's *'full'* scope of practice on a global scale (Box 8.1). However, the scope of practice of a midwife varies from country to country.

In addition, the *Global Standards for Midwifery Education* (ICM 2013) and the *Global Standards for Midwifery Regulation* (ICM 2011) provide a professional framework that can be used by midwifery associations, midwifery regulators, midwifery educators and governments to strengthen the midwifery profession and raise the standard of midwifery practice in their respective country. Furthermore, as discussed in Chapter 2, the ICM's three pillars of a strong midwifery profession – namely *education*, *regulation* (which sets the scope of professional practice) and *association* – collectively support the strengthening of the world's midwifery workforce (United Nations Population Fund and ICM 2016). The purpose of such a framework

---

BOX 8.1 ■ International Definition of the Midwife: Scope of Practice (International Confederation of Midwives 2017)

The midwife is recognized as a responsible and accountable professional who works in partnership with women:

- to give the necessary support, care and advice during pregnancy, labour and the postpartum period
- to conduct births on the midwife's own responsibility
- to provide care for the newborn and the infant.

This care includes preventative measures, the promotion of normal birth, the detection of complications in mother and child, the accessing of medical care or other appropriate assistance and the carrying out of emergency measures.

The midwife has an important task in health counselling and education, not only for the woman but also within the family and the community.

This work should involve antenatal education and preparation for parenthood and may extend to women's health, sexual or reproductive health and childcare.

A midwife may practise in any setting, including the home, community, hospitals, clinics or health units.

Adopted at Brisbane Council meeting, 2005.

Revised and adopted at Durban Council meeting, 2011.

Revised and adopted at Toronto Council meeting, 2017.

Due for next review 2023.

ensures midwives are supported and enabled to fulfil their role and contribute fully to the delivery of maternal and neonatal care in their country. These standards and founding values subsequently are the basis for the midwife's scope of practice and are central to the discussions within this chapter.

The Global Context of the Midwife's Scope of Practice

The ICM global standards for midwifery education (ICM 2013) were developed in 2010 to strengthen midwifery worldwide by preparing fully qualified midwives to provide childbearing women, their babies and their families with high-quality, evidence-based health care. However, these standards represent the *minimum* expected from a quality midwifery programme with emphasis on competency-based education rather than academic degrees; that is, as detailed in *Essential Competencies for Basic Midwifery Practice* (ICM 2018). It is therefore the responsibility of all midwifery educationalists to ensure that the curriculum content aligns with but does *not* exceed the regulatory authority for midwifery practice in the specific country where the programme is delivered. This could include knowledge and skills that the ICM would identify as *additional*, and consequently means that the midwife acquires the knowledge and skill set that might be particularly important depending on the environment in which the individual midwife practises (e.g. *lifesaving*), ultimately enhancing their scope of practice. The scope of practice is influenced by factors such as the demand for midwifery care and the requirement to respond to changing population needs, the education of midwives, national and local regulations and licensure and midwifery advocacy (Phillippi and Barger 2015).

In determining an international framework for quality maternal and newborn care to improve global health and well-being, Renfrew et al (2014) mapped the ICM (2018) essential competencies for basic midwifery practice to four practice categories that define the full scope of midwifery practice of all trained, licensed and regulated midwives; namely:

1. education, information and health promotion
2. assessment, screening, and care planning
3. promoting normal processes and preventing complications
4. first-line management of complications.

A fifth practice category – *management of serious complications* – for collaborative working with colleagues is also included (Fig. 8.1).

Under European Union law, midwifery and nursing are defined as sectoral professions, and through the Professional Qualifications Directive (2005/36/EC amended by Directive 2013/55/EU) are part of the automatic recognition regime across European Union member states. These directives specify the training requirements of midwives, including the theoretical and clinical components and the professional activities that each student midwife should undertake during their programme of study in order to take on the scope of the role of the midwife on successful completion.

UNITED KINGDOM

Because of the significant legislative and regulatory changes that took place in March 2017 necessitating a change in the Nursing and Midwifery Order 2001, leading to the Nursing and Midwifery (Amendment) Order 2017 (see Chapters 2 and 10), midwives in the United Kingdom (UK) must uphold *The Code* (NMC 2018a) in order to remain on the professional register and continue practising. *The Code*, which has superseded the *Midwives Rules And Standards*

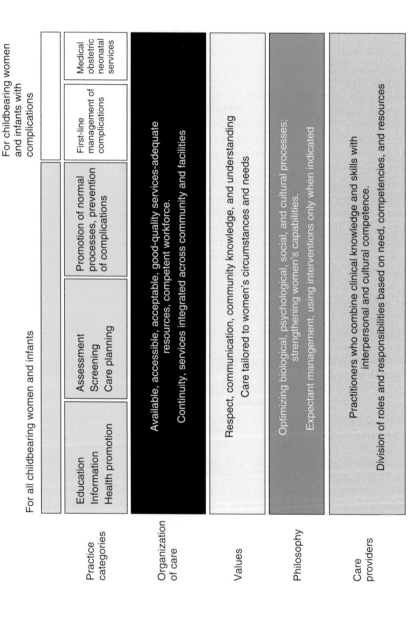

Fig. 8.1 The framework for quality maternal and newborn care: maternal and newborn health components of a health system needed by childbearing women and newborn infants. (Renfrew et al 2014)

(NMC 2012), requires midwives to uphold the relevant laws of the country in which they practise, including those relating to the notification of births, stillbirths and deaths. The NMC's publication *Practising as a Midwife in the UK* (NMC 2018b) specifies the regulatory framework for midwifery following the changes to legislation. The framework is not a regulatory standard but it describes the NMC's approach to the regulation of midwives and contains sections relating to each of the NMC's statutory functions: *the education of midwives, registration and revalidation, standards and guidance*, and *fitness to practise*. It should be read in conjunction with *The Code* and other standards and guidance. The NMC (2018b) states the scope of practice as shown in Box 8.2, which emphasizes that a midwife must not practise outside their skills, knowledge and competence.

Currently, in the UK, *Standards for Pre-registration Midwifery Education* (NMC 2009) guides the education, training and scope of midwifery practice; the standards are under review, with the anticipated implementation of new standards by 2021. The new competencies required of the future midwife in 2025 are expected to build on the professional values set out in *The Code* (NMC 2018a), be informed by best midwifery practice from the UK and internationally and be unambiguous, transparent and succinct.

The standards for competence for registered midwives (NMC 2014) require midwives to demonstrate knowledge and competence across four areas:

- effective midwifery practice
- professional and ethical practice,
- developing the individual midwife and others
- achieving quality care through evaluation and research.

BOX 8.2 ■ Midwife's Scope of Practice and Protected Function

Scope of Practice

The term *scope of practice* is frequently used in relation to professions such as midwifery, but health professionals in the United Kingdom tend not to be regulated with reference to a specified '*scope of practice*'.

The proficiency standards and *The Code* are important factors in thinking about the scope of practice. A midwife's scope of practice may change depending on the nature of their roles and the learning they have undertaken.

The Code requires midwives *not* to practise outside their skills, knowledge or competence. It is important that providers of maternity services are mindful of this professional duty when they deploy midwives.

A midwife's '*scope of practice*' might be taken to mean *the range of things that the midwife has the skills, knowledge and competence to do* and it should not be confused with *protected function*, which means *something that only midwives can legally do* as seen below.

Protected Function

There is a protected function associated with the title *midwife*. Only the following people may attend a woman in childbirth:

- a midwife
- a registered medical practitioner
- a student undergoing training with a view to becoming a midwife or a medical practitioner, as part of an approved course of practical instruction.

The exception to this is in a case of '*sudden or urgent necessity*'.

From Nursing and Midwifery Council (2017: 8–9).

Midwives must demonstrate their knowledge and competence in all four areas (formerly known as *domains*) to register as a midwife; these form the basis of the standards for preregistration midwifery education (NMC 2009). On registration all midwives will:

- assume full responsibility and accountability for their practice as midwives
- practically apply sound, evidence-based knowledge of facilitating childbirth and caring for the newborn
- act on their understanding of psychological, social, emotional and spiritual factors that may positively or adversely influence normal physiology, and be competent in applying this in practice
- use appropriate interpersonal skills to support women and their families
- use skills in managing obstetric and neonatal emergencies, underpinned by appropriate knowledge
- be autonomous practitioners and lead carers to women experiencing normal childbirth and be able to support women throughout their pregnancy, labour, childbirth and postnatal period, in all settings, including midwife-led units, birthing centres and the home
- be able to make critical decisions to support the appropriate referral of either the woman or the baby to other health professionals or agencies when they recognize that normal processes have been adversely affected and compromised.

The context of childbirth refers to the antenatal, intrapartum and postnatal periods.

CANADA

Although only recently established over the past 20–30 years, the model of midwifery care in Canada supports the full scope of midwifery practice. The Canadian Midwifery Regulators Council sets and maintains standards for midwifery education and practice; however, midwifery practice is regulated at the provincial level, and provincial regulators (midwifery colleges) uphold the national standards. Midwifery was first regulated in British Columbia in 1998, and demand for midwives continues to grow. In 2015, 21% of women had maternity care with a midwife (Perinatal Services BC 2016). Midwives provide care for women in the place of their choice and accompany them to hospital should they wish to give birth there. Hospitals employ maternity nurses, rather than midwives, to provide care for women who are admitted for antenatal care and following operative childbirth, as well as support midwives, family doctors and obstetricians facilitating labour and births.

The model of midwifery care in Canada is one of the most progressive models worldwide (Canadian Midwifery Regulators Council 2016). Midwives work as autonomous primary care providers, either as solo practitioners or in groups of up to four, with each midwife having a caseload of around 60 women per year. They are fully responsible for the provision of primary health services within their scope of practice. Midwives are paid per course of maternity care through the universal health care insurance model and provide personalized care from early pregnancy to 6 weeks postpartum, including the care during childbirth at home or in the hospital.

Midwifery practice is regulated by the College of Midwives of British Columbia using parameters defined in the Health Professions Act, Midwives Regulation (British Colombia Government 2009). They define the scope of practice as *midwifery*, which is the health profession in which a person provides the following services during normal pregnancy, labour, birth and the postpartum period:

- assessment, monitoring and care for women, newborns and infants, including the carrying out of appropriate emergency measures when necessary
- counselling, supporting and advising women, including advice and information regarding care for newborns and infants

- conducting internal examinations of women, performing episiotomies and amniotomies and repairing episiotomies and simple lacerations.
- contraceptive services for women during the 3 months following birth.

These regulations require the midwife to consult with a medical or nurse practitioner regarding any deviations from the normal and to transfer responsibility for care to another health professional when necessary or appropriate.

UNITED STATES OF AMERICA

In the United States of America (USA) there are variations from state to state in terms of the qualifications of midwives (e.g. certified midwives [CMs], certified nurse midwives [CNMs]), the types of midwifery education programmes offered, the degree of autonomy of the midwife (whether the midwife requires physician supervision or contractual practice agreements) and whether midwives are authorized to deliver expanded professional health care. King (2000) affirms the four factors that establish the scope of practice for midwives in the USA:

1. individually defined boundaries for safe practice
2. local service practice guidelines or policies
3. college documents and guidelines – for example the American College of Nurse-Midwives (2012) core competencies for basic midwifery practice and guidelines for incorporation of new procedures
4. legal authority to practise as defined by statutes and regulations.

In some states, such as Maine, CNMs are primary health care providers and licensed independent practitioners. In other states, such as Nebraska, CNMs must have physician supervision and complete written practice agreements that identify practice settings and medical functions that can be performed by the CNM in collaboration with the physician (Yang et al 2016). An analysis of the variations in scope of practice laws across the USA undertaken by Yang et al (2016) found that more CNMs were practising per 1000 births (an average of 4.85) in states with autonomous practice laws compared with those engaged in collaborative agreements (an average of 2.17 per 1000 births).

Now undertake Activity 8.1.

ACTIVITY 8.1 ■

Consider the midwife's scope of practice from the international, national and local perspective.
- What are the benefits of midwives practising the full scope of practice?
- In your own jurisdiction, what are the factors that have influenced the scope of midwifery practice?
- How does this compare with other countries?
- What impact does this have on your own practice as a midwife?

Health systems and cultural barriers often limit the full scope of midwives' practice within the country in which they are registered to practise (Renfrew et al 2014). In Australia, Homer et al (2009) identified a number of challenges that midwives face in practising their role and scope of practice and which relate to the health system and the culture within the system as well as within the midwifery profession, such as the lack of a clear image and consistent standards of education and practice. Furthermore, Homer et al (2009) highlighted personal factors affecting a midwife's scope of practice that included family responsibilities and social commitments that influenced to what extent midwives were able to work in a caseload practice model. This suggests that the scope of practice within a jurisdiction depends on a number of extrinsic and intrinsic factors as shown in Table 8.1.

TABLE 8.1 ■ Factors Influencing Midwifery Scope of Practice

Extrinsic	Intrinsic
• Demand for midwifery care and the need to respond to change • Legal authority to practise • National and local regulations and licensure • Organizational or institutional barriers • Dominance of medicine • Political context – invisibility of midwifery, lack of midwifery advocacy • Education and training available; lack of consistent standards of education and practice • Lack of opportunities to practise across the full scope of practice • Lack of a clear understanding of what midwifery is	• Preparation and training of the midwife • Philosophy of care • Willingness to negotiate scope of practice with other professionals • Motivation to practise within the limits of scope of practice • Personal, family or social commitments • Lack of understanding of what the full scope of practice is

Extending, Expanding/Advancing the Scope of Practice

Midwives have a clearly defined scope of practice and are accountable for that practice in whatever setting they practise, ensuring that the safety of mother and fetus/baby remains paramount and their knowledge and skill set remain contemporary. There may, however, be situations when a midwife wishes to develop their existing scope of practice, and therefore the principles and framework for incorporating a new skill into their skill set become relevant. The midwife should always consult the code of practice relevant to the country in which they practise, for example in the UK this would be *The Code* (NMC 2018a), as well as the employing organization with regard to the preparation and experience required, before any adjustment is made to the midwife's role. At this juncture, the definitions of *expanded practice* and *extended/advanced practice*, which are associated with developing a midwife's scope of practice and role, will be presented to help clarify their appropriateness in midwifery practice. Often the terms are used interchangeably and consequently can create some confusion among professionals.

EXPANDED PRACTICE

Expanded practice is a change to the role of an individual midwife that includes areas of practice that have not previously been within the scope of practice, but *are* within the overall scope of practice of the midwifery profession. It is organic in nature and considered more developmental than *extended* practice. Expanded practice involves taking on new roles, such as intravenous cannulation, midwife prescribing of medicines and newborn and infant physical examination, or delegation of roles and responsibilities. There are also clearly defined expanded roles of clinical midwife specialists in areas such as perinatal mental health, bereavement and diabetes.

Expanded practice should occur in the context of quality, safe, woman-centred care, maternity service needs and national policy. There is no specific stage in the midwife's clinical career at which expansion of practice occurs. The individual midwife's educational preparation and professional competence, rather than the nature or degree of difficulty of the task, should determine role expansion. Midwives who expand their roles must assume the associated responsibility, just as employers and managers must share the responsibility to facilitate role expansion, such as enabling access to further education, allocation of necessary resources, policy development and assessment of competence.

> **BOX 8.3 ■ The Canadian Midwife's Scope of Practice: Advanced Competencies (Canadian Midwifery Regulators Council 2008)**
>
> ■ Epidural monitoring.
> ■ Application of scalp electrodes.
> ■ Pharmacological augmentation of labour.
> ■ Induction of labour for postdates pregnancy.
> ■ Performing vacuum extraction
> ■ First surgical assist at caesarean sections.
> ■ Suturing of third-degree tears.
> ■ Evacuation of the uterus.
> ■ Fitting barrier methods of contraception.
> ■ Inserting intrauterine contraceptive devices.
> ■ Prescribing contraceptives.
> ■ Providing well-baby care to healthy newborns and after 6 weeks.
> ■ Providing well-woman care to healthy women and after 6 weeks.

EXTENDED/ADVANCED PRACTICE

Extension of a midwife's scope of practice could be viewed as mechanistic and task based, with little use of clinical judgement, and is often associated with doctor substitute roles. The shortages in medical establishments, especially in staffing junior doctor rotas (Department of Health [DH] et al 2002), and the European Working Time Directive (DH 1998) led to further discussion of advanced practitioner roles to cover some of the medical role.

Whilst these roles are evident in nursing, the Royal College of Midwives (2016) further tested their applicability to midwifery and did not find them appropriate in UK midwifery practice. Extending the midwife's role into obstetrics, nursing or other areas of practice does not demonstrably improve the quality of, or access to, midwifery expertise. Consultant midwives are already fulfilling the requirement of an experienced clinical expert with a wider scope of practice. Such a role encompasses expert practice, service development, clinical leadership, education and training.

In Canada, the scope of practice of a midwife is set out in *Canadian Competencies for Midwives* (Canadian Midwifery Regulators Council 2008); the competencies include *entry level* and *advanced* competencies. The advanced competencies are listed in Box 8.3. However, a number of these advanced competencies are considered to be entry level in some provinces. The midwife's scope of practice in individual provinces is outlined in provincial by-laws, and the extent of full scope differs from province to province depending on the scope negotiated with provincial governments.

Acquisition of New Skills

Whether midwives expand their midwifery skills or extend their skill set to the skills associated with medical colleagues, the fundamental issue is that they are *competent* and *safe* to undertake the task that requires such a skill. However, in determination of the feasibility of developing competence in a new skill, the skill should always be *integral* to the midwife's role, be reflective of the context in which the midwife works and be of benefit to mothers and babies. Fundamental to the debate of a midwife developing competence in a new skill is the issue of them being *responsible* and *accountable* (answerable) for their own actions or omissions. It is acknowledged that the concepts of *accountability* and *responsibility* are often used interchangeably and synonymously: accountability cannot exist without responsibility having been granted, accepted and assumed. A midwife cannot be held accountable for an action or have accountability imposed on them unless they are given and accept the responsibility on the basis of their professional preparation (i.e. through appropriate education and experience).

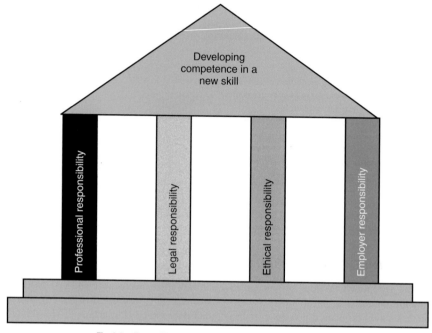

Fig. 8.2   Four pillars of responsibility. (From Marshall 2010)

MARSHALL'S (2010) FRAMEWORK OF RESPONSIBILITY

Frameworks of accountability such as Bergman's (1981) *preconditions of accountability*, Kitson's (1993) *dimensions of accountability* and Caulfield's (2005) *four pillars of accountability*, which were originally developed for the nursing profession, can be transferred to midwifery practice and support midwives in realizing their accountability through exploring the different components affecting their practice. Marshall (2010) adapted Caulfield's (2005) framework for midwives for use when developing competence in a new skill, specifically addressing the four pillars of responsibility (Fig. 8.2).

The four pillars provide a collective sense of responsibility for the midwife to address: namely, *professional, legal, ethical* and *employer responsibility.*

Professional Responsibility

The function of all professional and statutory regulatory bodies (PSRBs) is to safeguard the health and well-being of persons using the services of its registrants: public protection. As a consequence, a minimum standard of entry to the professional register is set that midwives must achieve, for them to perform their role safely and effectively within their professional boundaries and thus be fit for practice and purpose. Student midwives and registered midwives are assessed as *competent,* having demonstrated capability in certain skills to a required standard at a particular point in time. No midwife should therefore undertake any activity for which they do not have the underpinning knowledge and expertise. Whenever advancements occur in midwifery practice that require the midwife to develop competence in new skills beyond those acquired in initial preparation, consideration should be given as to whether these skills are fundamental to *every* midwife, to then be integrated into all preregistration midwifery education programmes.

Midwives are responsible for maintaining and developing the competence they achieved during initial and subsequent midwifery education, which in the UK is fundamental to the principles of *The Code* (NMC 2018a); that is, their knowledge and skills are contemporary. Should the midwife be found to be lacking in competence, as in situations of misconduct and ill health, they are likely to be referred to the NMC's Fitness to Practise Committee. This is to ensure that the standard of a midwife's practice and the midwifery care that is delivered is of the highest quality, and is reflective of local and national guidelines.

It is a midwife's personal responsibility to maintain their professional registration by going through a process of revalidation every 3 years. This includes maintaining a portfolio of evidence to demonstrate that their continuing professional development meets the standards required by the regulatory body (see Chapters 2 and 15) and an indemnity arrangement is in place when they apply to register or renew their registration. The indemnity arrangement must provide appropriate cover for their role and scope of practice, be relevant to the risks involved in their practice, and be sufficient to meet an award of damages if a successful claim is made against them. This requirement includes midwives employed as educators and midwives undertaking voluntary work. Midwives may obtain indemnity cover from an employer or a professional association (e.g. The Royal College of Midwives).

Legal Responsibility

A society determines rules and penalties to provide a common framework by which each member should live through the system of law. In the UK, law covers all aspects of a person's life, including health care, such that health professionals must have an understanding of how the law relates to their practice. The fundamental legal issues that have significance to midwifery practice and the role of the midwife when developing competence in new skills are *negligence* and *consent*, which are discussed in more detail in Chapter 7.

Each midwife has a duty of care to ensure the care they provide to mothers and babies is of a *reasonable* standard that does not cause any harm to the recipients for which they would become liable. Where a midwife develops competence in skills beyond initial midwifery preparation, they will be judged by the law according to the standard expected by other midwives/health professionals who are skilled in that particular area of practice. The midwife would be deemed *negligent* if they do not maintain this standard and as a consequence the mother or baby is harmed. This also applies to student midwives undertaking further training in skill development as they will be judged by the standards expected of an experienced midwife as the courts uphold that all members of society are entitled to receive maternity care that is deemed competent. It is vital that where a student midwife/midwife is unclear about a procedure they act responsibly and seek advice and supervision from more experienced colleagues until they have been assessed as competent. Such a process should be clearly reflected in the maternity records.

The midwife is also legally responsible for ensuring that consent is obtained from childbearing women before any physical contact with the body of that individual is undertaken, otherwise such contact would be deemed as *trespass to the person*. As with a student midwife, the midwife who is undertaking further skill development would also be considered to be in a *learner* capacity and should always ensure the woman is fully aware of their capabilities/limitations. This would provide the woman with the opportunity to make an autonomous decision to either give or refuse consent to the midwife undertaking the procedure in such circumstances. The maternity records should reflect such a decision. Furthermore, it is always good practice for the colleague supervising the midwife in developing competence in a new skill to countersign any entry that is made in relation to that particular skill until such time as the midwife is assessed as competent.

Ethical Responsibility

When midwives contemplate developing competence in new skills, they have a responsibility to assess what impact the ethical theories and principles of *respect for autonomy, justice, beneficence* and *non-maleficence* will have on themselves, their colleagues and childbearing women and their babies to whom they provide care and the organizations in which they work (see Chapter 6). Although midwives may determine the course of their continuing professional development/skill development that they wish to pursue, this would be considered by managers alongside the incurred costs to the organization in terms of the time and financial costs involved. The role and responsibility of the manager is to ensure that there is fairness (*justice*) when apportioning resources among staff, and consequently midwives should be respectful of the decisions that are made, which is associated with being an *autonomous* person.

The benefit to women and babies of the midwife developing competence in a new skill is also fundamental to their responsibility in acquiring such a skill. It is well documented that continuity of midwifery care and midwife-led contexts improve maternal satisfaction and birth outcomes (DH 1993; NHS England 2016). Marshall (2010) recognizes that midwives who are competent in skills such as perineal repair, newborn and infant physical examination, vaginal breech birth and uncomplicated vacuum or forceps birth can further enhance the continuity of midwifery care by avoiding transfer to medical colleagues and the resulting fragmentation of care. However, the context in which these skills are to be practised and maintained needs careful consideration to justify whether midwives should undergo further training to acquire the required competence. Where there is 24-hour obstetric cover within the hospital setting, there would be little benefit for midwives to be trained to undertake vacuum or forceps births, as opposed to in a stand-alone birth centre. In the latter context, the midwife ventouse practitioner is able to maintain continuity of care with the woman whilst retaining some degree of normality and without a transfer to an obstetric unit.

Employer Responsibility

The fourth and final pillar of the framework relates to the responsibility of the employer in supporting midwives acquiring new skills beyond initial midwifery preparation. Each National Health Service (NHS) Trust in the UK has a statutory duty in ensuring that its employees deliver quality care and systems are in place for clinical governance, with the Chief Executive Officer being ultimately accountable. *Skills for Health*, a not-for-profit organization, is committed to supporting employers across the UK in the development of an improved and sustainable workforce through appropriate employer-led qualifications and raising skills and training to maximize quality, productivity and health outcomes.

Where midwives plan to acquire new skills to improve maternity and neonatal care, it is important that NHS Trust policy clearly defines the midwife's role and responsibilities in such a skill to avoid any confusion over role ambiguity. If this detail is not apparent, the employer would not be held responsible should any harm result in the woman or baby as a result of a midwife contravening Trust policy. If a midwife who is competent in an extended/advanced skill moves to another Trust, they would only be able to continue practising such a skill if the NHS Trust policy of the new employer permits them to do so. It is also good practice that such policies and regulations make it clear that a midwife must have completed a certification programme for specific activities included in the scope of practice (e.g. complementary therapies, prescribing, newborn and infant physical examination, vacuum extraction). This would indicate that the midwife has been assessed as knowledgeable and competent by experts in that particular area of practice.

The employer is responsible for assessing the health and safety risk for its employees as well the clinical risk to the public which applies to midwives developing new skills; both being key components of *risk management* (see Chapter 9). The employer may be held responsible not only for negligence against the employee but also for negligence caused by the employee. It is vital therefore that the employer ensures all employees are competent as they can be directly liable in negligence for allowing an inexperienced employee to undertake tasks which they are not competent to perform without supervision. Should there be a case of alleged negligence, it is highly unlikely that an employer would refuse to accept responsibility for a midwife's practice providing the midwife has undertaken an approved education and training programme to develop competence in a new skill, has followed guidelines and risk management procedures and has evidence that the skill has been maintained. The doctrine of *vicarious liability* applies so that compensation can be paid to individuals who have suffered harm caused by a midwife in the course of their employment (see Chapter 7).

Now undertake Activity 8.2.

ACTIVITY 8.2 ■

You have developed an interest in the use of moxibustion as an intervention for facilitating cephalic version and improving the physiological vaginal birth rate of pregnant women who have a breech presentation. You would like to develop competence in this skill with the aim of introducing it into midwifery practice within the birthing environment in which you work.

- *Using the four pillars of responsibility*, consider the specific issues you would need to address in relation to developing competence in this new skill.
- What do you perceive would be the benefits of acquiring such a skill?
- Compile an action plan to present to your manager/employer to support your case.
- How do you envisage acquiring the skill and subsequently maintaining it?
- What evidence would you need to provide to demonstrate you are competent and continuing to develop this particular aspect of practice?

Delegation of Care

Delegation is the act of giving someone authority to act for another, and carries legal and safety issues in midwifery practice. The ability to delegate has been reserved for professionals because they hold the licence that sanctions the entire scope of practice for professions such as midwifery. Midwives may therefore delegate any independent midwifery activity as well as medical functions that may have been delegated to them, such as intravenous cannulation and newborn and infant physical examination, to other midwives. The delegating midwife, however, is responsible for determining that the individual to whom they have delegated the activity is competent to perform the delegated act and the activity is also *within* their scope of competence (NMC 2018a: Standard 11). Likewise, the person undertaking the delegated act is responsible for carrying out the delegated act safely. The midwife remains legally accountable for the midwifery acts delegated to others unless that individual is also a registered midwife, who would then assume that accountability by the nature of their licence to practise. A midwife can assign an activity to a student midwife or a maternity support worker (MSW), providing they have been appropriately trained and are deemed competent (e.g. taking vital signs, baby care/baby bath, assisted washes, breastfeeding support). The student midwife or MSW, however, cannot reassign this responsibility to any other person. Furthermore, in terms of data collected by a MSW, it is the midwife who is accountable for these data and their interpretation in order to determine any subsequent action. The National Council of State Boards of Nursing (1997) in the USA has defined *five rights of delegation* (Box 8.4) that midwives may also find useful when considering the appropriateness of delegating midwifery activities to others.

BOX 8.4 ■ The Five Rights of Delegation

- *Right task*: Is the task appropriate for delegation in a given care situation?
- *Right circumstances*: Is delegation appropriate in this case?
  - Health of woman/baby.
  - Care setting.
  - Complexity of the activity.
  - Delegates' competence.
  - Available resources.
- *Right person*: Can the midwife verify that the person delegated to do the task is competent to complete the task?
- *Right direction/communication:* Has the midwife given clear specific instructions?
  - Identifying the woman/baby.
  - Identifying the objective of the task.
  - Identifying the time frame.
  - Identifying the expected results.
- *Right supervision/evaluation*: Can the midwife provide supervision and evaluation of the woman/baby and the performance of the task?

Adapted from National Council of State Boards of Nursing (1997).

Record Keeping

Good record keeping is the mark of a skilled and safe health professional that reflects the extent of their role and level of competence. It is a core aspect of midwifery practice, providing a record of the information obtained from a woman about her needs and preferences, and assessments and evaluations made by the midwife and other care providers. These records can be paper based or electronic in format and should include details of the issues discussed, any consultations and advice sought, the decisions made and actions taken, including their rationale and timing, over the course of care provision. Most jurisdictions have clear regulatory requirements for midwives and other health care providers to document all aspects of the care that they provide, including confidentiality and information sharing, data protection, safe storage and disposal of records and the necessity of signatories for validation purposes in whatever form the records take (e.g. NMC 2018a: Standard 10).

Documentation is vital to support continuity of care, to ensure the accuracy of decision making, to enable peer review, to uphold professionalism to a licensing board, to protect midwives from litigation and to collect and collate statistics (Lieberman 2005). Furthermore, the accuracy and quality of documentation is instrumental to its use in midwifery care as a communication tool, to inform decisions, and to facilitate continuity of care (see Chapter 3). The quality of documentation is associated with the quality of patient care and patient outcomes (Bailey et al 2015).

TABLE 8.2 ■ The SOAP Documentation Notation

Subjective	What the individual is experiencing: can be written in their own words
Objective	Data collected by the health professional (e.g., vital signs, laboratory test results)
Assessment	What the health professional thinks is occurring, needs to be treated or has to rule out before being able to make a diagnosis
Plan	How the health professional plans to deal with what has been assessed

Adapted from Lieberman (2005).

Incomplete or poor records contribute to errors and substandard care (Wright 2013). In the UK courts of law, it is generally viewed that if something is not recorded, it has not been done (Unite the Union in Health 2012). A helpful model to guide a consistent approach to documentation is the *SOAP* model, recommended by Lieberman (2005), which provides a logical format for succinct information sharing (Table 8.2).

Midwife Prescribing

Midwife prescribing has been introduced in a number of countries in recent years, aimed at increasing the range of aspects of care that a midwife can provide without having to consult another practitioner, ultimately enhancing the quality of care that a woman receives and reducing delays in medicine administration or in transfer home from hospital. This usually requires midwives to undertake additional training and certification, to be entered into a special register for prescribers and to obtain prescriber status/posts from their employers. Usually, the range of medicinal products that they prescribe is limited to that contained within a specific formulary.

New standards for nurse and midwife prescribing programmes in the UK have been approved by the NMC (2018c) that adopt the Royal Pharmaceutical Society's competency framework for all prescribers (Royal Pharmaceutical Society 2016) as the foundation for registrants to receive a recordable qualification in nurse and midwife prescribing. Registrants must prescribe only from the formulary linked to their recorded qualifications, comply with statutory requirements related to their prescribing practice and only ever prescribe within their own level of experience and competence. Nurse and midwife prescribers are professionally accountable for prescribing decisions, actions and omissions, and cannot delegate this accountability.

The Code (NMC 2018a: Section 18) sets the professional standards regarding advising on, prescribing, supplying, dispensing and administering medicines within the limits of a registrant's training and competence, the law, PSRB guidance and other relevant policies, guidance and regulations. The prescribing of medicines should always be in line within local and national guidelines and be evidence based, with the midwife prescriber's knowledge and skills of prescribing remaining up to date. It is vital that all midwife prescribers are cognizant of the range of medicines they are able to prescribe in accordance with the legal and PSRB requirements (e.g. complementary and alternative therapies, controlled drugs and midwives' exemptions). Similarly, in British Columbia, midwives are permitted to independently prescribe, order and administer medicines from a list of specific antibiotics, local anaesthetics, analgesics, antiemetics, inhalational agents, intravenous fluids, uterotonic agents, vitamin and mineral supplements, etc. that are pertinent to the scope of midwifery practice. Midwives with additional certification may also independently prescribe, order and administer cervical ripening and induction/augmentation agents or after consultation with, and on the order of, a medical practitioner. The College of Midwives of British Columbia (2017) provides the standards and guidance for prescribing, ordering and administering drugs and controlled substances for midwives to adhere to in their prescribing role and consequently ensure public safety is always paramount.

Newborn and Infant Physical Examination

The *healthy* newborn baby undergoes an initial examination by the midwife following birth as a means of observing its successful adaptation to extrauterine life as well as any deviations, such as physical signs of birth trauma or malformations. Babies who are born prematurely, are small or are ill, however, should always be referred to a paediatrician to undertake this initial assessment. Student midwives undertake this examination of the healthy term baby as part of the requirements of their initial preparation to enter the midwifery profession (NMC 2009). A second and more thorough physiological examination is undertaken within 72 hours of the baby's birth (this was traditionally undertaken by a paediatrician), with a further examination between 6 and 8 weeks that is undertaken by the general practitioner. These assessments constitute the NHS newborn and infant physical examination screening programme (Public Health England 2018), which is under the direction of the UK National Screening Committee. The examination includes:

- examination of the eyes
- examination of the heart
- examination of the hips
- examination of the testes/external genitalia.

As stated earlier, changes in staffing junior doctor rotas (DH et al 2002) and the European Working Time Directive (DH 1998) contributed to an increasing number of midwives acquiring the knowledge and skills to undertake this function, but ultimately the impact of enhancing continuity of midwifery care and improving maternal satisfaction were the key reasons. To develop the skill of undertaking newborn and infant physical examination, each midwife is required to undertake a university-accredited examination of the newborn programme of study and undertake a locally agreed competency assessment by a practising newborn and infant physical examination examiner. Furthermore, the midwife is responsible for maintaining their own competence to carry out the examination to the highest standard and for the identification of any deficits in their knowledge and training needs (NMC 2018a).

Some universities in the UK have included the theoretical elements of the newborn and infant physical examination in their initial midwifery education programmes, with others providing both theoretical and practical elements. This means that an increasing number of student midwives are equipped to undertake the examination, once they are deemed both knowledgeable and competent, much earlier in their midwifery careers.

Now undertake Activity 8.3.

ACTIVITY 8.3 ■

Consider the principles of the professional code of practice pertinent to the jurisdiction in which you are training to become a midwife/practise as a midwife and their relevance to developing your knowledge and skill to safely undertake the newborn and infant physical examination.
Identify the level of your existing knowledge and skills, including any deficits and the training needs you require to undertake the physical examination of the healthy newborn, with reference to your code of conduct.

Conclusion

The scope of practice of the midwife enables midwives to be flexible and professionally challenging in their role to meet the demands of a dynamic maternity and health care service. Professional codes of practice provide guidance for midwives to use when contemplating situations of skill development that may not be within their current scope of practice and level of competence or, indeed, the scope of midwifery practice *per se*. In addition, use of a framework of responsibility for developing competence in a new skill identifies four pillars of responsibility (namely, *professional, legal, ethical* and *employer*) that can assist midwives in determining the value of developing their skill set. The wider implications of any adjustment to their scope of practice must be considered and whether any formal education and training programme is required to certify their competence and eligibility to practise beyond their role. As a result, decisions made about developing the scope of practice should always be discussed with the midwife's line manager and supported by the employer, ensuring that public protection always remains at the forefront of the midwife's practice and ultimately the maternity services.

KEY POINTS

- A midwife should be cognizant of their own scope of practice and its limitations and consequently should perform activities only for which they have been assessed as competent.
- All childbearing women are legally entitled to receive maternity care that is competent and safe, including care from those in a *learner* capacity.
- The rationale for any development in the scope of midwifery practice should be based on improved maternal and neonatal health outcomes, rather than convenience or professional preference.
- Comprehensive education and training programmes should always be at the forefront of the development of a midwife's scope of practice, discussed with the line manager and reviewed during the appraisal process.
- The *four pillars of responsibility* can provide a working framework for midwives to use in planning their continuing professional development and acquisition of new skills.
- Careful consideration of the act of delegating midwifery care to others is essential as it carries legal and safety issues, for which the midwife would be legally accountable (unless the activity has been delegated to another practising midwife).
- The midwife's role and responsibilities in tasks that have commonly been undertaken by medical staff should be clearly defined in policy documents within the employing organization.

References

American College of Nurse-Midwives. (2012). *The core competencies for basic midwifery practice*. Silver Spring: American College of Nurse-Midwives.

Bailey, S., Wilson, G., & Yoong, W. (2015). What factors affect documentation by midwives? A prospective study assessing relationship between length of shift, workload and quality of note keeping. *Midwifery, 31*, 787–792.

Bergman, R. (1981). Accountability: definitions and dimensions. *International Nursing Review, 28*(2), 53–59.

British Columbia Government. (2009). *Health Professions Act: Midwives Regulation, BC Reg. 155/2009*. Victoria: Queen's Printer.

Canadian Midwifery Regulators Council. (2008). *Canadian competencies for midwives, revised 10/11/2008*. Available at: http://cmrc-ccosf.ca/sites/default/files/pdf/National_Competencies_ENG_rev08.pdf.

Canadian Midwifery Regulators Council. (2016). *Midwifery in Canada*. Available at: http://www.cmrc-ccosf.ca.

Caulfield, H. (2005). *Vital notes for nurses: accountability*. Oxford: Blackwell.

College of Midwives of British Columbia. (2017). *Professional standards and guidelines for prescribing, ordering and administering drugs and controlled substances*. Vancouver: College of Midwives of British Columbia.

Department of Health. (1993). *Changing childbirth: Report of the Expert Maternity Group*. London: HMSO.

Department of Health. (1998). *European Working Time Directive*. London: HMSO.

Department of Health, National Assembly for Wales, National Health Service Confederation, & British Medical Association. (2002). *Guidance on working pattern for junior doctors*. London: HMSO.

Directive 2013 /55/EU of the European Parliament and of the Council of 20 November 2013 amending Directive 2005/36/EC on the recognition of professional qualifications and Regulation EU No 1024/2012 on administrative cooperation through the Internal Market Information System ('the IMI Regulation').

Homer, C. S. E., Passant, L., Brodie, P. M., Kildea, S., Leap, N., Pincombe, J., et al. (2009). The role of the midwife in Australia: views of women and midwives. *Midwifery, 25*, 673–681.

International Confederation of Midwives. (2011). *Global standards for midwifery regulation*. Available at: https://www.internationalmidwives.org/assets/files/general-files/2018/04/global-standards-for-midwifery-regulation-eng.pdf.

International Confederation of Midwives. (2013). *Global standards for midwifery education*. Available at: https://www.internationalmidwives.org/assets/files/general-files/2018/04/icm-standards-guidelines_ammended2013.pdf.

International Confederation of Midwives. (2017). *International definition of the midwife.* Available at: https://www.internationalmidwives.org/assets/files/definitions-files/2018/06/eng-definition_of_the_midwife-2017.pdf.

International Confederation of Midwives. (2018). *Essential competencies for basic midwifery practice.* Available at: https://www.internationalmidwives.org/our-work/policy-and-practice/essential-competencies-for-midwifery-practice.html.

King, T. (2000). Clinical boundaries: what parameters determine a midwife's scope of practice? *Journal of Midwifery and Women's Health, 45*(6), 448–449.

Kitson, A. (1993). Accountability for quality. *Nursing Standard, 8*(1), 4–6.

Lieberman, L. (2005). The business of midwifery: documentation for success II. *Midwifery Today, 76,* 46.

Marshall, J. E. (2010). The midwife's professional responsibilities in developing competence in new skills. In Marshall, J., E. & Raynor, M., D. (Eds.), *Advancing skills in midwifery practice* (pp. 7–18). Edinburgh: Churchill Livingstone.

National Council of State Boards of Nursing. (1997). *The five rights of delegation.* Available at: https://www.ncsbn.org/Delegation_joint_statement_NCSBN-ANA.pdf.

NHS England. (2016). *Better Births: Improving outcomes of maternity services in England. A five year forward view for maternity care.* Available at: https://www.england.nhs.uk/wp-content/uploads/2016/02/national-maternity-review-report.pdf.

Nursing and Midwifery (Amendment) Order. (2017). *Statutory Instruments No 321.* London: The Stationery Office.

Nursing and Midwifery Council. (2009). *Standards for pre-registration midwifery education.* London: Nursing and Midwifery Council.

Nursing and Midwifery Council. (2012). *Midwives rules and standards.* London: Nursing and Midwifery Council.

Nursing and Midwifery Council. (2014). *Standards for competence for registered midwives.* London: Nursing and Midwifery Council.

Nursing and Midwifery Council. (2018a). *The Code: Professional standards of practice and behaviour for nurses, midwives and nursing associates.* London: Nursing and Midwifery Council.

Nursing and Midwifery Council. (2018b). *Practising as a midwife in the UK: an overview of midwifery regulation.* London: Nursing and Midwifery Council.

Nursing and Midwifery Council. (2018c). *Realising professionalism: Standards for education and training. Part 3: Standards for prescribing programmes.* London: Nursing and Midwifery Council.

Nursing and Midwifery Order 2001 Statutory Instrument 2002 No 253. London: The Stationery Office.

Perinatal Services, B. C. (2016). *Midwifery report: Deliveries in BC 2014/15.* Vancouver: Perinatal Services BC.

Phillippi, J. C., & Barger, M. (2015). Midwives as primary care providers for women. *Journal of Midwifery and Women's Health, 60*(3), 250–257.

Public Health England. (2018). *Our approach to newborn and infant physical examination screening standards.* London: HMSO. Available at: https://www.gov.uk/government/publications/newborn-and-infant-physical-examination-screening-standards.

Renfrew, M. J., McFadden, A., Bastos, M. H., Campbell, J., Amos Channon, A., Cheung, N. F., et al. (2014). Midwifery and quality care: findings from a new evidence-informed framework for maternal and newborn care. *The Lancet, 384,* 1129–1145.

Royal College of Midwives. (2016). *Getting the midwifery workforce right.* London: Royal College of Midwives. Available at: https://www.rcm.org.uk/sites/default/files/Getting%20the%20Midwifery%20Workforce%20Right%20A5%2024pp_2_1.pdf.

Royal Pharmaceutical Society. (2016). *A competency framework for all prescribers.* London: Royal Pharmaceutical Society.

Unite the Union in Health. (2012). *Record keeping guidelines.* London: Unite the Union.

United Nations Population Fund & International Confederation of Midwives. (2016). *Comprehensive midwifery programme guidance.* Available at: http://www.unfpa.org/sites/default/files/resource-pdf/Midwifery%20Programme%20Guidance.pdf.

Wright, K. (2013). Ensuring best practice in clinical record-keeping. *Nursing Times, 109*(35), 20–21.

Yang, Y. T., Attanasio, L. B., & Kozhimannil, K. B. (2016). State scope of practice laws, nurse-midwifery workforce, and childbirth procedures and outcomes. *Women's Health Issues, 26*(3), 262–267.

Further Reading

Marshall, J. E., & Raynor, M. D. (Eds.). (2010). *Advancing skills in midwifery practice*. Edinburgh: Churchill Livingstone.

This text provides a guide to the continuing professional development needs of midwives, which can also be transferred across interprofessional boundaries, embracing interprofessional working and learning. A framework for assessing the responsibilities associated with developing new skills and advancing clinical skills is presented alongside the challenges of stepping outside the traditionally defined boundaries of the midwifery scope of practice.

Royal College of Midwives. (2016). *Getting the midwifery workforce right*. London: Royal College of Midwives.

This guidance paper explains the role of the midwife, the limits and scope of the role and its relationship with other professionals and care givers. It explores the challenges of policy initiatives and the changing context of maternity service delivery that advocates more flexibility in the focus and emphasis of the role and consequently presents approaches that can lead to safe and effective staffing decisions.

Useful Websites

American College of Nurse-Midwives: http://www.midwife.org/

Canadian Midwifery Regulators Council, Canadian Midwifery Regulators Council: http://www.cmrc-ccosf.ca

College of Midwives of British Columbia, College of Midwives of British Columbia: http://cmbc.bc.ca

International Confederation of Midwives: https://www.internationalmidwives.org

The *Lancet* series on midwifery: https://www.thelancet.com/series/midwifery

National Council of State Boards of Nursing: https://www.ncsbn.org

Nursing and Midwifery Board of Australia: https://www.nursingmidwiferyboard.gov.au

Nursing and Midwifery Council: https://www.nmc.org.uk

Public Health England: https://www.gov.uk/government/organisations/public-health-england

Royal College of Midwives: https://www.rcm.org.uk

Royal Pharmaceutical Society: https://www.rpharms.com

Skills for Health: http://www.skillsforhealth.org.uk

United Nations Population Fund: https://www.unfpa.org

CHAPTER 9

Facilitating Safety in Midwifery Education and Practice

Hannah G. Dahlen ▪ Lindsay J. Gillman

CONTENTS

LEARNING OUTCOMES

By the end of this chapter the reader should:
- have an overview of the concepts of risk and safety as applied to midwifery practice
- understand how to assess risk appropriately
- be able to reflect on the influence of midwifery and obstetric philosophy in the provision of care that supports physiological birth
- gain an understanding of how to facilitate safe birth in a risk-averse environment
- have an awareness of how international organizations can support safe childbirth

Overview

This chapter explores the concepts of risk and safety and how managing risk is not the same as facilitating safety. The fears that women and health providers may have about birth are presented along with determination of how midwives can empower women to trust in their ability to give birth and be mothers. The existing research that supports physiological birth, including ways of instilling confidence about normal birth in both women and midwives, is also examined. Exposure to environments in which safe physiological birth is facilitated is an important aspect of midwifery education which will impact on the development of a midwife's individual philosophy and future practice. The place of birth, the impact that various models of care have on birth, and the importance of effective relationships are also critically explored.

Introduction

Facilitating safety for women and babies during pregnancy, birth and early motherhood should always be the top priority for all maternity health care providers. However, there are often differences of opinion in defining what constitutes safety, and how to best facilitate it. In reality, it is usual that when health care providers discuss safety, what is often discussed is the concept of *risk*, and as Dahlen (2014) purports, *safety* and *risk* are not the same thing. Risk represents a threat to well-being, whilst safety represents the modification of threat and return to equilibrium of well-being. *Risk* is a fear-inducing concept, and so easily can turn into 'shroud waving' that can coerce vulnerable women into making choices they do not want to make, or have not fully understood the implications of (Dahlen 2011). *Safety*, on the other hand, is a concept of hope, positivity and possibilities, but most critically it encompasses not just physical safety but psychological, social, cultural and spiritual safety as well, and so positions the person as central to care, exploring the individual needs of that person. Managing risk therefore is not the same as facilitating safety.

Facilitating Safety Versus Managing Risk

Dahlen and Gutteridge (2015) use the analogy of an adult teaching a child to ride a bicycle to show how highlighting the risk of hitting the wall ahead increases the child's anxiety and reduces their enjoyment such that there is a higher possibility of them riding into the wall. Once the child has been alerted to the wall, they tend to focus on it and begin to concentrate on avoiding the wall and not riding on the path. The result of this is that they are no longer riding safely; their joy decreases, their anxiety increases and the chances of actually riding into the wall escalate. They will most probably avoid the wall but the extent to which they have enjoyed the experience and may consider continuing to master the skill could be questioned. In maternity care the message constantly sent to women and maternity care professionals is to avoid such 'a wall' (Dahlen and Gutteridge 2015). When important aspects of safety (psychological, social, cultural and spiritual factors) are subsumed under a fixation of risk, the result is so often traumatized women and dehumanized care, and this in itself creates additional risks (Jackson et al 2012).

PERSONAL PERCEPTION OF RISK

The perception of risk is very much an individual and unique concept. Even where there appears to be shared understandings of risk (such as within clinical policies and guidelines) there is rarely a similar understanding between health care providers, women and their families. Risk perception is a subjective assessment that is made by individuals and is informed by what matters most to them, their past experiences, how trusting they are of those providing information and choice, and how much they perceive they have to lose or gain. The example in Box 9.1 of the *three little*

> **BOX 9.1** ■ *'Little Pig, Little Pig I Will Blow Your House Down'*: Assumptions and Reality
>
> The story of the three little pigs tells of a brick house that could not be blown down by the big bad wolf. The implied wisdom in the story is that the third little pig managed the risk of having his house blown down by the big bad wolf through ensuring that his house was made of brick. To the human, the thought of a wolf blowing down a house would appear impossible. The story of Anna (a pseudonym), told by one of the authors (HD), illustrates how risk perception is uniquely personal.
>
> *After many days of trying to find housing for Anna, a pregnant woman in my caseload who was homeless and emerging from a violent relationship, I was so excited to tell her we had found a place for her to live. Expecting joy and gratitude I watched her impassive face as she received this news. After a long pause she asked, 'Do you know if it is a brick house?' I felt my impatience rise. How ungrateful, I thought, after all the effort we had gone to. It was a house and she surely did not have the right to be fussy. As I calmed myself down and thought of how to answer diplomatically, Anna went on to explain, 'You see, the bullets from drive-by shootings go right through the walls of the fibro house we had, and I was hoping a brick wall might stop them better.' Anna's violent life had not ended when her husband was charged with domestic violence, because he was now ordering hits on her from jail. I felt ashamed and I learned a valuable lesson; there are big bad wolves out there, and the fact I never have to worry about this does not mean this is not a high priority on someone else's list. Talking to Anna about diet and quitting smoking, when stopping the bullets is the only thing that currently matters to her, is slightly ridiculous. Being alive had become Anna's priority. Being alive for me is just an assumption. The way we could facilitate safety for Anna was by finding her a house with brick walls.*

pigs illustrates how perceptions about what is risky and how safety is defined are deeply personal, utterly individual and very hard to anticipate without relationship-based care that puts the woman and her needs at the centre.

A personal understanding of risk is equated with the potential for loss or damage, and the response to risk is therefore more context driven, understandably related to social and situational experiences (Carolan 2008). Exposure to elements in life and the areas in which personal expertise lies will influence the way an individual makes judgements about what is risky and what is safe. Although the personal concept of risk may include multiple variables, organizational risk assessment processes use the concept of *probability* and *consequence* to determine relative risk, or a statistical calculation of *odds and ratios*.

HEALTH PROFESSIONALS' PERCEPTION OF SAFETY AND RISK

Health professionals are not immune to their own view of what safety and risk comprise, and this will impact on the advice and care they provide. A commonly cited study from the United Kingdom (UK) (Al-Mufti et al 1997) showed that 31% of female obstetricians would opt for a caesarean section for their own births. Obstetricians have used this study to argue that this indicates the choice an informed group of women would make regarding the mode of birth if given the option (Thornton and Lubowski 2006). However, studies from countries where the caesarean section rate is low, such as Norway, Denmark and the Netherlands, have shown that a lower proportion of obstetricians (1.1–2%) would choose caesarean section for themselves or their partners (Backe et al 2002; Bergholt et al 2004).

Differences in risk perception between women and professionals have also been identified (Turner et al 2008). The study explored the level of morbidity that woman would be willing to accept from a vaginal birth before requesting an elective caesarean section. Their views were compared with those of clinicians providing care to childbearing women (midwives, obstetricians, urogynaecologists and colorectal surgeons). The women in this study were willing to accept higher risks than clinicians for all 17 complications presented to them. The views of midwives were

---

BOX 9.2 ■ Tips for Midwives to Deal With Fear

- Identify the fears.
- Share your fear/s with someone you trust.
- Take responsibility for your fears: most are a creation in your mind.
- Breathe and slow everything down so you can think.
- Watch the self talk and practice stopping negative thoughts.
- Use positive visualization.
- Have a cup of tea.
- Knit or crochet at births: it reduces adrenaline levels.
- Undertake an obstetric emergency skills course.
- Write about your fear and reflect on what influences it.
- Centre yourself with affirmations such as 'trust in the process'.
- Be sceptical when others fuel fear: gather information, think carefully.
- Beware the language of fear as it has many forms.
- Remember the loudest voice in the room usually indicates the most frightened.
- Balance your fear with faith in human female physiology.
- Reassure each other, so that you can reassure women that birth is *normal*.
- Facilitate women to trust in their ability to handle the outcome, whatever it may be.
- Retell the positive stories about birth to each other and to women.
- Most importantly, shed the fear and do not carry it to the next birth.

From Dahlen and Caplice (2014).

---

closest to those of the pregnant women, whilst urogynaecologists and colorectal surgeons were the most risk averse. The differences in the results from both studies suggest that the participants were informed of risk through the knowledge and experience obtained through their own professional practice, which was subsequently reflected in their personal choice regarding perception of risk and mode of birth.

It is therefore likely that midwives who are repeatedly exposed to situations in which childbirth is viewed as potentially pathological perceive birth to be risky unless it is medically managed. This has the potential to create a vicious cycle creating a fear of birth that midwives (and student midwives) may be completely unaware of, until they are exposed to other models and ways of working. Dahlen and Caplice (2014) provide helpful tips for midwives to support them in dealing with fear (Box 9.2).

Place of Birth and Safety

Reviewing the history of risk perception in childbirth is useful when one is considering the way in which maternity services have been shaped over the centuries, with fluctuating acceptance and rejection of the social and medical models of care. The concept of improving safety in childbirth is usually considered to be the main driver for the provision of maternity services. The evidence, however, does not support the view that the current medical model of maternity care is the safest option; and yet it remains the predominant model in the developed world. The reality of the medical model is often a depersonalized reductionist approach, which gained acceptance as the cultural norm in the 1970s and 1980s, influencing the development of an industrialized system in which pregnant women were viewed as baby-carrying units that needed to be monitored, investigated, measured and delivered on time (Walsh 2006; Gould 2011).

Before this era of the scientific-technocratic approach, maternity care provision in the UK was largely based on a social model of care in which local midwives and family doctors worked in partnership. However, this model was disrupted with the publication of the Peel report (Department of Health and Social Security 1970), built on the earlier foundations of the Cranbrook report (Ministry of Health 1959), which stated that maternity beds should be available to all women regardless of risk. This recommendation, however, was quickly adopted as a directive, and the provision for home- and community-based birth diminished. This position remained largely unchallenged for decades, even in the presence of evidence that refuted this model as the safest or preferred option for women (Tew 1985; De Jonge et al 2009; Brocklehurst et al 2011; Sandall et al 2015). The findings of national maternity service reviews in England over the past three decades have recommended that the provision should be more woman centred, and that continuity of care, rather than an increase in surveillance and medical intervention, is the critical factor for safe maternity care provision (Department of Health 1993, 2007; NHS England 2016).

Most births in middle- and high-income countries take place in a hospital setting. A report into the safety of childbirth in England reported that births outside an obstetric unit are relatively uncommon, amounting to just 8% of women (Brocklehurst et al 2011), which is not representative of women's preferences. In a recent survey of 5500 women, only 25% would choose to give birth in hospital, 10% would prefer a home birth and 65% would prefer to give birth in a midwifery-led unit (NHS England 2016). In the United States of America the proportion of women giving birth in an obstetric environment is even higher, at 98.6%, with only 1.4% of births occurring outside hospital (Martin et al 2015).

The National Institute for Health and Care Excellence (NICE) (2014) evidence-based guideline for intrapartum care recommends a return to holistic, community-based woman- and family-centred care, supporting out-of-hospital environments for women without identified risk factors. This reflects the recognition of the short-term and long-term health benefits of physiological birth for both women and their babies. The recommendations in the National Maternity Review *Better Births* report (NHS England 2016) recognize the importance of personalized care in the provision of *safe* maternity services, with the vision being the provision of a kinder, family-friendly service focused around women's individual needs and circumstances.

These recommendations have been informed by a number of other national reviews concerning the safety of the current medical model of maternity care. The underlying theme that was identified as a significant risk was the presence of the two *'necessarily different'* approaches to or philosophies of birth, exemplified in the two professions responsible for care provision. The report acknowledged the need for *respectful partnership working*, and that when there is too little understanding or appreciation of the other's contribution; debate between the professions is destructive and puts women and babies of adverse outcomes (King's Fund 2008).

Philosophies of Maternity Care Provision

The *'necessarily different'* approaches to childbearing identified in the report as a risk to safe care (King's Fund 2008) have evolved as a result of the development of the medical and midwifery professions over the last century. It is important to consider the philosophical position and paradigm within which midwifery and obstetrics operate to understand how the approaches have developed, and how tensions between the professions have arisen. The turbulent history of the relationship between the professions is well documented, and it is clear to see where certain historical events have shifted the power dynamic and the control over childbirth (Donnison 1988; Mander 2002; Allotey 2010). Before the introduction of the man-midwife in the 17th century, women and their female attendants held *authoritative knowledge* in the domain of childbirth. As medicine developed into a scientific discipline, the profession gained a position of *cultural authority*, economic power and political influence that led to the medicalized approach to childbearing becoming the accepted norm, upheld as the authoritative knowledge system (Jordan 1997). A more detailed overview of the history and professionalization of midwifery is provided in Chapter 1.

Previous experiences of and exposure to different approaches to birth will shape an individual's understanding and perspective and their view on the authority of knowledge systems. An understanding of how the different professional groups may identify and facilitate safety is important and may be conducive to creating partnerships based on trust between the professions. *Midwifery philosophy* is based on the social model of pregnancy and birth, recognizing that these are normal physiological life events and that overall well-being is an important aspect of the outcome. *Obstetric philosophy* supports the medical model, in which pregnancy is viewed as a potentially pathological state to be monitored and managed, with success measured in physical health outcomes.

Obstetricians, midwives and women will perceive risk and safety differently depending on their philosophical view and their personal experiences. As previously discussed, this individual perspective will affect what constitutes acceptable levels of risk and will influence how decisions about managing pregnancy and birth are made (Hunter 2004; Hunter 2008; MacKenzie Bryers and van Teijlingen 2010; Lokugamage 2011; Carlson and Lowe 2013).

Hunter (2004) identified two midwifery ideologies of '*with institution*', a model of care dominated by meeting service needs through a medicalized approach, and '*with woman*', which supports an individualized, natural approach to maternity care. Those who have witnessed physiological undisturbed birth and observed the midwifery art of *watchful waiting* (see the next section) may be more likely to support the social model of '*with woman*' maternity care. Conversely, if personal experience is limited to that of intervention when pathology is identified, the medical model may be viewed as the one with the least risk, and therefore the preferred option. Dahlen (2010) stresses that a fear of childbirth and the view that it is a risky process will have a strong influence on the type of care health professionals are willing to provide.

Midwives who are confident in the physiological processes of birth may use strategies to protect women from the risk of medicalization, often as a *risk-negotiator*, balancing both scientific and intuitive knowledge to inform their clinical decision-making. The concept of *risking normality*, defined by Dove and Muir-Cochrane (2014), encompasses the activities that midwives undertake to mitigate the risk of obstetric practices that do not facilitate physiological birth, and are not evidence based. This role of risk-negotiator is vital if midwives are to facilitate care that contributes to safe birthing outcomes for women. The trusting relationship between the childbearing woman and the midwife, gained through the provision of continuity of care, are key elements that enable this to happen.

Midwives working in both obstetric-led and out-of-hospital environments have described the practice of protecting women from unnecessary medical intervention through regulating the physical environment and through mediation with medical colleagues (Crabtree 2008; Priddis et al 2011). These midwives reported that they actively encouraged women to surround themselves with protective buffers and reinforced this with knowledge of instinctive birthing practices.

MacKenzie Bryers and van Teijlingen (2010) assert that the case may be that health care professionals do not confine their practice within a totally dualistic world where one philosophy or model is dominant but find that their practice is somewhere on a continuum, recognizing elements of the knowledge systems that underpin them both as partially or wholly valid. The process of clinical decision-making and the assessment of risk and safety rely on the multifaceted skills of the health care professional, the interpretation of the information they have and the experience and expertise they possess. This variation may be seen within the professions as well as between them. Priddis et al (2011) recognize that organizational culture with its compliance with accepted cultural norms can influence the way in which individual health care professionals practise.

WATCHFUL WAITING

In any setting, if there are fundamentally differing points of view of a concept, this in itself has the potential to create misunderstanding and miscommunication. An example of this can be seen with the concept of *watchful waiting*. Carlson and Lowe (2013) describe how midwives and obstetricians use this term to describe a fundamentally different activity. From a midwifery perspective the term is used to describe a period in which calm, non-invasive therapeutic support is provided to facilitate a woman to labour and give birth to her baby physiologically; Borelli (2013) refers to the term as "masterful inactivity" to describe this. For obstetricians, the term *watchful waiting* is a risk-based strategy usually defined as a period of intrapartum observation undertaken to avoid immediate intervention whilst undertaking active surveillance of the woman and fetus. Eason and Feldman (2000: 617) also describe the difficulty that the art of watchful waiting during the second stage of labour may present, depending on the perspective of the professional attending the birth:

> For those of a more 'surgical personality,' watchfully waiting for the perineum to stretch and verbally guiding a mother through the end of the second stage is much more difficult than just getting the infant out. 'Don't just do something, sit there!' requires discipline and assurance.

Such fundamental difference in perspective has the potential to create misunderstanding, compromise safety and create tensions in professional relationships. In an effort to reduce this, engagement in activities in which the professions can learn with, and about, each other should be embedded into the culture of maternity service models and in undergraduate programmes for midwives and obstetricians (NHS England 2016). The professions of midwifery and obstetrics are not exclusive but are complementary to each other; a mutual understanding of the expertise and knowledge each brings to childbirth can only lead to safer care for childbearing women and their babies.

Developing and Instilling Confidence in Physiological Birth

It may seem a peculiar concept that there is a need to instil confidence in the normal physiological process of giving birth as it is rare that an individual loses confidence in other physiological bodily functions. In 21st century society, being pregnant and giving birth are viewed as an inherently risky activity, and yet as observed in the latter half of the last century by Montgomery (1958: 706)

> '...there is no more need to interfere with the course of normally progressing labour than there is to tamper with good digestion, normal respiration and adequate circulation.'

In countries where there is a health infrastructure and women are cared for by trained and qualified birth attendants, it is recognized that childbirth is generally a safe event. Although this is the case, maternity care provision remains predominantly technocratic, driven by the underlying principle that birth is a potentially pathological process viewed only as normal in retrospect (Dahlen 2010; Coxon et al 2014; Dove and Muir-Cochrane 2014). To provide care based on a more social model, midwives need to engage in activities that restore their confidence in the physiology of birth and the importance of birth as a sociological life event. Box 9.3 provides suggestions of ways in which midwives may develop confidence to facilitate physiological birth that complement the top ten tips for safety and survival during home birth produced by Dahlen (2012).

The importance of situating midwifery care within community-based models has been recognized as a key factor in normalizing birth (Chief Nursing Officers of England, Northern Ireland, Scotland and Wales 2010, NHS England 2016), and is crucial in the future education

---

BOX 9.3 ■ Ways to Develop Confidence in Facilitating Physiological Birth

■ Engage with story-telling and the use of narrative to expand your experience of physiological births.

■ Spend time with midwives who are confident in facilitating physiological birth in a variety of settings, such as home birth, birth centres and independent practice.

■ Use language that supports a physiological and holistic approach to care: replace *delivery* with *birth* in your vocabulary and think about making other changes to the language that you use.

■ Engage with groups who recognize the importance of holistic care and respect women's knowledge as authoritative and valid (e.g. Positive Birth Movement, Birth Without Fear, National Childbirth Trust).

■ Nurture authentic relationships with women, do not be fearful of connection: remember that such connection is key to providing safe care.

---

of midwives to ensure early professional socialization into midwifery. Historically the student learning experience for midwives has been dominated by a hospital-based system, with opportunities for working within a caseloading model or independent midwifery practice seen as the exception rather than the norm. However, gaining experience of a woman-centred way of working positively impacts on student midwives' perceptions of childbearing, promotes confidence and competence in midwifery skills and enables them to build emotional trusting relationships with women (Aune et al 2011; Rawnson 2011; Dawson et al 2015). Embedding this approach to learning and consolidation into pre-registration midwifery curricula is important in enabling newly qualified midwives to maintain a midwifery philosophy and preserve a woman-centred approach.

Facilitating Safe Labour in a Risk-Averse Environment

The scientific-technocratic approach to risk management in childbirth has increased the rate of intervention without improving maternal or perinatal outcomes and is rarely critically examined. Hunter et al (2008) highlight that research findings which support the social model have been largely ignored, particularly qualitative research exploring women's experiences of their care during pregnancy and birth. The iatrogenic risk of unnecessary intervention, particularly operative birth, had been largely ignored and unchallenged until the publication of the epigenetic remodelling EPIIC (Epigenetic Impact of Childbirth) hypothesis (Dahlen et al 2013a). However, there are numerous examples of practices that have not been shown to bring benefit to childbearing women or babies yet remain part of the medicalized pattern of maternity care. Some of the practices that occur during the management of labour in obstetric-led maternity units are a prime example of this and are explored in the following sections. Repeated exposure to these ways of working without critical appraisal can lead to an acceptance of such practice as the norm, resulting in a skewed view of the elements that constitute safe care.

USE OF THE PARTOGRAM

Guidelines and policies for the management of labour and birth within the medical model are usually based on the progress of labour being measured by, and confined within, the numerical parameters of time, cervical dilatation and fetal descent. The use of a partogram or partograph to document progress is recommended by NICE (2014) and the World Health Organization (WHO) (2014) to visually assess progress and identify when intervention is required. It is also acknowledged that the evidence to support the use of the partogram is poor and that unnecessary intervention can negatively affect childbirth outcomes (Lavender et al 2012). NICE (2014), however, has since acknowledged that the progress of labour is not always linear and that the duration of labour differs from woman to woman.

The preoccupation with time and measurement is driven by the underlying fear that the length of labour, particularly the second stage, is detrimental for both the woman and the baby. However, there is limited high-quality evidence to suggest that this is the case. The collective available evidence suggests that the normal parameters for the second stage of labour may be 3 hours from the start of the active phase for a primigravida and 2 hours from the start of the active phase for a multigravida (NICE 2014). Interventions to shorten both stages of labour, however, continue to be used in the management of birth in the absence of evidence to support their use and even where there is evidence that they may cause harm.

VAGINAL EXAMINATIONS IN LABOUR

Regular vaginal examinations to assess progress in labour continue to be a standard component of maternity care. However, although the NICE (2014) guidelines for intrapartum care state vaginal examinations should be offered every 4 hours, they also acknowledge that the evidence on which this recommendation is based is of low quality. A Cochrane review (Downe et al 2012) found there was no evidence to support routine vaginal examination, which is extraordinary considering how routine this has become. Walsh (2012) acknowledges that midwives know that women's bodies do not fit a standard template for progress in labour and may use strategies to avoid documenting progress in the prescribed way. Midwives who work in out-of-hospital environments and within continuity-of-care models appear to undertake vaginal examination less routinely, based solely on need; however, they have described being viewed as *rebels* (Winter 2002; Dahlen et al 2013b). As Scammell and Stewart (2014) note, practising in a *'with woman'* rather than a *'with institution'* way may involve a complex system of managing risk and time, engaging in covert activities that reduce the risk of unnecessary medical intervention.

BIRTH POSITIONS

The position that women adopt for birth is a classic example of how the optimal position and the culturally accepted position differ, with the evidence for optimal birth positions frequently not translated into practice. It has been accepted for a long time that there are both psychological and physical benefits for women when they are able to choose an upright position during labour and birth; however, in many obstetric units the bed is the focus of the birthing room and the woman is expected to use it. If the woman's ability to choose the position she gives birth in is compromised, care provision may be considered disempowering, abusive and humiliating (Gupta et al 2012). There is also flagrant disregard for the woman as an autonomous and active participant in the birth process.

Surveillance interventions such as continuous fetal heart rate monitoring may shift the focus of attention from the woman to the machine, and her autonomy to move around as she wishes may not be respected (Priddis et al 2012). In environments where women are protected from unnecessary surveillance by a strong sense of midwifery autonomy and advocacy, Priddis et al (2012) also acknowledge that they are more likely to be able to adopt positions that enable them to labour and birth instinctively and avoid intervention.

PERINEAL PROTECTION

Perineal protection during birth is a controversial topic, debated widely by obstetricians and midwives because the recorded cases of severe perineal trauma (third- and fourth-degree tears) have

TABLE 9.1 ■ Risk Management: Basic Questions

What could go wrong?	Risk identification.
What are the chances of it going wrong and what would be the impact?	Risk analysis and evaluation
What can we do to minimize the chance of this happening or to mitigate damage when it has gone wrong?	Risk treatment: the cost of prevention is compared with the costs of getting it wrong
What can we learn from things that have gone wrong?	Risk control: sharing and learning

From Royal College of Obstetricians and Gynaecologists (2009).

increased over the past decade (Gurol-Urganci et al 2013; Dahlen et al 2015). From the data analysed, the risk of sustaining severe perineal trauma was six times more likely with an instrumental (forceps) birth and an episiotomy than during a physiological birth. However, it has been suggested that a change in midwifery practice to not use the hands to flex the fetal head and support the perineum at birth as routine may also be a factor causing an increase in the incidence of severe perineal trauma (Trochez et al 2011; Gurol-Urganci et al 2013).

The application of warm packs to the perineum has been shown to achieve the most significant reduction in the incidence of severe perineal trauma of all known techniques (Aasheim et al 2012). In addition to this, Dahlen (2007) and Dahlen et al (2009) have also found that warm packs applied to the perineum provide women with significant comfort in the second stage of labour that is equal to that provided by an epidural, but without the side effects. It is interesting that although this simple intervention would appear to improve a woman's experience and reduce the risk of severe perineal trauma, it is has not been widely adopted in practice.

The most recent guidelines from the Royal College of Obstetricians and Gynaecologists (2015) advocate the use of manual perineal protection to minimize perineal trauma; however, the evidence-based NICE (2014) guideline for intrapartum care does not make a recommendation for either the 'hands-on' or the 'hands-poised' approach, supported by further systematic reviews (Bulchandani et al 2015; Petrocnik and Marshall 2015). The recommendation for a 'hands-on' approach from the Royal College of Obstetricians and Gynaecologists (2015) reflects the medical lens through which birth is viewed. Such an approach presupposes that women are giving birth in a position which makes observation and manipulation possible and that they will be passive recipients of such an intimate and uncomfortable intervention. It also reinforces the discourse that women's bodies need to managed and manipulated in order to deliver them of their babies rather than supporting them to give birth (Dahlen et al 2015).

As discussed throughout this chapter, perception of risk is highly individual and influenced by a number of factors, particularly personal experience, knowledge and philosophy. However, to make objective judgements about risk, it is important to consider the likelihood of something happening in relation to the consequence of that outcome happening. Table 9.1 illustrates the basic questions used within the concept of relative risk determination using *probability* and *consequence*.

Making the Change: Facilitating Safety Rather Than Managing Risk

Making the transition from a maternity system that culturally views pregnancy and birth as risky and frightening to one that facilitates safety and sees birth as a physiological, emotional and spiritual process that can be powerful, beautiful and life-affirming is a challenge for all midwives to fulfil. Pregnancy and birth are more than just clinical episodes for women; they are periods of social and psychological transition of tremendous significance. However, the risk-averse climate often creates fear in both the health care professional providing maternity care and the woman receiving it. De Vries (2012) suggests that to provide safe maternity care there must be a professional balance to create an optimal environment where the key elements of *fear* and *trust* are in equilibrium.

There are numerous examples in which the professions of midwifery and obstetrics have not worked harmoniously, where the result has been that fear has overwhelmed trust, either between the health care professional groups involved or between the woman and her care provider. The investigation into the series of events at the University Hospitals of Morecambe Bay NHS Foundation Trust reported that there was a culture of pursuing normal birth at any cost, culminating in a situation that tragically led to avoidable harm and death of women and babies (Kirkup 2015). It was reported that working relationships were extremely poor, particularly between different staff groups, such as obstetricians, paediatricians and midwives. In the high-profile case of Elizabeth Montgomery (*Montgomery v Lanarkshire* [2015]) a reluctance to intervene by the obstetrician in the presence of risk led to poor outcomes for both the mother and the baby (see Chapter 7). In Ireland, the policy for midwifery attendance at home birth beyond term created a breakdown of trust between a pregnant mother and the maternity care system, causing her to leave her home for fear of being hospitalized for induction against her will (O'Boyle 2015). In each of these examples, a domination of one discourse occurred, leading to poor outcomes.

The balance between fear and trust can be created only when the root of fear is identified and a relationship of trust nurtured. Understanding and valuing the contribution of both midwifery and obstetrics in childbirth is the key to beginning to make the change.

Relationships: The '*Glue That Holds It Together*'

It is acknowledged that for women to be in a position to really choose where and how to give birth they need to be able to exercise high levels of personal autonomy and agency and have support from those who trust their judgements and decisions. Even with this support, women's choices are often constrained by the dominant discourse of risk (Coxon et al 2014). Women who are vulnerable and do not have such support are less able to exercise personal autonomy.

The latest review of the triennial confidential enquiry into maternal deaths in the UK indicates that women from vulnerable populations have a disproportionate risk of dying prematurely (Knight et al 2018). Vulnerability can present in a variety of ways and may be as a result of women being in particularly difficult social situations, such as being a refugee or seeking asylum. Other factors include poverty, homelessness, substance misuse, difficulty in speaking or understanding the language of the country in which care is provided, or being very young (NICE 2010). These factors may lead to compromise in personal autonomy and agency and a feeling of powerlessness for such women, who particularly require continuity of care from a midwife with whom they can develop a trusting relationship to improve their childbirth outcomes.

A Cochrane systematic review of midwife-led continuity-of-care models by Sandall et al (2015) affirmed there is no better way to facilitate safety for women and babies than through such an approach. Relationship-based care is safe physically, psychologically, socially, culturally and spiritually. The woman–midwife relationship has been identified as the '*glue that holds it together*' (Leap et al 2011), or the '*hidden threads in the tapestry of maternity care*' (Hunter et al 2008). Sandall et al (2015) found that women who get to know their midwives have less birth intervention, are more satisfied and have fewer adverse perinatal outcomes. Tracy et al (2013) demonstrated that for women of any risk, caseload midwifery is cost-effective and safe. The evidence is now so strong that it could be considered unethical not to offer all women this model of care, and for governments to prioritize funding towards this. The latest National Maternity Review (NHS England 2016) recommended more continuity of midwifery care, more midwife-led out-of-hospital births and even a new personal maternity care budget worth £3000 so that women can choose their maternity care providers. Despite the overwhelming evidence that midwife-led continuity-of-care models are the safest option for women, their babies and their families, it still is a phenomenon that many women throughout the world do not have access to.

Global Strategies to Promote Safety in Low-Resource Countries

A number of organizations provide vital health care work and advocacy to promote safer maternal and newborn health around the world, particularly in low-resource countries; for example the *Partnership for Safe Motherhood and Newborn Health* and the *White Ribbon Alliance.*

SAFE MOTHERHOOD CAMPAIGN

Every year hundreds of thousands of women die of complications related to pregnancy and birth. Sadly, the burden of mortality is carried by the developing world, and most deaths are avoidable (Islam 2007). To address this, the WHO along with other international agencies launched the Safe Motherhood Initiative in 1987. In 2004 this was expanded to form the *Partnership for Safe Motherhood and Newborn Health*. Safe motherhood focuses on six key factors:

- family planning
- antenatal care
- obstetric care
- postnatal care
- postabortion care
- sexually transmitted infection/HIV control.

WHITE RIBBON ALLIANCE

The White Ribbon Alliance is a global network of maternal health advocates and was convened to unite people from around the world to demand the right to safe birth for all women in all countries. The White Ribbon Alliance was launched in 1999 as an informal coalition of non-governmental organizations, donors and global partners to generate worldwide attention about the importance of making safe motherhood a priority for all. Today there are more than 13 national alliances in countries all over the world. The goal of the White Ribbon Alliance is to ensure all women realize their rights to be safe and healthy before, during and following birth, with a focus on holding governments accountable, and to campaign for them to deliver on their commitments. Campaign activities include:

- advocating for free contraception
- increasing the numbers of births attended by skilled birth attendants
- recognizing women's rights during childbirth.

Conclusion

When the evidence unequivocally points to birth as a predominantly safe event in the presence of a trained birth attendant in countries with developed health infrastructures, it is difficult to justify the problematization and medicalization of childbearing. The dominant discourse is that of risk, which creates fear. Wagner (2007) suggests that this has occurred in a number of ways, one of which is by redefining pregnancy and birth as a problem for which the medical profession can create and provide a solution. This scientific approach to risk emphasizes that pregnancy and birth is an event that must be managed by experts, with constant monitoring and investigation to detect and manage any perceived abnormality.

There is overwhelming evidence that supports the concept of physiological birth as a safe process where skilled midwives are an integral part of the woman's pregnancy and childbearing, especially through continuity-of-care models, of which student midwives *must* be a part of. As a consequence, the woman is less likely to experience unnecessary intervention, with subsequent physical and emotional outcomes improved in both the short term and the long term. This model of care allows finite resources to be used appropriately and rationally where they are required for specialist services. The dominant medical discourse must be replaced by a holistic biosocial one in which women are encouraged and supported to recognize the power of physiology and to trust in their body's ability to give birth. Coxon et al (2014) purport that a revolution in which a sociocultural repositioning of childbirth, with birth outside a medical setting being viewed as normative and acceptable practice, has to take place.

KEY POINTS

- Managing risk is not the same as facilitating safety.
- *Risk* is a fear-inducing concept, *Safety*, on the other hand, is a concept of hope, positivity and possibilities.
- The perception of risk is very much an individual and unique concept. Personal responses to risk are related to social and situational experiences.
- Working within woman-centred social models of care can enhance perceptions of childbearing as a physiological process and promote confidence and competence in midwifery skills.
- Professional partnerships between midwives and obstetricians based on mutual trust and respect are integral to the provision of safe, woman-centred care.
- Midwifery-led continuity-of-care models are the safest option for women of all risks: *all* women need a midwife, and *some* will need an obstetrician.

References

Aasheim, V., Nilsen, A. B. V., Lukasse, M., & Reinar, L. M. (2012). Perineal techniques during the second stage of labour for reducing perineal trauma. *Cochrane Database of Systematic Reviews.* https://doi.org/10.1002/14651858.CD006672.pub2.

Allotey, J. C. (2010). English midwives responses to the medicalisation of childbirth (1671-1795). *Midwifery, 27,* 532–538.

Al-Mufti, R., McCarthy, A., & Fisk, N. M. (1997). Survey of obstetricians' personal preference and discretionary practice. *European Journal of Obstetrics, Gynaecology and Reproductive Biology, 73*(1), 1–4.

Aune, I., Dahlberg, U., & Ingebrigtsen, O. (2011). Relational continuity as a model of care in practical midwifery studies. *British Journal of Midwifery, 19*(8), 515–523.

Backe, B., Salvesen, K. A., & Sviggum, O. (2002). Norwegian obstetricians prefer vaginal route of delivery. *The Lancet, 359*(9306), 629.

Bergholt, T., Ostberg, B., Legarth, J., & Weber, T. (2004). Danish obstetricians' personal preference and general attitude to elective caesarean section on maternal request: a nation-wide postal survey. *Acta Obstetrica et Gynecologica Scandinvica, 83,* 262–266.

Borelli, S. E. (2013). What is a good midwife? Some historical considerations. *Royal College of Midwives, Evidence Based Midwifery, 11*(2), 51–59.

Brocklehurst, P., Hardy, P., Hollowell, J., Linsell, L., Macfarlane, A., McCourt, C., & Birthplace in England Collaborative Group. (2011). Perinatal and maternal outcomes by planned place of birth for healthy women with low risk pregnancies: the Birthplace in England national prospective cohort study. *British Medical Journal, 343,* d7400.

Bulchandani, S., Watts, E., Sucharitha, A., Yates, D., & Ismail, K. M. (2015). Manual perineal support at the time of childbirth: a systematic review and meta-analysis. *BJOG: An International Journal of Obstetrics and Gynaecology, 122*(9), 1157–1165.

Carlson, N. S., & Lowe, N. K. (2013). A concept analysis of watchful waiting among providers caring for women in labour. *Journal of Advanced Nursing, 70*(3), 511–522.

Carolan, M. C. (2008). Towards understanding the concept of risk for pregnant women: Some nursing and midwifery implications. *Journal of Clinical Nursing, 18,* 652–658.

Chief Nursing Officers of England, Northern Ireland, Scotland and Wales. (2010). Midwifery 2020: Delivering expectations. Available at: https://www.gov.uk/government/uploads/system/uploads/attachment_data/file/216029/dh_119470.pdf.

Coxon, K., Sandall, J., & Fulop, N. J. (2014). To what extent are women free to choose where to give birth? How discourses of risk, blame and responsibility influence birth place decisions. *Health, Risk and Society, 16*(1), 51–57.

Crabtree, S. (2008). Midwives constructing 'normal birth'. In Downe, S., (Ed.), *Normal childbirth: Evidence and debate* (pp. 97–113). Edinburgh: Churchill Livingstone.

Dahlen, H. G. (2007). *Reduction of perineal trauma and improved perineal comfort during and after childbirth: The Perineal Warm Pack Trial. PhD thesis.* Sydney: University of Technology Sydney.

Dahlen, H. G. (2010). Undone by fear? Deluded by trust? *Midwifery, 26,* 156–162.

Dahlen, H. G. (2011). Perspectives on risk or risk in perspective? *Essentially MIDIRS, 2*(7), 17–21.

Dahlen, H. G. (2012). Homebirth: ten tips for safety and survival. *British Journal of Midwifery, 20*(12), 774–778.

Dahlen, H. G. (2014). Managing risk or facilitating safety? *International Journal of Childbirth, 4*(2), 66–68.

Dahlen, H. G., Homer, C. S. E., Cooke, M., Upton, A., Nunn, R. A., & Brodrick, B. S. (2009). "Soothing the ring of fire". Australian women and midwives experience of using perineal warm packs in the second stage of labour. *Midwifery, 25,* 39–48.

Dahlen, H. G., Kennedy, H. P., Anderson, C. M., Bell, A. F., Clark, A., Foureur, M., et al. (2013a). The EPIIC hypothesis: Intrapartum effects on the neonatal epigenome and consequent health outcomes. *Medical Hypothesis, 80*(5), 656–662.

Dahlen, H. G., Downe, S., Duff, M., & Gyte, G. (2013b). Vaginal examination during normal labour: Routine examination or routine intervention? *International Journal of Childbirth, 3*(3), 142–152.

Dahlen, H. G., & Caplice, S. (2014). What do midwives fear? *Women and Birth, 27*(4), 266–270.

Dahlen, H. G., Priddis, H., & Thornton, C. (2015). Severe perineal trauma is rising, but let us not overreact. *Midwifery, 31,* 1–8.

Dahlen, H. G., & Gutteridge, K. (2015). Stop the fear and embrace birth. In Byrom, S., & Downe, S., (Eds.), *The roar behind the silence: Why kindness, compassion and respect matter in maternity care* (pp. 98–104). London: Pinter and Martin.

Dawson, K., Newton, M., Forster, D., & McLachlan, H. (2015). Exploring midwifery students' views and experiences of caseload midwifery: A cross-sectional survey conducted in Victoria, Australia. *Midwifery, 31*(2), e7–e15.

De Jonge, A., van der Goes, B., Ravelli, A., Amelink-Verburg, M., Mol, B., Nijhuis, J., et al. (2009). Perinatal mortality and morbidity in a nationwide cohort of 529,688 low-risk planned home and hospital births. *BJOG: An International Journal of Obstetrics and Gynaecology, 116,* 1177–1184.

Department of Health. (1993). *Changing childbirth: Report of the Expert Maternity Group.* London: HMSO.

Department of Health. (2007). *Maternity matters: Choice, access and continuity of care in a safe service.* London: Department of Health.

Department of Health and Social Security. (1970). *Welsh Office. Domiciliary midwifery and maternity bed needs.* Report of the subcommittee. London: HMSO.

De Vries, R. G. (2012). Midwives, obstetrics, fear, and trust: a four-part invention. *The Journal of Perinatal Education, 21*(1), 9–10.

Donnison, J. (1988). *Midwives and medical men - a history of the struggle for the control of childbirth.* London: Historical Publications.

Downe, S., Gyte, G. M. L., Dahlen, H. G., & Singata, M. (2012). Routine vaginal examinations for assessing progress of labour to improve outcomes for women and babies at term. *Cochrane Database of Systematic Reviews.* https://doi.org/10.1002/14651858.CD010088.

Dove, S., & Muir-Cochrane, E. (2014). Being safe practitioners and safe mothers: A critical ethnography of continuity of care midwifery in Australia. *Midwifery, 30*(10), 1063–1072.

Eason, E., & Feldman, P. (2000). Much ado about a little cut: is episiotomy worthwhile? *Obstetrics & Gynecology, 95*(4), 616–618.

Gould, D. (2011). *Welcoming baby: Reflections on perinatal care.* Chester-le-Street: Fresh Heart Publishing.

Gupta, J. K., Hofmeyr, G. J., & Shehmar, M. (2012). Position in the second stage of labour for women without epidural anaesthesia. *Cochrane Database of Systematic Reviews.* https://doi.org/10.1002/14651858. CD002006.pub3.

Gurol-Urganci, I., Cromwell, D., Edozien, L., Mahmood, T., Adams, E., Richmond, D., et al. (2013). Third- and fourth-degree perineal tears among primiparous women in England between 2000 and 2012: time trends and risk factors. *BJOG: An International Journal of Obstetrics and Gynaecology, 120*, 1516–1525.

Hunter, B. (2004). Conflicting ideologies as a source of emotion work in midwifery. *Midwifery, 20*, 261–272.

Hunter, B., Berg, M., Lundgren, I., Ólafsdóttir, Á., & Kirkham, M. (2008). Relationships: The hidden threads in the tapestry of maternity care. *Midwifery, 24*, 132–137.

Hunter, L. (2008). A hermeneutic phenomenological analysis of midwives' ways of knowing during childbirth. *Midwifery, 24*, 405–415.

Islam, M. (2007). The Safe Motherhood Initiative and beyond. *Bulletin of the World Health Organization, 85*(10), 735.

Jackson, M., Dahlen, H. G., & Schmied, V. (2012). Birthing outside the system: Perspectives of risk amongst Australian women who have high risk homebirths. *Midwifery, 28*(5), 561–567.

Jordan, B. (1997). Authoritative knowledge and it's construction. In Davis-Floyd, R., & Sargent, C. F., (Eds.), *Childbirth and authoritative knowledge* (pp. 55–79). Berkeley: University of California Press.

King's Fund. (2008). *Safe births: Everybody's business: An independent inquiry into the safety of maternity services in England.* London: King's Fund.

Kirkup, B. (2015). *The report of the Morecambe Bay Investigation.* London: The Stationary Office. Available at: https://www.gov.uk/government/publications.

Knight, M., Bunch, K., Tufnell, D., Jayakody, H., Shakespeare, J., Kotnis, R., Kenyon, S., & Kurinczuk, J. J., (Eds) on behalf of MBRRACE-UK. (2018). *Saving Lives, Improving Mothers' Care- Lessons learned to inform maternity care from the UK and Ireland Confidential Enquiries into Maternal Deaths and Morbidity 2014-16.* Oxford, National Perinatal Epidemiology Unit, University of Oxford.

Lavender, T., Hart, A., & Smyth, R. M. (2012). Effect of partogram use on outcomes for women in spontaneous labour at term. *Cochrane Database of Systematic Reviews.* https://doi.org/10.1002/14651858. CD005461.pub3.

Leap, N., Dahlen, H. G., Brodie, P., Tracy, S., & Thorpe, J. (2011). Relationships-the glue that holds it together': midwifery continuity of care and sustainability. In Davis L., Daellenbach R., & Kensington M., (Eds.), *Sustainability, midwifery and birth* (pp. 61–74). New York: Routledge.

Lokugamage, A. (2011). Fear of home birth in doctors and obstetric iatrogenesis. *International Journal of Childbirth, 1*(4), 263–272.

MacKenzie Bryers, H., & van Teijlingen, E. (2010). Risk, theory, social and medical models: A critical analysis of the concept of risk in maternity care. *Midwifery, 26*, 488–496.

Mander, R. (2002). The midwife and the medical practitioner. In Mander R., & Fleming V., (Eds.), *Failure to progress: The contraction of the midwifery profession* (pp. 170–188). London: Routledge.

Martin, J. A., Hamilton, B. E., Osterman, M. J. K., Curtin, S. C., & Mathews, T. J. (2015). Births: Final data for 2013. *National Vital Statistics Reports, 64*(1), 1–65.

Ministry of Health. (1959). *Report of the Maternity Services Committee.* London: HMSO.

Montgomery, T. (1958). Physiologic considerations in labor and the puerperium. *American Journal of Obstetrics and Gynecology, 76*(4), 706–715.

Montgomery v Lanarkshire (2015). UKSC 11. Available at: https://www.supremecourt.uk/decided-cases/docs/UKSC_2013_0136_Judgment.pdf.

National Institute for Health and Care Excellence. (2010). *Pregnancy and complex social factors: A model for service provision for pregnant women with complex social factors (CG110).* Available at: https://www.nice.org.uk/guidance/cg110.

National Institute for Health and Care Excellence. (2014). *Intrapartum care for healthy women and babies (CG190).* Available at: https://www.nice.org.uk/guidance/CG190.

NHS England. (2016). *Better births: Improving outcomes of maternity services in England. A five year forward view for maternity care.* Available at: https://www.england.nhs.uk/wp-content/uploads/2016/02/national-maternity-review-report.pdf.

O'Boyle, C. (2015). Writing of one's own culture: an autoethnography of home birth midwifery in Ireland. In Dykes F., & Flacking R., (Eds.), *Ethnographic research in maternal and child health* (pp. 53–72). Abingdon: Routledge.

Petrocnik, P., & Marshall, J. E. (2015). Hands-poised technique: the future technique for perineal management of second stage of labour? A modified systematic literature review. *Midwifery, 31*(2), 274–279.

Priddis, H., Dahlen, H. G., & Schmied, V. (2011). Juggling instinct and fear: an ethnographic study of facilitators and inhibitors of physiological birth positioning in two different birth settings. *International Journal of Childbirth, 1*(4), 227–241.

Priddis, H., Dahlen, H. G., & Schmied, V. (2012). What are the facilitators, inhibitors, and implications of birth positioning? A review of the literature. *Women and Birth, 25*(2), 100–106.

Rawnson, S. (2011). A qualitative study exploring student midwives' experiences of carrying a caseload as part of their midwifery education in England. *Midwifery, 27*, 786–792.

Royal College of Obstetricians and Gynaecologists. (2009). *Improving patient safety: Risk management for maternity and gynaecology: Clinical governance advice 2*. London: RCOG Press.

Royal College of Obstetricians and Gynaecologists. (2015). *The management of third- and fourth-degree perineal tears. Green-top guideline no. 29 June 2015*. London: Royal College of Obstetricians and Gynaecologists. Available at: https://www.rcog.org.uk/globalassets/documents/guidelines/gtg-29.pdf.

Sandall, J., Soltani, H., Gates, S., Shennan, A., & Devane, D. (2015). Midwife-led continuity models versus other models of care for childbearing women. *Cochrane Database of Systematic Reviews* (9), CD004667.

Scammell, M., & Stewart, M. (2014). Time, risk and midwife practice: The vaginal examination. *Health, Risk and Society, 16*(1), 84–100.

Tew, M. (1985). Place of birth and perinatal mortality. *Journal of the Royal College of General Practitioners, 35*, 390–394.

Thornton, M. J., & Lubowski, D. Z. (2006). Obstetric-induced incontinence: A black hole of preventable morbidity. *Australian and New Zealand Journal of Obstetrics and Gynaecology, 46*, 468–473.

Tracy, S. K., Hartz, D. L., Tracy, M. B., Allen, J., Forti, A., Hall, B., et al. (2013). Caseload midwifery care versus standard maternity care for women of any risk: M@NGO, a randomised controlled trial. *The Lancet, 382*, 1723–1732.

Trochez, R., Waterfield, M., & Freeman, R. M. (2011). Hands on or hands off the perineum: A survey of care of the perineum in labour (HOOPS). *International Urogynecology Journal, 22*, 1279–1285.

Turner, C. E., Young, J. M., Solomon, M. J., Ludlow, J., Benness, C., & Phipps, H. (2008). Vaginal delivery compared with elective caesarean section: The views of pregnant women and clinicians. *BJOG: An International Journal of Obstetrics and Gynaecology, 115*(12), 1494–1502.

Wagner, M. (2007). Birth and power. In Savage, W., (Ed.), *Birth and power: A Savage enquiry revisited* (pp. 35–44). London: Pinter and Martin.

Walsh, D. (2006). Subverting the assembly-line: childbirth in a free-standing birth centre. *Social Science and Medicine, 62*, 1330–1340.

Walsh, D. (2012). *Evidence and skills for normal labour and birth: A guide for midwives*. Abingdon: Routledge.

Winter, C. (2002) *Orderly chaos: How do independent midwives assess the progress of labour (Masters dissertation)*. London: London South Bank University.

World Health Organization. (2014). *WHO recommendations for augmentation of labour*. Geneva: World Health Organization.

Further Reading

Schiller, R. (2017). *Why human rights in childbirth matter*. London: Pinter and Martin.

    This text discusses the human rights of women in the context of childbearing and the concept of risk. It includes information and support for women and midwives with the aim of improving birth practices and experiences for women.

Symon, A. (2006). *Risk and choice in maternity care: An international perspective*. Edinburgh: Churchill Livingstone.

    This text explores the complex interrelationship between risk and choice in maternity care. The concepts of 'high' and 'low' risk are explored along with the effect this labelling of women has on their ability to exercise informed choices throughout pregnancy.

Useful Websites

The Royal College of Midwives Better Births Initiative: http://betterbirths.rcm.org.uk/
   This website provides digital resources, case studies, webinars and pilot projects for maternity care and focuses on the three themes of facilitating normal births, increasing access to midwifery-led continuity of carer and raising awareness to reduce maternal and newborn health inequalities.

Transforming Maternity Care: http://transform.childbirthconnection.org/reports/physiology/
   This is the website of the United States of America-based organization Childbirth Connections. The website contains improvement tools and information for professionals to deliver the 2020 vision of a high-quality, high-value maternity care system which is consistently and reliably woman centred, safe, effective, timely, efficient and equitable.

Women's Views About Safety in Maternity Care: https://www.kingsfund.org.uk/sites/files/kf/field/field_document/womens-view-safety-maternity-care-qualitative-study-maternity-services-inquiry.pdf
   The full-text publication of the King's Fund-commissioned report into women's views about safety in maternity care is available on the King's Fund website.

Assessing and Managing Risk (NHS Scotland): http://www.sehd.scot.nhs.uk/publications/ifms/ifms-05.htm
   The webpage forms part of the strategy for 'implementing a framework for maternity services in Scotland'. It contains useful information to inform policy in relation to managing risk and improving safety in maternity care. The strategies recognize that women have to make difficult decisions about their maternity care, taking into account their previous experience, personal circumstances, expectations and needs.

White Ribbon Alliance: https://www.whiteribbonalliance.org
   The website contains current news stories, information about campaigns, video resources and tools to support the provision of safe and respectful care for women and their babies.

CHAPTER 10

Employer-Led Models of Midwifery Supervision

Sarah Purdy ■ Jessica Read

CONTENTS

LEARNING OUTCOMES

By the end of this chapter the reader will:

- have a greater understanding of the history of supervision of midwifery within the United Kingdom (UK) and the role it has played in protecting the public and supporting midwives in practice
- appreciate the rationale for a change in legislation and its impact on redefining clinical supervision and support for midwives in the UK
- understand the main differences between the new models of employer-led supervision of midwives across the four UK countries that support the delivery of high-quality midwifery care
- articulate the midwife's responsibilities in relation to clinical supervision, revalidation and peer review.

Introduction and Overview

The UK has a long history of providing midwifery supervision since it was enshrined in the 1902 Midwives Act. Over the years the mode by which supervision of midwives has been enacted has changed considerably. In recent years and up to March 2017, supervision of midwives was described in the Statutory Instrument 2002 No. 253 (Nursing and Midwifery The Order 2001). The Nursing and Midwifery Council (NMC) set out the rules which governed the practice of supervision of midwives within the former *Midwives Rules and Standards* (NMC 2012). Following the publication of reports by the Parliamentary and Health Service Ombudsman (PHSO) (2013) and by the King's Fund (Baird et al 2015), the NMC accepted the recommendations that midwifery supervision and regulation should be separated, with the NMC solely being in direct control of the regulation of midwives.

Statutory supervision of midwives was removed from statute in 2017, removing the midwives rules and standards (NMC 2012), and all four UK countries were tasked with establishing a time-limited task force to ensure that processes of good clinical governance and support for professional practice were put in place (Department of Health 2016).

This chapter will describe the historical context of supervision of midwifery, including case studies of effective and ineffective supervision. The chapter will also outline the catalyst for change which resulted in the disestablishment of statutory supervision of midwifery. The emergence of new models of employer-led midwifery supervision, particularly the A-EQUIP model in England, will be explored, with a description of the key themes within the models and the ensuing roles of the professional midwifery advocates (PMAs)/supervisors. Throughout the chapter there will be reflective activities to give the reader an opportunity to gain greater understanding of how the new models will benefit them in their practice.

Historical Context of Midwifery Supervision

Supervision of midwifery is intrinsically linked to the regulatory history of midwifery as a profession, which is explored in detail in Chapter 2. With the passing of the 1902 Midwives Act (England and Wales), the term *midwife* became protected under the law in England and Wales, with registration and regulation of midwives seen as the best way to safeguard women from uncertified practitioners. Scotland enacted similar legislation in 1915 and Ireland did so in 1918.

The Midwives Act 1902 (England and Wales), the Midwives (Scotland) Act 1915 and the Midwives (Ireland) Act 1918 led to the formation of the Central Midwives Board in the respective nations, which certified midwives and maintained a roll of accredited practitioners. Additionally, the Acts required local authorities to issue licences to certified midwives working in their neighbourhood. It is here that the system of midwifery supervision can be first identified, with midwives required to notify their intention to practise and abide by rules and conditions of practice in order to maintain their right to work. The supervising authorities were required to investigate accusations of a midwife's malpractice and make a report to the Central Midwives Board. They were also required to report midwives convicted of any criminal offence. Failure of the midwife to notify their intention to practise was punishable by a fine, whereas attempts to falsify certification or to practise without the necessary accreditation could result in imprisonment.

This authoritarian model of midwifery supervision was maintained for decades with the emphasis on compliance and the circumscription of the midwife's role within the organizational hierarchy of the National Health Service (NHS) and the increasing medicalization of birth. Midwifery autonomy and women's choice were inevitably curtailed and supervisors of midwives (SoMs) were widely regarded as part of the establishment, *policing* midwifery practice, rather than proactively supporting the development of the profession. Allison and Kirkham (1996) highlighted this view of the role of the SoM as punitive, with midwives reporting their efforts to hide practice concerns from the SoM.

The historical role of the SoM as custodian of the status quo is demonstrated by Osborne (2007). Her interviews with midwives who were practising in the late 1970s reveal the SoM as an enforcer of the prevailing orthodoxy, reminding midwives not to make trouble by offering women choice. It is worth noting that these same midwives acknowledged the development of supervision into the later model of proactive support for women and midwives. The model of statutory supervision which evolved following the Nursing and Midwifery Order 2001 is discussed in the next section.

The Model of Statutory Supervision of Midwifery 2004–2017

Up to 2017, the Nursing and Midwifery [The Order] 2001, which describes the NMC as a regulatory body whose role is to regulate nurses and midwives in the UK, contained the primary legislation relating to statutory supervision of midwifery. The Nursing and Midwifery [The Order] 2001 requires the NMC to set standards of education, training, conduct and performance and to provide a system of assurance to the public that those standards are met.

The Nursing and Midwifery [The Order] 2001 discharges additional powers to the NMC to set rules and standards of practice specific to midwives. Up to 2017, the rules provided midwives with a secondary layer of regulation defined as *statutory supervision of midwives* and they articulated the establishment of local supervising authorities (LSAs), which were responsible for the function of statutory supervision. This system of secondary regulation for midwives was unique to midwifery, and as acknowledged by Baird et al (2015), no other health profession in the UK or internationally operated such a model.

The key aim of statutory supervision of midwives was to protect the public by improving standards of midwifery practice, thereby resulting in positive outcomes for women and their families. This was undertaken through investigation of incidents where poor midwifery practice had been highlighted and supporting midwives in practice through reflection, development and formal assessment. The structure of statutory supervision of midwifery can be seen in Fig. 10.1 and is discussed in the following sections. However, in 2015, as a consequence of the recommendations by the King's Fund (Baird et al 2015) to separate midwifery regulation and statutory supervision

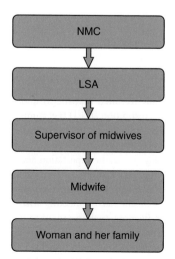

Fig. 10.1 Structure of statutory supervision of midwifery (before 2017). *LSA*, Local supervising authority; *NMC*, Nursing and Midwifery Council.

of midwifery, the NMC commenced proceedings with the Department of Health to amend legislation, resulting in statutory supervision of midwifery being disestablished in 2017.

LOCAL SUPERVISING AUTHORITIES

LSAs sat within health service organizations throughout the UK and were responsible for delivering the function of statutory supervision of midwifery in accordance with the rules and standards set out the former *Midwives Rules and Standards* (NMC 2012). Article 43 of the Nursing and Midwifery Order 2001 articulated the primary legislation with regard to the LSA function. LSAs were based within different health care organizations across the four countries in the UK:

- In England, NHS England was the LSA and distributed the LSA function across four regions: North, Midlands, South and London.
- In Wales the LSA function was held by Health Inspectorate Wales.
- In Northern Ireland the Public Health Agency oversaw the LSA function.
- In Scotland the LSA function was held within the 14 NHS Scotland Health Boards.

LOCAL SUPERVISORY AUTHORITY MIDWIFERY OFFICERS

The *Midwives Rules and Standards* (NMC 2012) stated that each LSA must appoint an adequate number of LSA midwifery officers (LSAMOs) to be responsible for exercising its function as the rules clearly defined. The LSAMOs had to meet the educational requirements as specified by the NMC. There were seven LSAMOs in England, two in Wales, one in Scotland and one in Northern Ireland. The LSAMO was responsible for recruiting and appointing an *adequate* number of SoMs to exercise supervision over the midwives practising within their LSA. Rule 9: 1.2 in the former *Midwives Rules and Standards* (NMC 2012) specified that each LSA should maintain a ratio of one SoM to 15 practising midwives.

SUPERVISORS OF MIDWIVES

SoMs were practising midwives with at least 3 years' experience who were nominated by their peers as possessing the qualities required to be an effective SoM. Those qualities were defined by the NMC (2014: 3) in *Standards for the Preparation of Supervisors of Midwives* and were grouped under four domains:

- professional values
- communication and interpersonal skills
- supervision in practice and decision-making
- leadership and team working.

The NMC required each successfully recruited midwife to undertake an approved education programme through a higher education institution (HEI) (i.e. a university) which prepared them to become a SoM, acquiring the required competencies to undertake the role. A newly qualified SoM was appointed to their role by the LSA and was accountable to the LSAMO. SoMs undertook the role in addition to their substantively employed role, the expectation being that they were provided with the necessary resources by their employing organization to undertake the role. This would include allocated time to fulfil the supervisory function, with locally agreed remuneration to cover this additional role.

The SoM supported midwives in practice by meeting with them at least annually, providing opportunities for debriefing and reflection, enabling them to develop their knowledge, skills and expertise. All SoMs had an important role to play in reporting and investigating clinical incidents where standards of midwifery practice had not been upheld. This was undertaken in close liaison with the LSA and the clinical governance departments within the health care organizations.

BOX 10.1 ■ A Proactive Model

Wales undertook a review of the model of statutory supervision in 2013 to improve the quality of statutory supervision throughout Wales. This resulted in the appointment of 18 full-time supervisors of midwives across Wales who would concentrate fully on fulfilling the function of statutory supervision. This increased the visibility and accessibility of supervisors of midwives to midwives and women. The model resulted in more efficient and proactive management of investigations and ensured timely remedial support for midwives. Wales established an all-Wales 24 hours a day on-call rota for regulatory advice and guidance, and the supervisors of midwives provided support through clinics and surgeries for midwives, students and women. The model was designed against eight key performance indicators, which were monitored by Health Inspectorate Wales (Ness and Richards 2014).

BOX 10.2 ■ A Model That challenged

North West Local Supervising Authority came under the scrutiny of the Public and Health Service Ombudsman (PHSO) in 2013 following investigation of three cases where the processes of statutory supervision of midwifery were found to have failed. The model was seen to create confusion between regulatory and supervisory processes. The PHSO found a perceived conflict of interest to be inherent within the model and a lack of sharing of information between supervisors of midwives and the employing organization. Supervisory investigation reports were found to be of poor quality and failed to answer important questions raised by families. The PHSO found the dual role of supervisor providing support and a regulatory function as a conflict of interest. The PHSO report *Midwifery Supervision and Regulation: Recommendations for Change* (PHSO 2013) was the catalyst for a major review undertaken by the King's Fund into statutory supervision and midwifery regulation in the United Kingdom.

In 2013, statutory supervision of midwives was reviewed by the PHSO when it was found that there was the potential for conflict between the supervisor's role of both supporter and regulator (investigating practice). As a result of this, Wales was the first nation to develop a new model of statutory supervision, as shown in Box 10.1.

The Catalyst for Legislative Change

The PHSO's investigation of complaints made by three families in the northwest of England in 2013 related to governance processes in the maternity services and the supervision of midwives at a local level (Box 10.2). The investigation resulted in the PHSO compiling a report that included recommendations for change. These were based on two key principles which consequently formed the premise for change to the system of midwifery regulation:

    1. that midwifery supervision and regulation should be separated
    2. that the NMC should be in direct control of regulatory activity (PHSO 2013).

The NMC accepted the PHSO findings, and in response commissioned the King's Fund to review potential models for the future of midwifery regulation, with particular reference to the principles outlined in the PHSO report. The King's Fund reported to the NMC in January 2015, and the key recommendation made by Baird et al (2015), as shown in Box 10.3, were subsequently accepted by the NMC in January 2016.

    The legislative amendments to the Nursing and Midwifery Order 2001 had the biggest impact on the midwifery profession in the UK since the passing of the Midwives Act 1902 (England and Wales), Midwives (Scotland) Act 1915 and Midwives (Ireland) Act 1918. Essentially the statutory function of supervision of midwifery was to cease, and it became vitally important that

> **BOX 10.3 ■ Kings Fund Recommendation**
>
> 'The NMC [Nursing and Midwifery Council] as the health care professional regulator should have direct responsibility and accountability for the core functions of regulation. The legislation pertaining to the NMC should be revised to reflect this. This means the additional layer of regulation currently in place for midwives and the extended role for the NMC over statutory supervision of midwives should end' (Baird et al 2015: p.23).

midwives and women were at the centre of designing the new model of non-statutory midwifery supervision.

Within the King's Fund report (Baird et al 2015) a number of functions were seen as beneficial and valued by midwives. These included supporting and developing individuals, leading the profession, and midwives having a strategic oversight of maternity services. As a result of this, the Department of Health established a UK-wide consultation with key stakeholders, including the four chief nursing officers from England, Wales, Scotland and Northern Ireland, the Royal College of Midwives, the NMC and the LSAMO Forum UK to develop a set of guiding principles which would be embedded in the new model of non-statutory midwifery supervision as published in the policy paper 'Proposals for changing the system of midwifery supervision in the UK' (Department of Health 2016). There were clear differences between statutory supervision of midwifery and the new models; these are outlined in Table 10.1.

As a consequence of the Department of Health's (2016) recommendation, each of the four UK nations established a Midwifery Supervision Taskforce to develop a new model of supervision. It was acknowledged that because of the variations in demographics and size, each nation would operationalize the model differently but would agree on a consistent set of principles. The Department of Health also requested that each taskforce address any risks associated with the removal of the LSA function, such as the provision of 24-hour advice and support to midwives and the advocacy role to maternity service users, as well as maintain the oversight of the transition across to an employer-led supervision model.

Introducing the New Employer-Led Model of Supervision in England

The Local Supervising Authority England National Taskforce was established in early 2016 following publication of the Department of Health's proposals for changing the system of midwifery supervision in the UK (Department of Health 2016). The new model A-EQUIP, *A*dvocating for *E*ducation and *Q*uality *I*mprovement, was co-produced with women, midwives, educationalists, nurse and midwifery leaders and managers, commissioners and the Royal College of Midwives. The model was developed following extensive stakeholder engagement, and the taskforce agreed that a supportive approach was required which was consistent, strategic and integrated (Gillman and Lloyd 2015).The feedback from stakeholder engagement required that the model would:

- have a supportive function
- build professional resilience
- support all midwives to provide high-quality care and seek to improve it
- support the advocacy role of the midwife
- include strategies that value, develop and invest in midwives
- allow flexibility for local organizational application
- not create additional financial pressure on providers.

TABLE 10.1 ■ Comparison Between Statutory Supervision of Midwives and the New Models

Statutory Supervision of Midwives	New Model
Statutory, therefore legislated for	Non-statutory, therefore loss of statutory lever
As secondary regulation, supervision of midwifery was accountable to the Nursing and Midwifery Council (NMC)	Supervision is now separated from the NMC and is employer led
Protection of the public was the main function	Public protection continues to be the responsibility of the NMC and the employer. New models will support high standards of midwifery practice
Every midwife was required to submit an intention to practice annually to a supervisor of midwives.	The NMC process of revalidation provides for 3-yearly review of the requirements for registration
The local supervising authority (LSA) provided a policy for the storage of health care records for self-employed midwives once they ceased to practise. The records had to be kept securely for 25 years	This responsibility does not exist in the new models
Each LSA across the United Kingdom (UK) appointed an LSA midwifery officer (LSAMO), who was responsible for exercising its functions in relation to the supervision of midwives	Each UK country has had to articulate a structure of professional midwifery leadership within their new model
Supervisors of midwives were appointed by the LSA following completion of an approved programme of education. The LSA had to ensure that the ratio of supervisors to midwives was not greater than 1:15	Facilitators of the new model need to be adequately prepared. Employers take the lead in designating suitable midwives to be prepared for the new role, ensuring there are adequate numbers to meet the requirements of the new model
The LSA published a policy for the reporting of, and investigation of, adverse incidents relating to midwifery practice. Supervisors of midwives investigated allegations of impaired fitness to practice on behalf of the LSA. Investigation findings were fed back to the employing organization. Provision was made for supporting the midwife concerned	Health care organizations are responsible for investigating serious incidents using guidance from national bodies such as the Heath Service Investigation Branch and NHS Resolution. The England model: A-EQUIP enables a system of support and development from a professional midwifery advocate
The LSA and/or the NMC had the authority to undertake visits and inspections of maternity services according to the Midwives Rules and Standards (NMC 2012)	The Care Quality Commission is the independent body which undertakes this role although it will not have a role in 'regulating' any new model of midwifery supervision
The LSA provided the NMC with an annual report containing specific information requested by the NMC pertaining to statutory supervision and maternity services	The LSA no longer exists, so the annual report will not be required
The LSA had the authority to suspend a midwife from practice following appropriate investigation and referral to the NMC	An employing organization has the authority to suspend a midwife from duty and refer the midwife to the NMC. The authority to suspend a midwife from practice sits with the NMC as the regulator
Each year every midwife was required to meet their named supervisor of midwives for an annual review to discuss their practice and identify any development needs	Revalidation is a requirement for every registered nurse and midwife with the NMC and occurs every 3 years. The new model may incorporate an annual review which can support the midwife with revalidation
The LSAMO structure provided professional midwifery leadership and advice which covered all midwives	Each UK country to provide a structure for professional midwifery leadership within their new model

For the new model the data are from Department of Health (2016).

Now undertake Activity 10.1

ACTIVITY 10.1 ∎

Consider the seven elements of the new model that were important to key stakeholders from page 164. Identify one which you can most identify with, and reflect on why that may be and how the new model should address this.

The Local Supervising Authority England National Taskforce based the A-EQUIP model on Proctor's (1986) three-function model of clinical supervision and Hawkins and Shohet's (2012) adaptation. The four functions are demonstrated in the model and described in Fig. 10.2.

CLINICAL SUPERVISION (RESTORATIVE)

Restorative clinical supervision (RCS) has been found to address the emotional needs of staff and to support the development of resilience. Pettit and Stephen (2015) state that RCS provides the creation of space, allowing the practitioner to physically and mentally slow down whilst restoring their thinking capacity and ability to understand and process thoughts, enabling them to consider different perspectives and inform decision-making. The RCS approach has been found to reduce stress, increase job satisfaction, have a positive impact on physical and emotional well-being and improve relationships with colleagues.

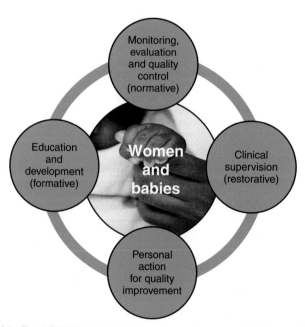

Fig. 10.2   The A-EQUIP model. (Modified with permission from NHS England 2017)

MONITORING, EVALUATION AND QUALITY CONTROL (NORMATIVE)

This element of the A-EQUIP model is focused on evaluation and quality control aspects of professional practice, referred to by Proctor (1986) as the *accountability* or *normative* function. This element benefits the midwife by promoting a sense of personal and professional accountability, becoming more self-aware, being involved in service improvement and being able to identify enhancements in performance.

PERSONAL ACTION FOR QUALITY IMPROVEMENT

Personal action for quality improvement should follow the midwife's progress through peer review and RCS. As the midwife identifies aspects of her practice which would benefit from improvement, the next step is to identify how such actions to improve her knowledge and skills will ultimately benefit women and their families. According to NHS England (2017), action to improve quality of care should become an intrinsic part of every health professional's role.

EDUCATION AND DEVELOPMENT (FORMATIVE)

This element of the A-EQUIP model is seen to support the NMC process of revalidation, employer-led appraisal and leadership development. The *formative* process can be guided by peer review and reflection and is seen to increase self-awareness and self-confidence.

The A-EQUIP model requires the role of Professional Midwifery Advocates (PMAs) to facilitate the model within provider organizations. The role of the PMA and details of the preparation for the role are presented in the following sections.

The Role of the Professional Midwifery Advocate

The PMA undertakes the non-statutory functions of supervision, which were maintained following disestablishment. The focus of the role is to implement the four domains of the A-EQUIP model as described above, with the PMA holding a facilitator role within health care organizations. The purpose of the PMA is primarily to support and guide midwives to maintain and improve high-quality, woman-centred practice, with an emphasis on resilience building, reflective practice and personal development. It is also recommended that the annual supervisory review (previously a statutory requirement) will continue within the context of good practice and to support the NMC revalidation process.

The responsibility for implementing the A-EQUIP model rests with the individual health care provider and NHS organization. Consequently, the role of the PMA is likely to differ slightly across England, with employers fulfilling their responsibilities as best suits the needs of the childbearing women, their babies and their families. Despite this variation, the essential functions of the PMA will be evident. The principles of supporting midwives to act as advocates for women demonstrates the concept of accountable practice where midwives manage their own professional development to achieve the highest standard of midwifery care.

The PMA is an important midwifery leader within the organization, with key responsibilities for quality improvement, interprofessional relationships and advocacy within maternity care. The A-EQUIP model operational guidance document (NHS England 2017) includes a template job profile. This comprehensively explores the activities that are appropriate for the PMA to undertake or facilitate within the provider organization. The profile emphasizes the extensive working relationships the PMA must foster, both within and outside the provider organization, to practise effectively.

Preparing Midwives to Be Professional Midwifery Advocates

The first cohorts of PMAs were drawn from former SoMs. Although there are clear distinctions between the remits of the two roles, the characteristics required of the post-holders are very similar. Additionally, it was acknowledged that the Preparation of Supervisors of Midwives (PoSoM) programme effectively facilitated the development of many of the competencies required of the PMA. In keeping with the characteristics of the SoM, the PMA is also required to demonstrate leadership, excellent interpersonal skills, strategic vision and professional integrity.

Midwives who had previously undertaken the PoSoM course were able to 'top up' their prior learning and experience with a shortened PMA 'bridging' programme of not less than 4 days' duration (NHS England 2017). This abridged course was designed to build on the previous learning and experience of the SoM, whilst providing an opportunity to develop the skills necessary to facilitate RCS. Midwives who did not have the SoM qualification were required to complete a longer preparation programme of at least 10 days' duration. It was stipulated by NHS England that this programme must be facilitated through HEIs at Framework for Higher Education Qualifications academic level 7 (master's degree level). Whilst the previously mandated eligibility criteria for the PoSoM course no longer apply, the person specification in the PMA role descriptor and the educational criteria applied to the PMA programme effectively create a similar entry threshold. On the basis of these descriptors, the PMA should be an experienced midwife who commands professional credibility and the respect of colleagues and external stakeholders, has excellent communication skills and has the ability to think strategically and effectively drive the quality improvement agenda within their workplace.

Both the bridging programme and full programme ensure the new PMA meets the competency requirements detailed in the NHS England (2017) guidance. The competencies have been modelled on those of the Care Quality Commission (2017) key lines of enquiry: 'safe', 'effective', 'caring', 'responsive' and 'well-led'. By alignment of the criteria, there is a clear acknowledgement of the PMA role in driving the NHS quality agenda. The programme uses a competency framework to ensure PMAs, by whichever route they qualify, are equipped to undertake the new role.

Now undertake Activity 10.2

ACTIVITY 10.2 ■

Consider the most recent Care Quality Commission report that was undertaken in your maternity unit.

Select one of the 'key lines of enquiry' domains and consider how the professional midwife advocate could address the issues raised in the report through the four elements of the A-EQUIP model.

Other Employer-Led Models of Supervision

Box 10.4 presents a summary and comparisons of the tenets of the employer-led models of clinical supervision adopted by the four nations.

WALES

The transition from statutory supervision to a new model was slightly different in Wales, as a full review and remodelling of services that was part of their 'future-proofing' process in 2014

> **BOX 10.4 ■ The Four Nations at a Glance**
>
> **England**
> - The professional midwifery advocate (PMA) role can be full-time or combined with clinical practice.
> - The ratio of PMAs to midwives is set by each employer according to local needs.
> - Mandated minimum of 1 hour of supervision a year.
>
> **Wales**
> - Full-time supervisors with 20% of their time working on labour wards.
> - Mandated ratio of 1:125 (supervisor to midwives).
> - Four hours of supervision a year, with 2 hours of this as group supervision. Further ad hoc sessions available as needed.
>
> **Scotland**
> - Supervisors combine role with clinical practice. All experienced midwives encouraged to consider becoming involved in supervision.
> - Individual boards to set the ratio of supervisors to midwives.
> - One mandatory group session a year with individual support as needed.
>
> **Northern Ireland (Interim Arrangements)**
> - Experienced, additionally trained midwives provide supervision.
> - Current ratio of 1:15 (supervisors to midwives) maintained.
> - Midwives entitled to at least one supervisory meeting a year, plus round-the-clock access to advice as needed.
>
> ------
> Modified from Royal College of Midwives (2017).

(Ness and Richards 2014) had already taken place. This had introduced the full-time supervisor, which had proved very popular with midwives. Following review in 2016, the decision was made to retain the elements of the future-proofing model which would meet the needs of the post-disestablishment supervisor remit.

Rather than devolve the implementation of the new model to the health care provider, the Welsh Government has mandated the provision of clinical midwifery supervision, with a ratio of one full-time supervisor to every 125 midwives. Supervisors are required to spend 20% of their time working clinically on labour wards, and midwives are entitled to 4 hours of supervision annually, half of which may be in group supervision.

Because of the small number of midwifery supervisors in Wales, bespoke development for the new role is not viable. The Welsh Government is looking to commission development from the current university provision for leadership and mentoring, as these align well with the new supervision role.

SCOTLAND

Following its review, the Scottish taskforce devised a model of supervision very similar to that adopted in England. The focus is on restorative supervision, with an emphasis on reflection and advocacy. An education programme for prospective supervisors similar to that already discussed for England has been developed, and the transition to the new model will be evaluated over 3 years by researchers at the University of Dundee.

NORTHERN IRELAND

The Northern Ireland Practice and Education Council for Nursing and Midwifery was tasked with producing an overarching framework of supervision which covers midwifery, nursing and children's safeguarding. The new arrangements are very similar in structure to the previous statutory supervision, with the exception of the investigatory function.

Northern Ireland has retained 24-hour access to experienced clinical midwifery advice from the original supervision model, and there is also the expectation that all midwives will retain a 'named midwifery supervisor' (Department of Health 2017), with whom they will meet at least annually. It is not specified that previous appointment as a statutory SoM is required, nor what suitable additional training might entail. Heads of midwifery are required to maintain a list of midwifery supervisors and allocated supervisees, aiming for a ratio of 1:15. Midwives are required to meet regularly with SoMs to discuss emerging issues and promote high standards.

Midwives Working in Education, Research and Management

Midwives who work in education and research historically had access to statutory supervision through the LSA, whereby a SoM would be allocated to them if none were available in their workplace. Since the removal of statutory supervision, HEIs and other employers of midwives have had to consider how they will provide this function to their staff. Some HEIs considered equipping a number of midwifery lecturers to become PMAs to be able to provide this support to midwifery staff; however, this provision has so far been variable, with no consensus on how midwives working outside institutional maternity providers will access the support of a PMA. In its policy paper, the Department of Health (2016) makes a distinction between the needs of midwives working in clinical roles and the needs of midwives in education, research and management settings, emphasizing the need for the provision of supervision to be proportional to the risk profile of the working environment. Whilst a form of clinical supervision is recommended for midwives who provide clinical care, the suggestion is that a system of peer review would be appropriate for those midwives whose roles are less exposed to the clinical practice setting.

HEIs in England have the additional consideration of how the move from statutory supervision to the A-EQUIP model impacts on the educational needs of student midwives. Historically, SoMs would support the student midwives based at their clinical site, ensuring they understood the role, with each student midwife having a named SoM as a point of contact in practice. The typical arrangement would be for a SoM to take responsibility for a specific cohort of students, often facilitating group discussions and opportunities to participate in activities undertaken as part of the SoM role, such as care planning for women and care quality audits. These practice-based activities enabled students to consolidate learning and explore how the underpinning theory of autonomous and accountable practice was applied in the clinical area and supported by supervision. This non-statutory aspect of the SoM role was generally undertaken in an informal way, in addition to the SoM's official duties. It is unclear whether the PMA will have such capacity to continue this beneficial and well-evaluated activity.

The Department of Health (2016) also postulated the need for HEIs to consider whether sufficient emphasis is placed within their midwifery education programmes on the advocacy role of midwives. Before disestablishment, SoMs could provide impartial support to women regarding their birth choices. The Department of Health (2016) highlighted concerns that in future midwives may be reluctant to act effectively as advocates for women in their care, fearful of employer censure. It is essential that students and registered midwives are effectively prepared to confidently act as advocates for women, especially those whose wishes deviate from recommended care pathways.

Now undertake Activity 10.3

ACTIVITY 10.3 ▪

Consider the following scenarios. How would you support the women involved? What does the Nursing and Midwifery Council expect from you as a registrant? Where could you access support for your advocacy?

Scenario 1

Jane, a 29-year-old woman, is pregnant for the third time. Her first baby, a boy, was born spontaneously and weighed 3.6 kg. Jane made an uneventful recovery and had a second baby 2.5 years later. This baby, a girl, was born by caesarean section as she was a breech presentation. The baby weighed 3.9 kg, and following the caesarean section Jane made a good recovery as before. This second child is now 3 years old.

Jane is now at 32 weeks' gestation and her pregnancy has been healthy. She is planning a home birth. The obstetrician caring for Jane has made it quite clear that this request is not supported and has informed her of the possible risk of uterine rupture and the need to closely monitor her on the labour ward to prevent any such problem arising.

Jane is not convinced of the obstetrician's arguments and the need for a hospital birth. She very much wants a vaginal birth and believes that with the support of her family and community midwife this is most likely to be achieved at home. She has accessed the Internet and has amassed information on vaginal birth after caesarean section (VBAC). She has also spoken to other women who have successfully had a VBAC.

She asks for your support during her routine antenatal visit.

Scenario 2

Marla, a multigravida, has been admitted to the birth centre in early labour. She is at term and has had an uneventful pregnancy. She has requested a physiological third stage of labour as part of her birth plan.

During your initial discussion with Marla, it becomes clear that her previous birth was complicated by a retained placenta, which required removal under anaesthesia. Marla is convinced the retained placenta was caused by the administration of an uterotonic drug, hence her request for physiological care this time.

Conclusion

For more than 100 years, midwives in the UK have worked within a system of regulation which included statutory supervision of midwifery, and this chapter has described how the statutory system came into being, with the catalyst for its final removal from legislation. The various models of employer-led midwifery supervision that have emerged within the four UK nations since disestablishment have been discussed to encourage the reader to consider how the new models may be relevant to their own contemporary midwifery practice, regardless of the setting.

It is worth noting that the transition from statutory supervision to an employer-led model of midwifery supervision has been implemented in various ways by maternity care providers across the four nations of the UK. However the principles-based nature of the models allows individual health care organizations to manage their delivery flexibly such that they ultimately benefit childbearing women, midwives and the maternity services. In particular, the A-EQUIP model operational guidance document clearly identifies potential issues for maternity providers to consider and mitigate, and the model itself provides a useful framework for maternity managers to use more broadly within their services, as it is based on sound professional development principles.

At times of immense change, great opportunities emerge, and the new models of employer-led supervision demonstrate the resilience of the midwifery profession to ensure that the support, advocacy and professional midwifery leadership that was exemplified in statutory supervision was retained in the new models for the benefit of future generations of midwives, childbearing women and their families. The efficacy of these approaches will need to be evaluated over the following years to ensure they do fulfil their intended purpose.

KEY POINTS

- For more than 100 years, statutory supervision of midwifery that included a regulatory, supportive and advocacy function for midwives and childbearing women was integral to professional practice.
- Following high profile maternity cases where supervision of midwifery was implicated in governance failures, the decision was taken to disestablish midwifery supervision from statute.
- There has been no other alteration in midwifery practice than the decision to disestablish midwifery supervision from statute that has had such a major impact in the history of professional midwifery within the UK.
- Following removal of the regulatory function of supervision, the need to maintain a supportive structure, that benefits midwives, maternity services and childbearing women, is key within the various employer-led models of supervision that have subsequently emerged.
- The employer-led model supports midwives in promoting reflective practice, self-efficacy, advocacy and professional leadership through clinical supervision, revalidation and peer review; elements that were exemplified in the former model of statutory supervision of midwifery.
- The efficacy of these approaches will need to be evaluated over the following years to ensure they do fulfil their intended purpose of ultimately providing safe, competent and high-quality midwifery care to childbearing women, their babies and their families in the UK.

References

Allison, J., & Kirkham, M. (1996). Supervision of midwives in Nottingham 1948-1972. In Kirkham M. (Ed.), *Supervision of midwives* (pp. 28–37). Trowbridge: Books for Midwives.

Baird, B., Murray, R., Seale, B., Foot, C., & Perry, C. (2015). *Midwifery regulation in the United Kingdom.* Available at: https://www.nmc.org.uk/globalassets/sitedocuments/councilpapersanddocuments/council-2015/kings-fund-review.pdf.

Care Quality Commission. (2017). *Key lines of enquiry, prompts and ratings characteristics for healthcare services.* Available at: http://www.cqc.org.uk/guidance-providers/healthcare/key-lines-enquiry-healthcare-services.

Department of Health. (2016). *Proposals for changing the system of midwifery supervision in the UK.* Available at: https://www.gov.uk/government/publications/changes-to-midwife-supervision-in-the-uk.

Gillman, L. J., & Lloyd, C. (2015). *Re-framing midwifery supervision: a discussion paper.* Available at: https://www.rcm.org.uk/sites/default/files/Re-framing%20supervision%20-paper%20for%20discussion%20final%2023%203%202015.pdf.

Hawkins, P., & Shohet, R. (2012). *Supervision in the helping professions* (4th ed.). Maidenhead: Open University Press.

(England and Wales). *Midwives Act.* (1902). London: HMSO.

Midwives (Ireland) Act. (1918). London: HMSO.

Midwives (Scotland) Act. (1915). London: HMSO.

Ness, V., & Richards, J. (2014). Future proofing supervision in Wales: improving the quality of statutory supervision. *British Journal of Midwifery, 22*(4), 276–280.

NHS England. (2017). *A-EQUIP a model of clinical midwifery supervision.* Available at: https://www.england.nhs.uk/wp-content/uploads/2017/04/a-equip-midwifery-supervision-model.pdf.

Nursing and Midwifery Council. (2012). *Midwives rules and standards.* London: Nursing and Midwifery Council.

Nursing and Midwifery Council. (2014). *Standards for the preparation of supervisors of midwives.* London: Nursing and Midwifery Council.

Nursing and Midwifery The Order. (2001). *Statutory Instruments 2002 No. 253.* London: The Stationery Office. Available at: http://www.legislation.gov.uk/uksi/2002/253/article/1/made.

Osbourne, A. (2007). Supervision of midwives: past and present. In Osbourne, A., Wallace, V., Moorhead, C., Jones, D., Thomas, N., Esson, P., Demilew, J., McElligot, M., Kirby, J., & Rogers, C. (Eds.), *Statutory supervision of midwives: A resource for midwives and mothers* (pp. 1.1–1.12). London: Quay Books Division.

Parliamentary and Health Service Ombudsman. (2013). *Midwifery supervision and regulation: Recommendations for change.* Available at: https://www.ombudsman.org.uk/sites/default/files/Midwifery%20supervision%20and%20regulation_%20recommendations%20for%20change.pdf.

Pettit, A., & Stephen, R. (2015). *Supporting health visitors and fostering resilience – literature review.* London: Institute of Health Visiting.

Proctor, B. (1986). Supervision: A co-operative exercise in accountability. In Marken, M., & Payne, M. (Eds.), *Enabling and ensuring - supervision in practice.* Leicester. National Youth Bureau Council for Education and Training in Youth and Community Work.

Further Reading

Kirkup, B. (2015). *The report of the Morecambe Bay Investigation,* Preston, Lancashire. The Stationery Office. Available at: *https://assets.publishing.service.gov.uk/government/uploads/system/uploads/attachment_data/file/408480/47487_MBI_Accessible_v0.1.pdf.*

> *This report commissioned by the Department of Health and written by Dr Bill Kirkup investigates failings in maternity and neonatal care at Furness General Hospital from 2004 to 2013 and makes recommendations for both the University Hospitals of Morecambe Bay NHS Foundation Trust and the wider National Health Service to prevent such failings happening in the future.*

National Advisory Group on the Safety of Patients in England. (2013). *A promise to learn – a commitment to act: improving the safety of patients in England.* London: Department of Health. Available at: https://www.gov.uk/government/uploads/system/uploads/attachment_data/file/226703/Berwick_Report.pdf.

> *The review into improving the quality and safety of care within the National Health Service was undertaken by Professor Don Berwick following the Francis report (2013) into the failings of Mid Staffordshire NHS Foundation Trust and makes a number of recommendations to improve patient safety, such as embracing a culture of learning within the National Health Service.*

Read, J., & Wallace, V. (2014). Supervision in action: An introduction. *British Journal of Midwifery, 22*(3), 59–62.

> *As a response to the recommendation of the Parliamentary and Health Service Ombudsman (2013) to review statutory supervision, this article provides examples of innovative and proactive supervision in action throughout the United Kingdom. It is the first in a series of articles that focuses on the impact of statutory supervision on the quality agenda, addressing the nine recommendations made by the Berwick report (National Advisory Group on the Safety of Patients in England 2013).*

Royal College of Midwives. (2017). Supervision: Rewriting the rule book. *Midwives, 20,* 66–67.

> *This article provides a useful overview of the employer-led models of supervision that have developed in each of the four nations since statutory supervision was disestablished. Specific website links are included to the respective national models.*

Useful Websites

Healthcare Safety Investigation Branch (an Independent patient safety investigation service): https://www.gov.uk/government/groups/independent-patient-safety-investigation-service-ipsis-expert-advisory-group

NHS Resolution: http://resolution.nhs.uk/

NHS England's webpage for A-EQUIP and midwifery supervision: https://www.england.nhs.uk/mat-transformation/midwifery-task-force/a-equip-midwifery-supervision-model/

New midwifery supervision New midwifery supervision model in Northern Ireland: https://www.health-ni.gov.uk/articles/changes-midwife-supervision-uk

New midwifery supervision model in Scotland: https://www.nmc.org.uk/globalassets/sitedocuments/standards/midwifery-supervision-scotland.pdf

New midwifery supervision model in Wales: http://gov.wales/docs/phhs/publications/170519clinical-supervisionen.pdf

Nursing and Midwifery Council: https://www.nmc.org.uk/

CHAPTER 11

Mentorship, Preceptorship and Coaching in Midwifery Education and Practice

Jayne E. Marshall ■ Claire McKellow ■ Crecious Mutinta Muleya

CONTENTS

LEARNING OUTCOMES

By the end of this chapter the reader will:

- have an understanding of the historical development of mentorship[*], preceptorship and coaching.
- appreciate the comparisons in the role and function of the mentor, preceptor and coach
- appreciate how individuals learn
- be cognizant of the Standards Framework for Nursing and Midwifery Education which inform student supervision and assessment in practice
- understand the factors that contribute to an effective learning environment in the university and practice settings
- be cognizant of the ways in which the knowledge and competence of learners can be assessed
- appreciate the strategies that can be adopted by mentors/practice supervisors and practice assessors, preceptors and coaches when facing various challenges in their respective roles.

[*]Please note that where the terms mentor and mentorship are used, it is in the general sense. In accordance with the Nursing and Midwifery Council (NMC) (2018) standards for student supervision and assessment, the roles with the assigned titles practice supervisor, practice assessor and academic assessor relate to the former midwife mentor/teacher roles. These titles will therefore be used within this chapter when reference is made specifically to the context of midwifery education and practice.

Overview

This chapter examines the concept of mentoring, preceptorship and coaching in midwifery education and practice and provides an overview of the context in which mentoring, preceptorship and coaching take place. The chapter commences with a historical perspective of mentoring and how this has developed into supporting the learning of health care professionals, such as midwives, through supervision and assessment. It discusses how the university and practice settings can be effective in facilitating student learning, including the challenges that mentors/practice supervisors and practice assessors, preceptors and coaches may face in their role, such as deciding to fail a student. The latter part of the chapter explores the role of the preceptor in supporting the transition of the new registrant into a confident practising midwife and how the act of coaching can enable midwives to reach certain goals within their careers.

Introduction

Education in the practice setting has remained an important aspect of midwives' and nurses' professional education. It provides students with real-life situations to which they can apply their knowledge and develop the skills necessary for registration and their subsequent future practice. Although clinical experience is integral to midwifery education and practice, initially it can be quite daunting for the new student who is unfamiliar with the socialization into the organizational environment (see Chapter 1). Various models of clinical education have been used to support students' acquisition of clinical skills, and the practice of *mentoring* has increased in popularity over the years as a beneficial approach to the clinical teaching and learning of health care professionals.

Mentorship

However popular this concept is, there remains a variation in defining *mentoring* and *mentorship*, and often the terms are used interchangeably, including the use of alternative terms such as *supervising*, *preceptoring* and *facilitating* (Chandan and Watts 2012). According to Morton-Cooper and Palmer (2000), a mentor is someone who provides an enabling relationship that facilitates another person's growth and development. Such a relationship should be dynamic and reciprocal, but can be emotionally intense as the mentor assists with career development and guides the mentee through the organizational, social and political networks.

HISTORICAL PERSPECTIVE

The term *mentor* originates from Greek classical mythological literature, specifically from the time when Odysseus set off for the Trojan War and entrusted his household, including his wife and son Telemachus, to his friend Mentor for the length of his absence. Mentor became a guide and counsellor to Telemachus, caring, encouraging and helping him to solve problems (Murray et al 2010). As a result of this relationship, the term *mentor* has been adopted in the English language to mean a *wise counsellor*, denoting a more experienced person who acts as a trusted friend, advisor or teacher (Murray et al 2010).

Traditionally associated with the professions of medicine, law and business, mentorship has increasingly become a popular approach for supporting professionals in various disciplines and has been applied in different ways according to the specific discipline. Examples include the master–apprenticeship model of instruction and mastery (Morris et al 1988; Clutterbuck 2004). The concept of modern mentorship began to appear in the nursing and midwifery literature in the 1960s (Maggs 1994).

In the United Kingdom (UK), the clinical learning in midwifery and nursing education programmes was traditionally based on an apprenticeship model where students not only learned on the job but, as an employee, also provided a service in the practice setting. As a result, as Melia (1987) affirms, the students' learning in practice was given less attention in such a model as the priority was to the maternity/health services in *getting the work done*. With the introduction of the Project 2000 programmes in nursing, the learning needs of students took precedence over their contribution to the demands of the services. Consequently the students acquired supernumerary status for most of the programme, and as they were no longer employees, formal mentorship was introduced as a means of supervising them (Murray et al 2010). To some degree, informal mentoring had taken place previously, but with the introduction of Project 2000 programmes, mentorship became integral to preregistration education in the 1990s (Andrews and Wallace 1999), becoming a mandatory requirement of all preregistration nursing and midwifery education programmes (NMC 2008, 2009a, 2010).

Over the years, mentorship has slowly evolved to include broader elements of learning and teaching with the expectations of both students and mentors increasing, acknowledging that the concept of mentorship is indeed complex (Andrews 2008). Although *mentorship* has been widely adopted as a way of supporting students in the practice setting (Suen and Chow 2001), there continues much ongoing debate as to the definition of the role and function of the mentor.

DEFINING MENTORING

Although numerous definitions and descriptions of mentoring exist, many refer to concepts such as *guiding, supporting, advising* and *career planning*. Anderson and Shannon (1988) describe mentoring as a *nurturing process* which involves an experienced and more skilled person who acts as role model who *teaches, encourages* and *counsels* another individual who is less skilled and less experienced so that the latter is able to develop professionally. This is further elaborated by Faure (2000: 3), who defines mentoring as

a supportive learning relationship between a caring individual who shares knowledge, experience and wisdom with another individual who is ready and willing to benefit from this exchange, to enrich their professional journey.

QUALITIES OF THE MENTOR

For mentors to be successful in their mentoring role, they need to possess certain qualities and skills that will help them meet the expectations of the mentoring role. Fisher (1994) believes that a good mentor should be *intelligent* and *have integrity, good professional attitude, high personal standards, enthusiasm* and *a willingness to share accumulated knowledge*. Huybrecht et al (2011) highlighted that mentors also consider the following as important to their role:

- ability to give constructive feedback
- experience
- availability of time
- positive attitude
- patience and enthusiasm.

Furthermore, NHS Education for Scotland (2013) identified the following desirable mentor qualities:

- *Commitment to student nurse and midwifery education:* advancement of the profession demonstrated through their willingness to educate the next generation of nurses and midwives.

- *Skills to facilitate learning:* being a good communicator, being able to provide feedback about performance, identifying every possible opportunity for learning, providing rationale for their practice, developing the student's confidence, empowering students by allowing them to practise and being able to focus on student learning in busy environments.
- *Personal characteristics and behaviours:* acting as a role model, being aware of their own practice, and having knowledge of the programme and styles of learning, clinical competence and a positive attitude towards students.

These qualities and characteristics of the mentor are valuable in facilitating the development of a meaningful relationship with the student/mentee, but do not necessarily correlate with the extent of the mentor's experience.

E-MENTORING

With the development of the Internet in the 1990s, *e-mentoring* has begun to increase in popularity, and includes the provision of a guided mentoring relationship using online software or email. Many early programmes used email communication to link mentors and mentees, including *telementoring* using telephone communication. One of the first e-mentoring programmes was developed in Canada in 1990, where teachers from schools in British Columbia were given online support and training by experienced peers: the teachers and peers never met face-to-face (Miller 2002).

Modern e-mentoring projects often rely on Web-based solutions, enabling both mentors and mentees to log into a secure online environment where they can converse under the supervision of moderators and coordinators. Online mentoring websites attempt to offer a knowledge base with access mechanisms so a mentee can acquire mentoring advice comparable to the advice from an experienced mentor, via their smartphone, tablet or computer, without having to communicate with a human, which is thus is less time-consuming than face-to-face mentoring. However, one of the limitations of online mentoring is that immediate feedback can be difficult. Because of the inability to pick up on visual or social cues, this mode can be seen as impersonal. Nevertheless, e-mentoring can retain face-to-face interaction through mediums such as FaceTime, Google Hangouts, and Skype.

The quality of the e-mentoring relationship is heavily influenced by the amount of common interests that the mentee and mentor have. It is generally accepted that any mentoring relationship is most effective during a transitional period in the mentee's life, such as applying to university or making decisions about future careers. An example of an e-mentoring organization is the American *MentorNet*, which focuses on women and under-represented minorities in the science, technology, engineering and mathematics fields (STEM). MentorNet is unique in that it uses an algorithm to match mentors and mentees, and since 1997 has matched more than 27 000 mentor relationships (see http://www.mentornet.net).

Brightside is a UK non-profit-making e-mentoring organization that works with businesses, charities and universities (see https://www.thebrightsidetrust.org/). It provides a secure online portal that includes interactive content and resources through which trained online mentors are connected with young people, providing them with information about education and employment. University careers departments are increasingly using e-mentoring platforms such as *Aluminati*, which is targeted at alumni and students of higher education institutions, to offer support in the making of career and employment decisions.

PEER MENTORING

Peer mentoring is a form of mentorship that usually takes place between a person who has lived through a specific experience (peer mentor) and a person who is new to that experience (peer mentee), and can be an effective activity in education, health care and the workplace. The peer mentor may challenge the mentee with new ideas, and encourage the mentee to move beyond the things that are most comfortable. Most peer mentors are selected for their sensibility, confidence, social skills and reliability (Bozeman and Feeney 2007). The frequency with which peer mentors and mentees meet differs according to the mentoring programme, and usually they meet more frequently at the beginning of the relationship to establish a good foundation. Mentors and mentees may maintain contact through email, telephone or face-to-face encounters.

Little is known of the peer mentoring relationship beyond good feelings and the development of friendships; however, peer mentoring led by senior students may discourage diversity and improve experiences within higher education. Peer mentoring can help new students adapt to a new academic environment, and mentors are chosen because they are academically successful and possess good communication, social and leadership skills. As a consequence, the mentor serves as a positive role model for students, guiding them towards academic and social success, and through their support, advice, encouragement and friendship, they may improve student retention rates (Andrews and Clark 2011).

Most peer mentoring programmes led by undergraduate students rarely have direct supervision of university staff full-time, and so it is essential that those who wish to act as peer mentors receive extensive training and supervision for their role to ensure they always offer reliable guidance to their peer mentee. At Kingston and St Georges, student midwives in their second year undergo additional training to take on the role as a peer mentor to support first-year student midwives assimilate knowledge of biological sciences. This provides new students with a good support network and allows a smooth transition to the volume of the workload required within the university and practice settings.

Now undertake Activity 11.1

ACTIVITY 11.1 ■

You are a second-year student midwife, enrolled on the peer mentor scheme at your university, and on completion of the student mentor training programme have been paired with Melissa, a first-year student, to support her transition into higher education.
You are to meet Melissa for the first time in the students' union building at the end of the week. Draw up a plan as to how you envisage facilitating this first meeting in terms of:
- environment
- establishing purpose
- setting clear goals and objectives
- ensuring your guidance is reliable and authentic
- planning subsequent meetings: type, frequency, venue etc.

Standards for Student Supervision and Assessment

The NMC (2008) *Standards to Support Learning and Assessment in Practice* (SLAiP) affirmed that mentors are a mandatory requirement for students undertaking pre-registration midwifery and nursing education programmes. However, in 2018, the NMC published its new radical education and training strategy entitled *Realising Professionalism: Standards for Education and Training*, based on *The Code* (NMC 2018a), which is to be implemented across all approved education institutions (AEIs) and practice learning partners by 2020, consequently replacing the NMC standards in *Standards to Support Learning and Assessment in Practice* (NMC 2008).

The standards for education and training consists of three parts, which should all be read in conjunction with each other:

- *Part 1: Standards Framework for Nursing and Midwifery Education* (NMC 2018b).
- *Part 2: Standards for Student Supervision and Assessment* (NMC 2018c).
- *Part 3: Programme Standards:* one for each programme that the AEI provides (e.g. nursing, midwifery, prescribing etc.) (Whilst *Standards for Pre-registration Nursing Programmes* [NMC 2018d] and *Future Nurse: Standards of Proficiency for Registered Nurses* [NMC 2018e] have been published, *Standards for Pre-registration Midwifery Programmes* and *Standards of Proficiency for Registered Midwives* were in the later stages of development at the time this text went to print).

The standards are all outcome focused, and compliance with *all three sets of standards* is required for an education institution to be approved and offer NMC-approved programmes.

Standards for Student Supervision and Assessment (NMC 2018c) defines the changes to the role that clinicians and academics play in supporting the learning and assessment of students in practice, and is divided into three parts:

- Section 1: *Effective practice learning.* This section describes what needs to be in place to deliver safe and effective learning experiences for the student in the practice setting and specifies that *all* midwives and nurses should contribute to practice learning in accordance with *The Code* (NMC 2018a).
- Sections 2–5: *Supervision of students.* These sections describe the principles of student supervision in the practice setting and the role of the *practice supervisor.*
- Sections 6–19: *Assessment of students and confirmation of proficiency.* These sections set out what is required from educators who are assessing and confirming students' practice and academic achievement. The roles of the *practice assessor* and *academic assessor* are described in these sections.

As a consequence of these changes, the titles of *mentor* and *sign-off mentor* have been replaced by *practice supervisor* and *practice assessor*, for which there are clearly defined roles and responsibilities, which are summarized in Box 11.1, noting that practice assessors are not simultaneously the practice supervisor and academic assessor for the same student. All students on an NMC-approved education programme are assigned to a *different nominated practice assessor* for *a practice placement or series of practice placements* and a *different nominated academic assessor* (e.g. a university midwifery lecturer) for *each part of the programme*; the latter may, however, prove challenging for academic teams to implement because of the volume of students this will apply to.

The NMC (2018c) specifies that AEIs, together with practice learning partners, must ensure that practice supervisors, practice assessors and academic assessors are effectively prepared for and supported in their roles to develop their professional practice and knowledge so as to contribute to student learning and assessment. In addition, this involves having a good understanding of the proficiencies and programme outcomes they are supporting students to achieve. Whilst the specific preparation for the role of *practice supervisor* is less defined (other than they have to be a health or social care registrant), it is expected that to become a *practice assessor* the midwife or nurse is expected to demonstrate achievement of the following outcomes as a *minimum* (NMC 2018c: 11):

- interpersonal communication skills, relevant to student learning and assessment
- conducting objective, evidence-based assessments of students
- providing constructive feedback to facilitate professional development in others
- knowledge of the assessment process and their role within it.

For the *academic assessor*, this also entails that the midwife or nurse is working towards or holds a relevant qualification as required by their employer (university/academic institution) and local and national policies.

BOX 11.1 ■ **The Role and Responsibilities of Practice Supervisor and Practice Assessor**

Approved Education Institutions, Together with Practice Learning Partners, Must Ensure That:

A Practice Supervisor:	*A Nominated Practice Assessor:*
■ is a Nursing and Midwifery Council (NMC)-registered nurse, midwife and nursing associate, or other registered health and social care professional, such as a physiotherapist or social worker	■ is always an NMC registrant with the equivalent experience to the student's field of practice: nurse (adult, child, mental health, learning disability), midwife or nursing associate
■ serves as a role model for safe and effective practice in line with their code of conduct	■ conducts assessments to confirm student achievement of proficiencies and programme outcomes for practice learning
■ supports learning in line with their scope of practice to enable the student to meet their proficiencies and programme outcomes	■ makes assessment decisions informed by feedback sought and received from practice supervisors
■ supports and supervises students, providing feedback on their progress towards, and achievement of, proficiencies and skills	■ makes and records objective, evidenced-based assessments on conduct, proficiency and achievement, drawing on student records, direct observations, student self-reflection and other resources
■ has current knowledge and experience of the area in which they are providing support, supervision and feedback	■ maintains current knowledge and expertise relevant for the proficiencies and programme outcomes they are assessing and receives ongoing support to fulfil their role
■ receives ongoing support to participate in the practice learning of students	■ has an understanding of the student's learning and achievement in theory
■ contributes to the student's record of achievement by periodically recording relevant observations on the conduct, proficiency and achievement of the students they are supervising	■ works in partnership with the nominated academic assessor as scheduled to evaluate and recommend the student for progression for each part of the programme, in line with programme standards and local and national policies
■ contributes to student assessment to inform decisions for progression	■ has sufficient opportunities to periodically observe the student across environments in order to inform decisions for assessment and progression
■ has sufficient opportunities to engage with practice assessors and academic assessors to share relevant observations on the conduct, proficiency and achievement of the students they are supervising	■ has sufficient opportunities to gather and coordinate feedback from practice supervisors, any other practice assessors and relevant people in order to be assured about their decision for assessment and progression
■ appropriately raises and responds to student conduct and competence concerns and is supported in doing so.	■ appropriately raises and responds to student conduct and competence concerns and is supported in doing so.

Adapted from Nursing and Midwifery Council (2018c).

Facilitating Learning: How Do Others Learn?

Illeris (2004) presents contemporary learning theory as an integration of three dimensions – *cognitive*, *emotional* and *social* – which occur simultaneously in the learning process. Although learning is a holistic human process, Illeris (2004) overlooks other possible dimensions of learning such as *physical* or *spiritual*. Nevertheless, the purpose of facilitating learning in any setting is to acquire, enhance or make changes in personal knowledge, skills, values, and world views. The Department of Health (2001) indicates that facilitation of learning should allow students to find opportunities to identify experiences that meet their specific learning needs.

Facilitation of adult learning transforms students through experiential learning in a supportive environment that enables them to make sense of and learn from the experiences gained, of which the mentor/practice supervisor is key and the student is at the centre. Shifting from a *teacher-centred (pedagogical)* approach to a more *learner-centred (andragogical)* approach involves putting the learners' needs at the centre of activities; however, facilitating learning can be a challenge for midwives to accomplish in busy practice settings with increasing service demands (Garrison and Kanuka 2004; Warren 2010).

To be an effective mentor/practice supervisor who can confidently optimize a student's learning, the midwife needs to have knowledge of different learning theories, such as the social learning theory developed by Bandura (1977), and learning styles of others (*visual*, *auditory* and *kinaesthetic*) as well as the facilitation skills to apply the principles/frameworks to their practice. It is, however, worth noting that although everyone has the capability of learning by all three styles, they are usually dominant in one and individuals retain *20%* of what they *see*, *40–50%* of what they *see and hear* and *90%* of what they *see, hear and do*, as shown in Fig. 11.1.

Selecting suitable teaching and learning methods is critical in assisting students to bridge the gap between theoretical and practical knowledge. The learning approach should be mutually agreed with the individual student, and it should facilitate reflection and autonomy to enable students to take responsibility for their own learning and make progress in their studies (Pritchard and Gidman 2012). Table 11.1 shows some of the methods that appeal to visual, auditory and kinaesthetic learners.

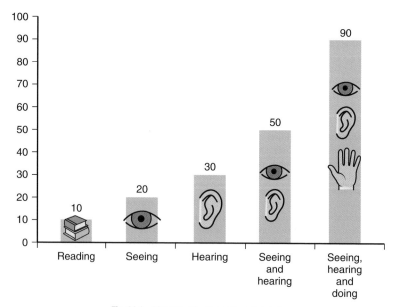

Fig. 11.1 How much do we learn/retain?

TABLE 11.1 ■ Learning Styles and Teaching Methods

Visual	Auditory	Kinaesthetic
Videos, slides	Lectures	Role play
Flip charts	Group discussions/seminars	Simulation
Records, documents, texts	Informal conversations	Practice demonstrations
Demonstrations	Case studies, stories	Writing/note taking

TABLE 11.2 ■ Knowles's (1984) Five Assumptions of Adult Learners

1. Self-concept	As a person matures, his/her self-concept moves from one of being a dependent personality towards one of being a self-directed human being
2. Adult learner experience	As a person matures, he/she accumulates a growing reservoir of experience that becomes an increasing resource for learning
3. Readiness to learn	As a person matures, his/her readiness to learn becomes oriented increasingly to the developmental tasks of his/her social roles
4. Orientation to learning	As a person matures, his/her time perspective changes from one of postponed application of knowledge to immediacy of application. As a result, his/her orientation towards learning shifts from one of subject centredness to one of problem centredness
5. Motivation to learn	As a person matures, the motivation is internal

THE ADULT LEARNER

The notion of the adult learner particularly underpins many aspects of postgraduate education and training, but also influences undergraduate education in that the learning has a purpose and participation is voluntary. Adult learners are characterized by maturity, self-confidence and autonomy, who bring their life experiences and self-awareness to learning, which younger learners do not. Assumptions about the characteristics of adult learners have been made by Knowles (1970) which can serve in supporting mentors/practice supervisors to direct appropriate learning activities in the practice setting and are shown in Table 11.2.

The adult learner should always be involved with the mentor/practice supervisor in the planning and evaluation of their learning, which includes setting clear learning goals and objectives. Past experiences, including any errors/oversights, should provide the basis for developing subsequent learning activities for the learner. Usually adults are most interested in learning about subjects that have immediate relevance to and impact on their job or personal life. In addition, Kearsley (2010) purports that adult learning is problem centred rather than content oriented.

Now undertake Activity 11.2.

ACTIVITY 11.2 ■

- Think about your various learning styles (*visual, auditory* and *kinaesthetic*) and consider which of these styles enables you to learn more effectively in your current role (student, midwife, educator). *(There may be more than one style.)*
- What specific teaching methods do you find effective to help you translate your knowledge into practice in the specific role you occupy (student, midwife, educator)?
- How can you transfer this knowledge and awareness of your own learning style to facilitate the learning of others as a peer mentor, midwife practice supervisor, practice assessor, preceptor, coach and educator/academic assessor?

'LEARNING BY DOING': BECOMING A PROFESSIONAL

Learning by doing is an educational theory that originated from the American philosopher John Dewey and is based on learning being relevant and practical, rather than passive and theoretical. Although its origins were in pedagogy, this approach has been adapted and applied to other types of education, such as apprenticeship and vocational training, including midwifery and nursing. Learning in the practice setting is also part of the socialization of becoming a professional, of which the mentor/practice supervisor plays a critical part (see Chapter 1).

Supporting students in the practice setting often involves seeking out opportunities for learners to practise clinical skills ranging from simple procedures, such as undertaking urinalysis, to much more complex activities, such as breaking bad news or undertaking perineal repair. In midwifery and nursing education, much of the learning is necessarily experiential, as there is a lot of *learning by doing* as well as *learning by observation* to become socialized into the workplace and the professional role. Benner (1984) observed that learning the clinical skills to become a health care professional develops in five stages throughout the career trajectory, progressing from *novice* to *advanced beginner* then *competent practitioner* at the point of registration to *proficient practitioner* and ultimately to *expert practitioner* (see Chapter 1). It is imperative that mentors/practice supervisors understand at what stage of learning the student is, to ensure they not only assign suitable activities for the student to undertake but also provide the appropriate level of guidance and supervision to facilitate their ongoing learning and development. This would range from *initial observation* to *direct supervision* and eventually *indirect supervision*.

Creating an Effective Learning Environment in the University and Practice Setting

For students to experience quality learning, educators and mentors/practice supervisors and practice assessors play a vital role in creating an environment that is conducive to learning, albeit the culture of the setting, be it in the university or in practice placements, can also play a considerable role in affecting a positive or negative learning experience. Edwards et al (2004) discuss that an effective learning environment is one that is supportive, has a good atmosphere, has excellent interprofessional working relationships and is perceived to produce positive learning outcomes. In the practice setting, this would be an environment where students are welcomed and practice-based staff are happy, are friendly, have a positive attitude and are willing to teach and guide students in providing quality health care (Papp et al 2003; Edwards et al 2004; Papastvrou et al 2010; Chuan and Barnett 2012). This builds the students' confidence as they are motivated to learn in an environment where they are respected, supported and identified as part of the care team (Chesser-Smyth 2005; Kelly 2007; Levett-Jones and Lathlean 2008; Henderson et al 2010). However, an unfriendly learning environment in any setting denies students the opportunity to learn, build their confidence and become knowledgeable and competent.

According to Jarvis and Gibson (1997), some of the characteristics of an effective learning environment include but are not limited to:

- having effective links with the university (AEI) or educational establishment
- having dedicated and uninterrupted time for group and individual seminars and tutorials where students can have time to participate
- use of an interprofessional team approach in the facilitation of learning and the assessment of the educational processes
- having adequate resources for students learning in the clinical environment
- having dedicated clinical staff who continually update their knowledge through research, are adequately prepared to undertake the roles as teachers and assessors and are also willing to share their knowledge with the students through a variety of processes.

All student midwives and nurses are *supernumerary* in the practice setting, and the NMC (2018c) further determines effective practice learning. This includes there being a nominated person for each practice setting to actively support students and address their concerns, empowering students to be proactive and take responsibility for their learning and providing opportunities for them to learn from a range of relevant people, such as service users, registered and non-registered individuals and other students as appropriate. The level of supervision should be tailored to the learning needs of the individual student and commensurate with the stage of their learning, proficiencies and programme outcomes. Learning experiences should be inclusive, supporting the diverse needs of individual students. This may include providing adjustments in accordance with relevant equalities and human rights legislation in all learning environments, as well as for supervision and assessment.

Assessing the Knowledge and Competence of the Learner

All student midwives must be supported and assessed by appropriately prepared practice supervisors, practice assessors and academic assessors (NMC 2018c). Aston and Hallam (2011) state that assessing a student's learning and application to practice is one of the most important roles of a registrant, for which they are accountable. It is the responsibility of the practice assessor to evaluate the total performance of students, including their knowledge, skills, attitudes and behaviours, and thus contribute to the overall decision made about their entry to the professional register.

The assessment should include both *formative* and *summative* elements. *Formative* assessments are diagnostic in nature and usually take place in an informal way throughout a practice placement to assess the extent of a student's progress (Kilgallon and Thompson 2012). They may not necessarily involve grading the performance, but they provide an opportunity of highlighting to the student their strengths and the areas for improvement, in a non-threatening manner and timely way, in order to guide future learning strategies. Such assessments are useful in preparing the student for *summative* assessments, which are undertaken towards the *end of a period of practice* and *before entry to the professional register,* usually involving the actual grading of the student's final performance in terms of knowledge and competence (Kilgallon and Thompson 2012).

Several methods and strategies can be used to assess a student's competence and may include:

- *direct observation* of care provision, simulation, objective structured clinical examination (OSCE).
- *written sources,* such as student self-assessment, portfolio of evidence, learning contracts
- *verbal sources,* including interactive reflective discussion, service user comments and through team mentorship.

MAKING THE DECISION TO FAIL A STUDENT

The assessment of students should always be objective. This can often prove a challenge where there is a mentor–mentee relationship that develops over an extended period, such that biases may creep into assessing/grading a student's performance. The personal friendship built during the course of the mentoring relationship should never hinder objective assessment of students' performance. Duffy (2015), however, refers to the emotional stress mentors experience with failing a student and the sense of personal failing regarding their mentorship skills. Assessing students' unsatisfactory performance in practice is a demoralizing experience, and mentors in Duffy's (2015) study identified feelings of self-doubt, anxiety, anger and sadness as they moved through the decision to fail a student in practice.

The introduction of the *Standards for Student Supervision and Assessment* (NMC 2018c) defining separate roles of the practice supervisor and the practice assessor aims to minimize the challenges mentors have experienced in the past and strengthen the objectivity of assessment. Should a mentor/

practice supervisor have concerns about a student's performance in that they feel they are unlikely to reach the required level of competence, it is good practice, in the first instance, to seek support from a colleague to provide an independent assessment of the student's ability. Informing the student's academic assessor/personal tutor/university link lecturer at the earliest opportunity and arranging a tripartite meeting is also important to explore ways in which additional support can be provided from a range of sources. Duffy (2015) supports the practice of an action plan, regular meetings and clear documentation of the areas of concern as a means of managing a failing student. However, should the student fail to demonstrate the required level of competence at the summative practice point despite the additional support, the university should respect the practice assessor's judgement and support their decision to fail the student. In addition, a number of studies have emphasized the importance of the university providing ongoing support for practice staff after they have made the decision to fail the student. This should include receiving feedback/debriefing from the academic team of the outcome and the academic processes, particularly in cases where a student has made an appeal against the decision (Basnett and Sheffield 2010; Duffy 2015).

Case Study 11.1 highlights just one scenario that a mentor/practice supervisor may be faced with in the practice setting – that of a student midwife who may be having difficulty in achieving both theoretical and practice outcomes – and suggests ways in which the mentor/practice supervisor can be facilitative towards the student's additional needs and contribute towards their progress.

CASE STUDY 11.1 ■

Student midwife Sarah has recently received a diagnosis of dyslexia at the end of the first year of her studies. She was referred for testing after failing some academic assignments and struggling with information and documentation whilst in clinical practice. She finds there is too much pressure to complete maternity health records quickly and accurately. She also finds it especially hard to remember lots of information given at once by different health professionals. There are a number of strategies that a mentor/practice supervisor and practice assessor can use to support Sarah's additional learning needs and facilitate her moving forward through her studies.
Strategies to support this may include:

- Completing learning contracts at the beginning of the placement to enable Sarah to discuss her learning objectives with her mentor/practice supervisor for this part of the programme. This discussion should provide an opportunity to explore how the mentor/practice supervisor can support Sarah's additional needs for her to achieve the required learning outcomes.
- In this particular case, the mentor/practice supervisor should allow Sarah more time to complete documentation and support her to slowly take on more recording of details as her experience grows. This should be reviewed as Sarah progresses throughout the programme towards the point of registration to enable her to complete records in a more timely fashion and in more depth.
- Consideration should be given as to how Sarah can assimilate the information discussed whilst in clinical practice, particularly during interprofessional conversations. To aid her memory, Sarah should be encouraged to take written notes or even audio record the information so that this can be reviewed at a later point. However, confidentiality of information regarding individual childbearing women and their babies must be maintained at all times.
- The mentor/practice supervisor should always liaise with the academic assessor, practice assessor and link lecturers to ensure that the best possible opportunities are given to students such as Sarah to achieve their learning outcomes and they are assessed without discrimination whilst in the practice setting.

However, it is important to remember that by the end of their studies, student midwives with additional learning needs must be able to demonstrate the *same level* of academic and clinical competence as *all students* to successfully complete the requirements of the midwifery education programme to register as a midwife with the respective country's professional statutory and regulatory body, such as the Nursing and Midwifery Council.

Challenges of Mentoring

Although there are many benefits of mentoring, there can also be challenges that may hinder the effectiveness of the role of the mentor. A study by Veeramah (2012) exploring the barriers to successful mentoring of pre-registration student nurses and student midwives revealed the following:

- Lack of time and the demands of health/maternity care are two key barriers to successful mentoring (Elcock and Sookhoo 2007; Gopee 2011).
- Inadequate preparation and support can result in mentors passing students they should otherwise fail.
- Mentors need more support and educational guidance in completing the practice assessment documentation from the higher education institution (McCarthy and Murphy 2008; Nettleton and Bray 2008).
- Mentors should have regular updates and relevant in-service training to remain contemporary in their mentorship skills (Myall et al 2008).
- Practice development managers and clinical practice facilitators should work with link lecturers to support mentors in practice.

It is essential that supervision and assessment of students is effective. The NMC (2018c) standards aim to facilitate innovative and creative approaches for supporting student learning in practice in a more collegial way that should reduce some of the challenges previously experienced with mentorship. To ensure that the public is protected by prevention of the registration of unsafe and incompetent midwives and nurses, registrants undertaking the role of practice supervisor and practice assessor require protected time away from their clinical duties to effectively support students in practice as well as to attend regular updates for their own supervising/assessing role. It is vital that AEIs and service providers continue to collaborate to ensure that registrants are appropriately supported in these vital roles.

Preceptorship

Deriving from the Latin *praecipere* meaning *to teach*, a *preceptor* is defined as a *teacher/instructor* or an *expert/specialist*. The concept of preceptorship as defined by the Department of Health (2010) is a structured period of transition that the newly qualified practitioner undertakes when they commence employment within the National Health Service (NHS), during which they will be supported by a preceptor to develop their confidence as an autonomous professional, refine skills, values and behaviours, and continue on their journey of lifelong learning.

In midwifery, the aim of preceptorship is to enhance the skills of the newly qualified midwife in relation to their clinical practice skills, developing their confidence and working relationships within a multiprofessional culture and ultimately improve the retention of midwives in the profession by providing the best start to their career journey. Hughes and Fraser (2011) express concerns regarding the high attrition of early-career midwives, due in part to their feelings of lack of support and the overwhelming feeling of inadequacy in not being experienced enough to deal with certain cases.

The Northern Ireland Practice and Education Council for Nursing and Midwifery (NIPEC) (2013) describes the provision of professional support and development within the nursing and midwifery professions as being part of a continuum, commencing with the support given to students undertaking pre-registration programmes and preceptorship for those newly qualified, those returning to practice or new registrants from outside the UK. Preceptorship should not be underestimated and needs to be firmly endorsed across the midwifery profession. Mason and Davies (2013) affirm that preceptorship programmes aim to bridge the gap between learner and accountable practitioner; support, nurture and retain newly qualified midwives; and enable them to develop into safe and effective practitioners of the future. At the point of entry to the NMC register, midwives are confirmed as safe, effective and proficient practitioners in supporting and promoting physiological childbirth (NMC 2009). As a consequence, Mason and Davies (2013) acknowledge that the newly qualified midwife will not necessarily be fully equipped with the range of skills associated with care for women who have complex health and social care needs and therefore require a structured programme and an additional period of support in their new role. This support should be designed to help the newly qualified midwife to develop confidence and enhance their competence, including their critical thinking and decision-making skills.

The transition from student to qualified midwife can, however, be a stressful time, where perceived lack of knowledge and support during this phase can be a cause of anxiety in coping with the complex demands of clinical practice for all staff (Robinson and Griffiths 2009; Park et al 2010). In recognition that the period after qualifying for newly qualified midwives is *pivotal*, the *Preceptorship Framework* (Department of Health 2010) was developed to ease the transition to the work environment. The delivery of programmes of preceptorship, however, is variable in both timing and content as they tend to remain a local responsibility for the employer to devise and implement. The NIPEC (2013) has devised its own preceptorship framework, which includes elements of teaching, role-modelling, socializing, assessing and orienting midwives into the practice setting in their new role.

Stewart et al (2010) highlighted the benefits of preceptorship programmes following an evaluation of their structured programme. It was found that new registrants felt more confident, had improved critical thinking ability, had increased knowledge and, as a consequence, stated they had more job satisfaction and felt valued by their employer.

THE PRECEPTOR

A preceptor is a registered practitioner who has been given a formal responsibility to support a newly qualified practitioner through a period of preceptorship. The benefits of preceptorship are experienced not only by the preceptee but also by those in the preceptor role who feel positive in having the opportunity to develop their colleagues professionally through acting as a good role model. As the NIPEC (2013) acknowledges, the ultimate outcome of preceptorship programmes is that service users benefit as a result of being cared for by safe, competent and confident practitioners.

The terms *preceptor* and *mentor* have often been used interchangeably, and consequently this has caused some confusion when attempting to compare the concept of mentorship with that of preceptorship. Mason and Davies (2013) suggest that protected learning time should be available in the first year of qualified practice, with access to a preceptor, with whom regular meetings are held. The role of the preceptor is to provide support, guidance and evaluation to allow the newly qualified autonomous practitioner opportunity to enhance and further develop their autonomy, rather than work closely with them, observing their practice as a mentor/practice supervisor would do with a student (Yonge et al 2007).

The Preceptorship Framework (Department of Health 2010) has a clear vision of what attributes a preceptor should have, including having the ability to act as an exemplary role model and to be a conduit to formalize and demonstrate continued professional development. However, there is no clear guidance as to what preceptor preparation should include (Panzavecchia and Pearce 2014).

Currently, in the UK there is no requirement for preceptors to have a teaching or assessing qualification. Panzavecchia and Pearce (2014) discuss that with the move to an all-graduate profession, this education paradigm requires experienced preceptors with sufficient knowledge to support preceptees in this crucial period to play a vital role in shaping professional attitude. This is also supported by DeWolfe et al (2010), who state that preceptors need knowledge of how students or preceptees learn in order to facilitate their development.

A preceptor training programme, devised in conjunction with the local AEI, would ensure that preceptors have the knowledge and skills required to enhance confidence to provide the appropriate developmental environment for their preceptees. It would give preceptors a formal *preceptor* status/qualification, which will enhance their own development. The Royal College of Midwives (2010) has devised a 5-day programme to support midwife preceptors who have a role in guiding newly registered midwives. The programme covers learning and developing leadership styles and aims to develop the preceptee's confidence in ongoing skills acquisition.

As there is little evidence in the UK on preceptorship, Lackey (2007) argues that if midwives are not to be lost to the profession, there is a need for more research in this area to assess how the initial period of practice can be effective in confidence building and support. It is also crucial to ascertain what factors may influence a midwife's decision to leave the profession after recently qualifying (Currie and Watts 2012).

EFFECTIVENESS OF PRECEPTORSHIP

Mason and Davies (2013) evaluated a 12–18-month preceptorship programme facilitated in one NHS Foundation Trust in the UK by individual interviews and focus groups with newly qualified midwives, preceptors and midwifery managers. All participants seemed highly focused on the issue of skills acquisition, which Mason and Davies (2013) suggested was reflective of a culture where newly qualified midwives/preceptees are expected to *hit the ground running* and that *ticking off* a list of competencies appeared to be linked with the development of confidence. However, both newly qualified midwives and preceptors felt that the practice-based education and support by members of the multidisciplinary team effectively facilitated the development of confidence, skills and decision-making expertise.

Feltham (2014) conducted a study on the value of preceptorship for newly qualified midwives and came to similar conclusions. Preceptorship provided the newly qualified midwife with the opportunity to learn and reflect in the clinical environment, which was important in enhancing and developing their clinical skills with support and guidance from an experienced midwife rather than being *dropped in at the deep end*.

Panzavecchia and Pearce (2014) describe comparisons between mentoring and precepting, with consensus that the preceptor role draws on the skills of coaching. This is further explored by Clutterbuck (2007) who discusses that the ability to use a variety of styles, skills and techniques should be appropriate to the context in which the coaching takes place.

Coaching

The notion of a coach provides an impression of some form of sports coach, *directing/pushing* an individual or group of individuals through instruction, giving advice and offering guidance to improve their performance by focusing on a particular aspect of their game. Thomson (2014: 10), however, highlights a *non-directive/pulling* approach to coaching that

> *is a relationship of rapport and trust in which the coach uses their ability to listen, to ask questions and to play back what the client has communicated in order to help the client to clarify what matters to them and to work out what to do to achieve their aspirations.*

Non-directive coaching creates a different relationship than if the coaching were directive and is about facilitating, not instructing, advising or guiding, but rather working with someone, not doing something to them. A coach is required to have the skills of *listening*, *questioning* and *paraphrasing* and the ability to establish rapport and trust in the relationship. The coach continually draws on their personal experiences and intuition to influence the next steps in the coaching relationship, which Thomson (2014) refers to as an art rather than a science. Downey (2003) lists different behaviours a coach might use in a conversation with an individual and places them on a continuum from directive behaviour, where the coach aims to solve an individual's problem for them, to non-directive behaviour of helping an individual to solve their own problem. These are shown in Fig. 11.2.

Coaching usually takes place through conversations, and a simple framework a coach can use is that of the *GROW* model (Whitmore 2002), which provides a powerful tool to highlight, elicit and maximize inner potential through a series of sequential coaching conversations.

GROW is an acronym standing for *goals*, *reality*, *options* and *will*, highlighting the four key steps in the implementation of the GROW model. By an individual working through these four stages, the GROW model raises an individual's awareness and understanding of:

1. their own aspirations
2. their current situation and beliefs
3. the possibilities and resources open to them
4. the actions they want to take to achieve their personal and professional goals.

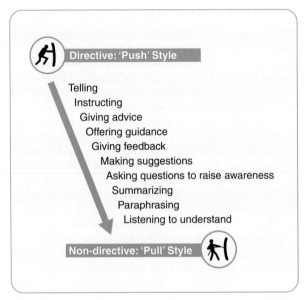

Fig. 11.2 The coaching continuum. (Adapted from Downey 2003)

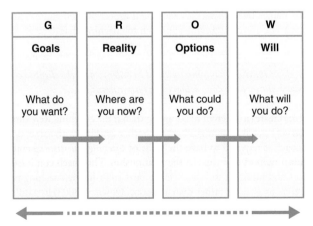

Fig. 11.3 The GROW model.

The GROW model as shown in Fig. 11.3 forms the most common basis of coaching in many organizations and universities globally. It is one of the most popular principal pillars used within the international coaching community as a whole because of its success in both problem solving and goal setting, helping to maximize and maintain personal achievement and productivity. It is a powerful leadership tool that is flexible, and its efficacy transcends boundaries of culture, discipline and personality.

By setting goals which are *inspiring* and *challenging* as well as specific, measurable and achievable in a realistic time frame (SMART), the GROW model successfully promotes confidence and self-motivation, leading to increased productivity and personal satisfaction. The *will* element of the fourth stage in the model is the barometer of success. It relates to volition, desire and intention. By using carefully structured questions, the GROW model promotes a deeper awareness and responsibility and encourages proactive behaviour, as well as resulting in practical techniques to accomplish goals and overcome obstacles.

The use of continuous and progressive coaching skills support provides the structure which ultimately helps to release an individual's true potential by increasing confidence and motivation, leading to both short-term and long-term benefits. Such a model has been seen to yield higher productivity, improved communication, better interpersonal relationships and a better quality working environment, and thus is a viable option to use in midwifery education and practice to enable midwives to achieve their career aspirations.

Now undertake Activity 11.3.

ACTIVITY 11.3 ■

You have successfully completed the pre-registration midwifery education programme and are now a registered midwife with the professional, statutory and regulatory body of the country in which you studied. You have been offered a post as a midwife in the local maternity unit and are due to commence employment in the next week.

- List the short-term goals you wish to achieve within the first year of employment.
- How would a *mentor, preceptor* and *coach* be effective in supporting you to achieve each of your personal career aspirations?

Conclusion

The lifelong learning of midwives throughout their career from students to newly qualified practitioners and subsequent experts in the field requires a nurturing and encouraging environment: in both the university and the practice setting. It is the role of mentors/practice supervisors and practice assessors, preceptors and coaches to provide vital nurturing and supportive environments and opportunities to ensure the development of a safe and effective workforce. Although each role is unique, their involvement at various stages and throughout the midwife's career trajectory is crucial. It is vital that midwives appreciate the way in which adults learn in an increasing technological society and value the attributes that each of these roles possess. Establishing the concepts of mentorship/supervising and assessing, preceptorship and coaching firmly within the organizational culture is key to enabling midwives to develop their confidence, enhance interprofessional working relationships and ultimately improve the retention of midwives within the profession.

KEY POINTS

- The concepts of *mentoring* and *preceptoring* are often used interchangeably, which can cause lack of clarity in the respective roles and function of *mentor* and *preceptor*.
- Midwives require an understanding of different learning theories and learning styles to be an effective mentor/practice supervisor, preceptor or coach to others.
- An effective learning environment in both the university and the practice setting is one that is supportive, has a good atmosphere, has excellent interprofessional working relationships and is perceived to produce positive learning outcomes.
- Where a mentor/practice assessor has made the decision to fail a student, they should be supported by the academic team throughout the entire process, including any appeal made against the decision and the subsequent outcome.
- Peer mentoring in higher education can be an effective strategy to improve student retention rates.
- Preceptorship programmes aim to bridge the gap from learners to safe and effective practitioners.
- The GROW model coaching tool is a viable option to use in midwifery education and practice to enable midwives achieve their career aspirations by highlighting, eliciting and maximizing an individual's inner potential through a series of sequential coaching conversations.

References

Anderson, E., & Shannon, A. (1988). Towards a conceptualization of mentoring. *Journal of Teacher Education, 39,* 38–42.

Andrews, J., & Clark, R. (2011). *Peer mentoring works! How peer mentoring enhances student success in higher education.* Birmingham: Aston University. Available at: https://www.heacademy.ac.uk/system/files/resources/aston_what_works_final_report_1.pdf.

Andrews, M. (2008). Contemporary issues in mentoring practice. In S. West, T. Clark, & M. Jasper (Eds.), *Enabling learning in nursing and midwifery practice; a guide for mentors.* Chichester: John Wiley and Sons.

Andrews, M., & Wallis, M. (1999). Mentorship in nursing: a literature review. *Journal of Advanced Nursing, 29*(1), 201–207.

Aston, L., & Hallam, P. (2011). *Successful mentoring in nursing.* Exeter: Learning Matters.

Bandura, A. (1977). *Social learning theory.* Englewood Cliffs: Prentice Hall.

Basnett, F., & Sheffield, D. (2010). The impact of social work student failure upon practice educators. *British Journal of Social Work, 40,* 2119–2136.

Benner, P. (1984). *From novice to expert: Excellence and power in clinical nursing practice.* Menlo Park: Addison-Wesley.

Bozeman, B., & Feeney, M. K. (2007). Toward a useful theory of mentoring: a conceptual analysis and critique. *Administration and Society, 39*(6), 719–739.

Chandan, M., & Watts, C. (2012). Mentoring and pre-registration nurse education. Available at: http://www.williscommission.org.uk/__data/assets/pdf_file/0009/479934/Mentoring_and_pre-registration_nurse_education.pdf.

Chesser-Smyth, P. A. (2005). The lived experiences of general student nurses on their first clinical placement: A phenomenological study. *Nurse Education in Practice, 5,* 320–327.

Chuan, O. L., & Barnett, T. (2012). Student tutor and staff perceptions of the clinical learning environment. *Nurse Education in Practice, 12,* 192–197.

Clutterbuck, D. (2004). *Everyone needs a mentor* (4th ed.). London: Chartered Institute of Personnel and Development.

Clutterbuck, D. (2007). *Coaching the team at work.* London: Nicholas Brealey International.

Currie, I., & Watts, C. (2012). *Preceptorship and pre-registration nurse education.* London: Department of Health.

Department of Health. (2001). *Working together-learning together: a framework for lifelong learning for the NHS.* London: Department of Health.

Department of Health. (2010). Preceptorship framework for newly registered nurses, midwives and allied health professionals. Available at: http://webarchive.nationalarchives.gov.uk/20130104212348/ http://www.dh.gov.uk/en/Publicationsandstatistics/Publications/PublicationsPolicyAndGuidance/ DH_114073.

DeWolfe, J. A., Laschinger, S., & Perkin, C. (2010). Preceptors' perspectives on recruitment, support and retention of preceptors. *Journal of Nurse Education, 49*(4), 198–206.

Downey, M. (2003). *Effective coaching*. London: Texere.

Duffy, K. (2015). Deciding to fail: nurse mentors' experiences of managing a failed practice assessment. *Journal of Practice Teaching and Learning, 11*(3), 36–58.

Edwards, H., Smith, S., Courtney, M., Finlayson, K., & Chapman, H. (2004). Impact of clinical placement location on nursing students' competency and preparedness for practice. *Nurse Education Today, 24,* 248–255.

Elcock, K., & Sookhoo, D. (2007). Evaluating a new role in mentoring the mentors. *Nursing Standard, 15*(6), 35–38.

Faure, S. (2000). Introduction to mentoring: IM/IT community. Available at: http://www.ciodpi.gc.ca/ orobgc/devprog/mentor/2000-09/mentoring/mentoring_e.pdf.

Feltham, C. (2014). The value of preceptorship for newly qualified midwives. *British Journal of Midwifery, 22*(6), 427–431.

Fisher, B. (1994). *Mentoring*. London: Library Association Publishing.

Garrison, D. R., & Kanuka, H. (2004). Blended learning: Uncovering its transformative potential in higher education. *The Internet and Higher Education, 7*(2), 95–105.

Gopee, N. (2011). *Mentoring and supervision in healthcare*. London: Sage.

Henderson, A., Twentyman, M., Eaton, E., Creedy, D., Stapleton, P., & Lloyd, B. (2010). Creating supportive clinical learning environments: an intervention study. *Journal of Clinical Nursing, 19*(1–2), 177–182.

Hughes, A. J., & Fraser, D. M. (2011). 'Sink or swim': The experience of newly qualified midwives in England. *Midwifery, 27*(3), 382–386.

Huybrecht, S., Loeckx, W., Quaeyhaegens, Y., de Tobel, D., & Mistiaen, W. (2011). Mentoring in nursing education: perceived characteristics of mentors and the consequences of mentorship. *Nurse Education Today, 31,* 274–278.

Illeris, K. (2004). A model for learning in working life. *Journal of Workplace Learning, 16*(8), 431–441.

Jarvis, P., & Gibson, S. (1997). *The teaching practitioner and mentoring in nursing, midwifery, health visiting and the social services*. Cheltenham: Stanley Thomas.

Kearsley, G. (2010). Andragogy (M. Knowles). The theory into practice database. Available at: http://tip. psychology.org.

Kelly, C. (2007). Students' perceptions of effective clinical teaching revisited. *Nurse Education Today, 27,* 885–892.

Kilgallon, K., & Thompson, J. (Eds.). (2012). *Mentoring in nursing and healthcare: A practical approach*. Chichester: John Wiley and Sons.

Knowles, M. S. (1970). *The modern practice of adult education: Andragogy vs. pedagogy*. New York: Association Press.

Knowles, M. S. (1984). *Andragogy in action: Applying modern principles of adult education*. San Francisco: Jossey Bass.

Lackey, T. (2007). Transition of the newly qualified. *RCM Midwives, 10*(6), 296.

Levett-Jones, T., & Lathlean, J. (2008). Belongingness: A prerequisite for nursing student clinical learning. *Nurse Education in Practice, 8,* 108–111.

Maggs, C. (1994). Mentorship in nursing and midwifery education issues for research. *Nurse Education Today, 14,* 22–29.

Mason, J., & Davies, S. (2013). A qualitative evaluation of a preceptorship programme to support newly qualified midwives. *Evidenced Based Midwifery, 11*(3), 94–98.

McCarthy, B., & Murphy, S. (2008). Assessing undergraduate nursing students in clinical practice: Do preceptors use assessment strategies? *Nurse Education Today, 28*(3), 301–313.

Melia, K. (1987). *Learning and working: The occupational socialization of nurses*. London: Tavistock Publications.

Miller, A. (2002). *Mentoring students and young people: A handbook of effective practice*. London: Kogan Page.

Morris, N., John, G., & Keen, T. (1988). Mentors: Learning the ropes. *Nursing Times, 64*(46), 24–26.

Morton-Cooper, A., & Palmer, A. (2000). *Mentoring, preceptorship and clinical supervision. A guide to professional support roles in clinical practice* (2nd ed.). London: Blackwell Science.

Murray, C., Rosen, L., & Staniland, K. (Eds.). (2010). *The nurse mentor and reviewer update book*. Maidenhead: Open University Press.

Myall, M., Levett-Jones, T., & Lathlean, J. (2008). Mentorship in contemporary practice: The experiences of nursing students and practice mentors. *Journal of Clinical Nursing, 17*, 1834–1842.

Nettleton, P., & Bray, L. (2008). Current mentorship schemes might be doing our students a disservice. *Nurse Education in Practice, 8*, 205–212.

NHS Education for Scotland. (2013). *National approach to mentor preparation for nurses and midwives.* (2nd ed.). Available at: https://www.nes.scot.nhs.uk/media/2066328/national-approach-to-mentor-preparation-2nd-edition.pdf.

Northern Ireland Practice and Education Council for Nursing and Midwifery. (2013). Preceptorship framework for nursing, midwifery and specialist community public health nursing in Northern Ireland. Available at: http://www.nipec.hscni.net/previous-work-and-projects/pro-prof-dev-of-nurs-mids/preceptorship/.

Nursing and Midwifery Council. (2008). *Standards to support learning and assessment in practice. NMC Standards for mentors, practice teachers and teachers.* London: Nursing and Midwifery Council.

Nursing and Midwifery Council. (2009). *Standards for pre-registration midwifery education.* London: Nursing and Midwifery Council.

Nursing and Midwifery Council. (2010). *Standards for pre-registration nursing education.* London: Nursing and Midwifery Council.

Nursing and Midwifery Council. (2018a). *The Code: Professional standards of practice and behaviour for nurses, midwives and nursing associates.* London: Nursing and Midwifery Council.

Nursing and Midwifery Council. (2018b). *Realising professionalism: Standards for education and training. Part 1: Standards framework for nursing and midwifery education.* London: Nursing and Midwifery Council.

Nursing and Midwifery Council. (2018c). *Realising professionalism: Standards for education and training. Part 2: Standards for student supervision and assessment.* London: Nursing and Midwifery Council.

Nursing and Midwifery Council. (2018d). *Realising professionalism: Standards for education and training. Part 3: Standards for pre-registration nursing programmes.* London: Nursing and Midwifery Council.

Nursing and Midwifery Council. (2018e). *Future nurse: Standards of proficiency for registered nurses.* London: Nursing and Midwifery Council.

Panzavecchia, L., & Pearce, R. (2014). Are preceptors adequately prepared for their role in supporting newly qualified staff? *Nurse Education Today, 34*, 1119–1124.

Papastavrou, E., Lambrinou, E., Tsangari, H., Saarikoski, M., & Leino-Kilpi, H. (2010). Student nurses experience of learning in the clinical environment. *Nurse Education in Practice, 10*, 176–182.

Papp, L., Markkanen, M., & von Bonsdorff, M. (2003). Clinical environment as a learning environment. Student nurses perceptions concerning clinical learning experiences. *Nurse Education Today, 23*, 262–268.

Park, J. R., Wharrad, H., Barker, J., & Chapple, M. (2010). The knowledge and skills of pre registration masters' and diploma qualified nurses: A preceptor perspective. *Nurse Education in Practice, 11*, 41–46.

Pritchard, E., & Gidman, J. (2012). Effective mentoring in the community setting. *British Journal of Community Nursing, 17*, 119–124.

Robinson, S., & Griffiths, P. (2009). *Preceptorship for newly qualified nurses: Impacts, facilitators and constraints.* London: National Nursing Research Unit, King's College.

Royal College of Midwives. (2010). Leadership programme for preceptor midwives. Available at: https://www.rcm.org.uk/news-views-and-analysis/news/leadership-programme-for-preceptor-midwives.

Stewart, S., Pope, D., & Hansen, T. (2010). Clinical preceptors enhance an online accelerated bachelor's degree to BSN program. *Nurse Educator, 35*(1), 37–40.

Suen, L. K., & Chow, F. L. (2001). Students' perceptions of the effectiveness of mentors in an undergraduate nursing programme in Hong Kong. *Journal of Advanced Nursing, 36*, 505–511.

Thomson, B. (2014). *First steps in coaching.* London: Sage Publications.

Veerumah, V. (2012). What are the barriers to good mentoring? *Nursing Times, 108*(39), 12–15.

Warren, D. (2010). Facilitating pre-registration nurse learning: A mentor approach. *British Journal of Nursing, 19*(21), 1364–1367.

Whitmore, J. (2002). *Coaching for performance.* London: Nicholas Brealey.

Yonge, O., Billay, D., Myrick, F., & Luhanga, F. (2007). Preceptorship and mentorship: Not merely a matter of semantics. *International Journal of Nursing Education Scholarship, 4*(1), 1–13.

Further Reading

Health Education England. (2017). *Preceptorship framework*. London: Health Education England, NHS England, & NHS Improvement. Available at: https://hee.nhs.uk/sites/default/files/documents/Capital-Nurse%20Preceptorship%20Framework.pdf.

This is a framework resource developed for organizations, preceptors and preceptees to support the practice of new health care registrants. This recommended 'best practice' was developed with stakeholders and practitioners across London. The approach recognizes the benefits to newly registered staff, where firmly established preceptorship is established in organizational culture.

Nursing and Midwifery Council. (2018). *Realising professionalism: Standards for education and training*. London: Nursing and Midwifery Council. Available at: https://www.nmc.org.uk/standards-for-education-and-training/.

These standards, fully implemented from 2020 across all approved education institutions, aim to provide a more modern and innovative approach to the way universities and their practice partners educate and train midwives and nurses in the United Kingdom. The framework should allow greater independence of assessment and greater innovation by practice providers. All parts should be read in conjunction with each other by both student midwives and registered midwives.

Thomson, B. (2014). *First steps in coaching*. London: Sage Publications.

This is an essential guide providing a practical introduction to the theory, skills and art of coaching that would be useful to any midwife starting out in the coaching profession. The text contains a wide selection of ideas, models and exercises to stimulate the reader's learning and reflect on and make sense of their experiences.

Useful Websites

Brightside: https://www.thebrightsidetrust.org/

Department of Health and Social Care: https://www.gov.uk/government/organisations/department-of-health-and-social-care

Health Education England: https://www.hee.nhs.uk/

MentorNet (mentoring in engineering and science): http://www.mentornet.net

NHS Education for Scotland: https://www.nes.scot.nhs.uk

NHS Employers: http://www.nhsemployers.org

Northern Ireland Practice and Education Council for Nursing and Midwifery: http://www.nipec.hscni.net

Nursing and Midwifery Council: https://www.nmc.org.uk

Royal College of Midwives: https://www.rcm.org.uk

CHAPTER 12

The Science of Midwifery and Evidence-Based Practice

Julie M. Harrison ■ Sima Hay

LEARNING OUTCOMES

By the end of this chapter the reader should be able to:

- discuss the relationship of the *art* and *science* of midwifery and how this informs the midwife's practice
- discuss the origins of research in midwifery and how evidence-based practice has evolved
- critique the concept of the hierarchy of evidence and how this pertains to midwifery practice
- appreciate the potential of scientific methodology in enhancing the quality of care for mothers, their babies and their families
- examine possible barriers to the implementation of evidence-based practice
- discuss the notion of developing research mindedness in midwifery education and practice.

Overview

This chapter examines the nature of the science of midwifery practice and explores the different types of evidence that can be described as having scientific methodologies. The origins of midwifery research are discussed, as is how midwifery research has developed into an evidence base for midwifery education and practice. The discussion is illustrated with examples of landmark publications that have contributed to the strengthening of the midwifery evidence base. The potential for enhancement of care provided for women and babies is emphasized. Finally, there is a discussion of the importance of research mindedness for current and future midwifery education and practice. Within the chapter are activities for the reader to undertake to apply the theory in a meaningful way that will ultimately inform their practice as a midwife.

Introduction

There has been much debate as to what constitutes the essence of midwifery practice. For some practitioners the concept of midwifery being associated with scientific methods might be thought contentious. Previous deliberations have revolved around the issue of whether midwifery is a *science* or an *art* or possibly both (Kennedy and Lowe 2001; Power 2015). This chapter could therefore be deemed controversial as *science* has been traditionally associated with technology and the biomedical model of care which focuses on risk rather than normality (Davis-Floyd 1992; Van Teijlingen 2005). Consequently, concerns have been expressed as to the appropriateness of becoming more scientific, and whether this could conflict with the holistic ethos of midwifery care. However, different types of science have been described, and this chapter will explore the nature of the science of midwifery in terms of building a midwifery evidence base and evidence-based practice (EBP). The chapter will also discuss how this has the potential to enhance not only the outcomes for mothers, babies and families but also the quality of the childbirth experience. The past, present and future of EBP in midwifery will be explored.

Evolution of Midwifery Research and Evidence-Based Practice

Research without practice is like building castles in the air.
Practice without research is like building castles on a slippery ground.

PARAHOO 2006: 7

The evolution of midwifery research and EBP traverses a fascinating journey in the history of childbirth. The origin of research in childbirth and EBP was very much within the obstetric biomedical model of care, with midwifery-specific research being very much a new emergence towards the latter part of the 20th century. Up to this time, medicalization had served as the dominant framework for the analysis of historical change in pregnancy and childbirth. However, with the increasing women's health movement and the developing interest in human rights, including female autonomy in childbirth in the 1980s, the debate on EBP was pushed into the political centre stage (Morgen 2002; Kline 2010). This prompted studies being undertaken on women's health care that influenced subsequent academic as well as popular writing on pregnancy and birth, such as Oakley's (1984) *The Captured Womb: A History Of The Medical Care of the Pregnant Woman*. This text explores the development of antenatal care and modern obstetric interventions as state-driven strategies aimed at controlling the childbirth process.

The pivotal role of the advances in obstetrics and technology, such as the development of ante-natal ultrasound scanning, further reinforced the trend to reduce pregnant women to being simply a passive bearer of the unborn fetus (Roberts 2012). Around the 1980s, midwives were beginning to question the impact of medicalization of physiological childbirth on the woman, her baby and her family, seeking the evidence that such policies and practices were based on.

The publication of *Effective Care in Pregnancy and Childbirth* (Chalmers et al 1989) was con-sidered by many to be the start of the journey towards change in childbirth and the development of EBP. Page (1996) was among many authoritative leaders in the midwifery profession who con-sidered this publication to be the catalyst of change that would legitimately question medicalized, obstetric-led birth. However, as Lomas et al (2005) claim, such a progressive observation was not made by all. Much of the midwife's practice at this time was based on accepted dogma rather than evidence-based theory, until midwives began questioning the effectiveness of their practice and the subsequent impact on the woman's or baby's health and well-being. Examples of studies that midwives undertook to evaluate routine practices, and which often led to a change in midwifery practice to the woman's benefit, involved perineal shaving (Romney 1981) and the performing of an episiotomy (Sleep et al 1984). The journey developing midwifery research had commenced, and midwives had begun to positively embrace EBP that ultimately supported women-centred care.

EARLY RESEARCH CENTRES

In 1993 the Cochrane Centre was set up in the United Kingdom to meet the growing awareness of the need to use good-quality evidence to inform practice in all fields of health care. The Centre for Evidence-Based Medicine was established in Oxford in 1993, along with the Centre for Evi-dence-Based Nursing at the University of York and the Centre for Evidence-Based Child Health at the Institute of Child Health in London. These centres were primarily focused on dissemi-nating their research results so they could be applied in clinical practice. The maternity services were the first health care specialty to have a comprehensive review of evidence to aid midwives in informing women of the available evidence and subsequently making informed clinical decisions.

Concurrently with the increasing development of midwifery-specific research was the move of mid-wifery education into higher education institutions (i.e. universities), where there is access to research centres to which midwifery lecturers have become affiliated. This has also provided opportunities for the midwifery lecturers to engage in research activities and develop their own research potential as well as undertake higher degrees and doctoral studies, ultimately strengthening the midwifery evi-dence base and academic profile of the midwifery profession. With such knowledge and research skills among the midwifery academic teams, the concept of research and EBP is now an integral part of all undergraduate pre-registration midwifery education curricula (Spiby and Munro 2010), with all stu-dent midwives developing their understanding and skills in the research process as shown in Box 12.1.

THE SCIENCE OF MIDWIFERY

The term *science* comes from the Latin word *scientia*, meaning *knowledge* (Trumble and Brown 2004). By definition, the term *scientific* refers to a system of acquiring knowledge which involves deductive reasoning to generate hypotheses, and according to Polit and Beck (2014) uses system-atic methods to test them in either an experimental or a real-life situation. In health care settings the use of scientific methods was traditionally associated with the practice of medicine, although this developed in the latter part of the 20th century to encompass other health care disciplines as well as those outside the medical/health care field, such as agricultural science, social science and educational science. Nevertheless, a common feature of them all is the relationship to the use of methodology which is designed to increase objectivity, reduce bias introduced by the researcher and so obtain valid and reliable evidence to advance the specific field of practice.

BOX 12.1 ■ The Stages of the Research Process

1. The research question
2. The literature review
3. Planning the study
4. The research design (methodology):
   - the sample
   - deciding on the data to be collected
   - methods of data collection
   - the method of analysis and presentation
   - ethical issues
5. The pilot
6. Data collection
7. Data analysis
8. Conclusion and recommendations
9. Communication of findings

From Rees (2011).

EVIDENCE-BASED PRACTICE

Albers (2001: 130) in an article on *evidence* and midwifery practice identified that the implementation of evidence-based care *'represented a paradigm shift as it involves a change in the way that clinicians work'*. Before this, care was based on expert opinion, which often lacked objectivity, rather than information gained from research studies. Research methodology is categorized by two main approaches or paradigms: quantitative and qualitative (Polit and Beck 2014). Moreover, research may be conducted on a local, regional, national or international level depending on the extent of impact the study is intended to have. Caution, however, is required in interpretation of the findings as data from one country cannot always be generalized to another country (Parahoo 2006).

In contemporary midwifery practice the *science* is the process of acquiring knowledge that can be used as evidence regarding an aspect of care being effective (Erickson-Owens and Kennedy 2001; Hoope-Bender and Renfrew 2014). Thus, evidence-based care is based on the unbiased evidence collected by scientific methods to inform the best practice (Polit and Beck 2014). However, supporters of EBP also recognize the value of clinical expertise, which is *the art* of midwifery as highlighted in Sackett's (1996) model shown in Fig. 12.1. Importantly this is not seen as an opposing entity, but rather as Kennedy and Lowe (2001: 91) suggest is an *'astute ability to meld the application of scientific evidence with clinical judgement.'*

Rees (2011) identified two perspectives of research: that of the individual undertaking research themselves or using research that others have done to inform personal practice. The concept of EBP is endorsed by the Nursing and Midwifery Council (NMC) (2018) in *The Code*, whereby all midwives and nurses must practise in line with the best available evidence to achieve high-quality care for members of the public. Furthermore, autonomous, evidence-based decision-making by members of an occupation who share the same values and education, such as midwives, is a key characteristic of professionalism (NMC 2017). Reflecting on and evaluating one's own practice, which could be undertaken as a self-audit or on a collective basis, such as intrapartum record keeping, is also recommended as good practice Such activity may also be viewed as being scientific as it involves setting criteria or standards against which an aspect of care can be measured.

The Hierarchy of Evidence

Not all research studies are considered to produce evidence of equal strength, and this is related to the level of possible bias. Consequently, a recognized hierarchy of evidence exists;

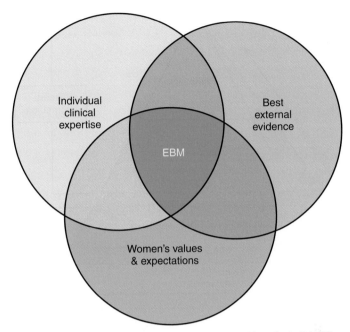

Fig. 12.1   Evidence-based midwifery *(EBM)*. (Adapted from Sackett 1996)

however, this favours quantitative data, positioning the randomized controlled trial (RCT) and systematic reviews of RCTs at the top as being the least biased research method that is most likely to have valid and reliable results (Aveyard 2014). It could be argued that the hierarchy of evidence as shown in Fig. 12.2 reinforces the biomedical model of care rather than humanistic philosophy of midwifery practice that is an essential part of being a midwife. McCourt (2005) argues that understanding the advantages and limitations of research methodology is important, and highlights that the evidence for midwifery practice is complex and does not always fit into such a hierarchical structure. Consequently, little consideration has been given to qualitative research approaches, such as exploring the thoughts, feelings and experiences of those receiving the care. One can claim that these approaches are essential to developing and delivering effective care strategies, but as Aveyard (2014) purports, they do not feature in the hierarchy of evidence.

RANDOMIZED CONTROLLED TRIALS

As shown in Fig. 12.2, because of their position in the hierarchy of evidence, RCTs and meta-analyses of systematic reviews of RCTs have been regarded as the *gold standard* of clinical research (Aveyard 2014). This means they are the most appropriate method for evaluating the effectiveness of an intervention or treatment as this provides the strongest evidence, being the least biased because of the randomization process. This is due to the removal of selection bias, and is particularly so when the randomized *double-blind* method is used with a placebo (Rees 2011). The first RCT was devised in the 1940s for investigation of the treatment of tuberculosis (Medical Research Council 1948). However, a disadvantage of RCTs is that the control is often so tight that it does not resemble the real-life situation. Another issue is that large samples are required, especially if the phenomenon under investigation is rare (hypoxia), and so the RCT can be expensive and difficult to conduct. However, RCT methodology has been used to investigate certain aspects of midwifery practice, as shown in the following examples:

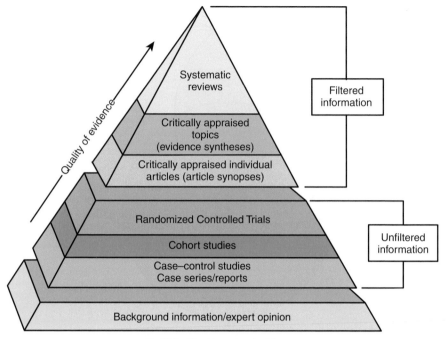

Fig. 12.2   The hierarchy of evidence.

- Carfoot et al (2005): 'A randomised controlled trial in the north of England examining the effects of skin-to-skin care on breast feeding'
- Downe et al (2015): 'Self-hypnosis for intrapartum pain management (SHIP) in pregnant nulliparous women: a randomised controlled trial of clinical effectiveness'
- Naughton et al (2017): 'A large multi-centre pilot randomized controlled trial testing a low cost, tailored, self-help smoking cessation text message intervention for pregnant smokers (MiQuit)'.

Now undertake Activity 12.1.

ACTIVITY 12.1 ■

- Select a clinical guideline from your maternity unit.
- With reference to the hierarchy of evidence shown in Fig. 12.2, review the guideline and explore what level of evidence the final recommendations are based on.

Emergence of the Qualitative Approach

From the holistic perspective, the traditional notion of testing a hypothesis is problematic as it is part of the quantitative research paradigm which is based on the analysis of numerical data, or data that can be translated into numbers such as rating or Likert scales (Rees 2011). Conversely, not all aspects of midwifery practice can be appropriately investigated in this way as the woman's experiences are not considered in any depth. As a result of improvements in maternity and neonatal care, Simpkin (1991) acknowledges that the importance of the quality of the birth experience for the woman, her baby and her family became increasingly recognized. As Lavender et al (2004) suggest, midwifery research should be undertaken in a more holistic manner to reflect and improve all aspects of the birth experience that are important to women and their families.

With a paucity of studies of women's views about childbirth and their experiences of maternity services, there has been an emergence and acceptance of qualitative research studies by midwives which integrated qualitative data to ensure the humanistic approach was evident (Cluett 2006). However, such types of inquiry have been long the subject of study by social scientists rather than midwives. The fascinating journey in the history of childbirth took another path towards placing women in the centre of research studies (Department of Health 1993, NHS England 2016), although challenges still continue today.

Aspects of Quality Of Care and Evidence-Based Practice

On an international level, Renfrew et al (2014) in their discussion of how midwifery care could be improved in low-income, medium-income and even high-income countries emphasized that poor-quality care relates not only to lack of interventions when needed but also to the use of unnecessary interventions that may consequently lead to iatrogenic complications. As a result of this, Renfrew et al (2014) developed an evidence-informed framework for the assessment of quality maternal and newborn care as part of *The Lancet* midwifery series as shown in Fig. 12.3. By use of scientific methods (analyses of existing reviews of women's views and experiences, practices and interventions, and workforce), a framework was developed that firmly places the needs of women and their babies at its centre that are fundamental to improving the quality of universal health. Furthermore, effective use of the scientific method in midwifery research not only aims to improve direct clinical *hands-on* care but also addresses other important issues, such as cost-effectiveness of services and educational and professional aspects for health care professionals.

Now undertake Activity 12.2.

ACTIVITY 12.2 ▪

Select one aspect of your role (practising midwife) or an aspect of care you need to demonstrate your competence in (student midwife).

With the use of the framework for quality maternal and newborn care (Renfrew et al (2014)) consider how you already/will incorporate the various elements to deliver midwifery/neonatal care to the highest standard:

- *Care providers:* What knowledge and skills do you require to undertake this particular role? Do you need any additional training and support?
- *Philosophy:* How can you optimize the biological, psychological and cultural processes to strengthen the woman's/baby's abilities without any intervention?
- *Values:* How do you ensure the care you provide is respectful and tailored to the individual woman's/baby's needs?
- *Organization of care:* What resources do you require to fulfil your role and provide a good-quality service?
- *Practice categories:* What specific evidence, knowledge and skills do you require to provide care to the woman/baby that is safe, competent and of quality?

Evidence from Multimedia/Social Media

With increasing advances in social media, it is acknowledged that there is greater access to data via mobile phones with multimedia resources such as videos, blogs, YouTube links, Google alerts and online publications. Furthermore, midwives need to be aware of the characteristics/personality traits

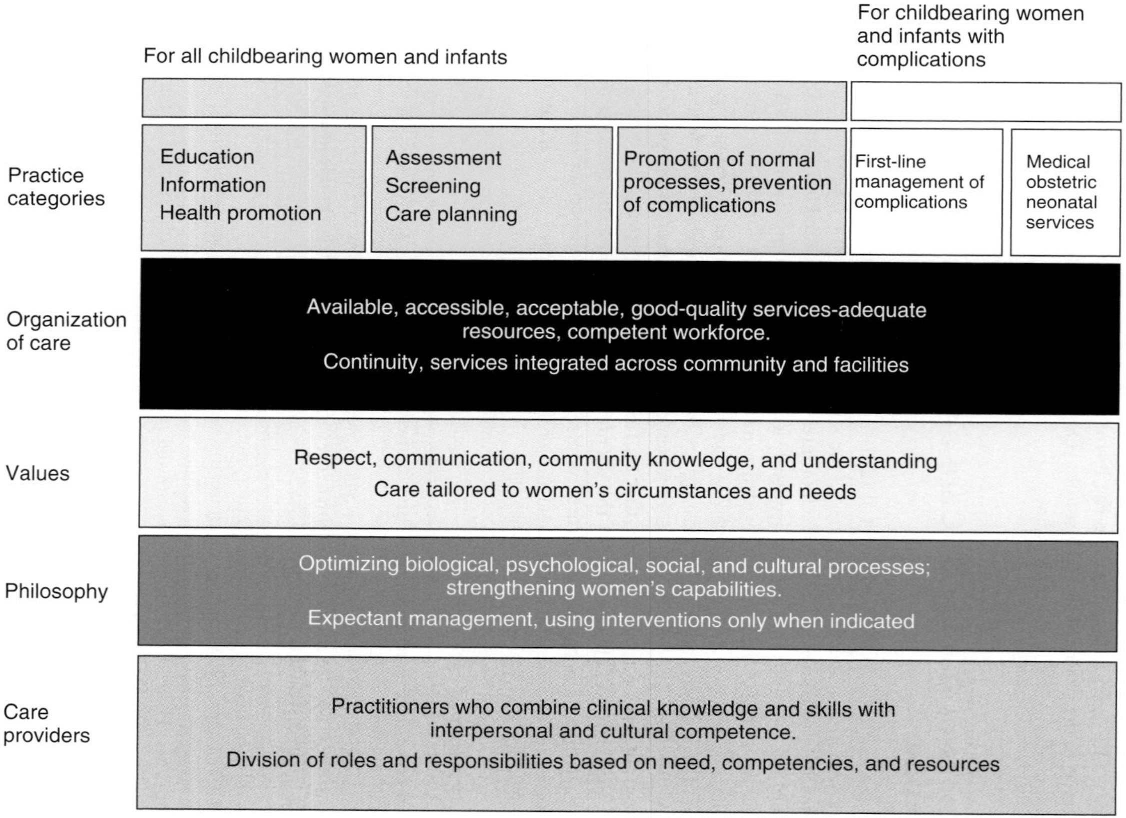

For all childbearing women and infants

For childbearing women and infants with complications

Practice categories	Education Information Health promotion	Assessment Screening Care planning	Promotion of normal processes, prevention of complications	First-line management of complications	Medical obstetric neonatal services

Organization of care
Available, accessible, acceptable, good-quality services-adequate resources, competent workforce.
Continuity, services integrated across community and facilities

Values
Respect, communication, community knowledge, and understanding
Care tailored to women's circumstances and needs

Philosophy
Optimizing biological, psychological, social, and cultural processes; strengthening women's capabilities.
Expectant management, using interventions only when indicated

Care providers
Practitioners who combine clinical knowledge and skills with interpersonal and cultural competence.
Division of roles and responsibilities based on need, competencies, and resources

Fig. 12.3 The framework for quality maternal and newborn care: maternal and newborn health components of a health system needed by childbearing women and newborn infants. (Renfrew et al 2014)

that student midwives and parents who are of the *Generation Z* group, born between 1995 and 2010, may have. According to a study undertaken by Jones et al (2015), *Generation Z* are those individuals born into the digital age and consequently are technological multitaskers who thrive on instant access to data that can be linked and mapped in seconds and arrive on their mobile phones. Consequently, they tend towards self-directed learning and appear to be well informed. However, health professionals should always check the various multimedia sources students or parents may be accessing to ensure the information is accurate, reliable and valid, and consequently is the *best* available evidence to inform their practice and decision-making. The hierarchy of evidence is always a useful framework to use as a starting point in assessing the quality of any *research* that is published on these multimedia resources.

Strengthening Midwifery Practice

Pregnancy is a normal physiological process and is not usually pathological, and therefore by definition pertains to the scope of midwifery practice as the autonomous role of the midwife relates to normality (International Confederation of Midwives 2017). The view of midwifery practice stated in *Midwifery 2020* (Chief Nursing Officers of England, Northern Ireland, Scotland and Wales 2010) emphasized the importance of the midwifery influence on maternal and neonatal well-being, and how the role of the midwife can be maximized. This is advantageous as midwives are influential and have the potential to implement practices which will improve the quality of care for women, their babies and their families (Renfrew et al 2014). Importantly, Horton and Astudillo (2014) highlight the pivotal role of the midwife in the reduction of mortality for women and children. They concluded that 80% of maternal and newborn deaths, including stillbirths, could be prevented if the evidence described in *The Lancet* midwifery series had been implemented in midwifery practice. Strengthening the midwifery research base in accordance with women's needs is important, and individualized care is central to the midwifery role and should be promoted as the hallmark of midwifery practice (Kennedy and Lowe 2001). This concept was previously supported by the Quality Assurance Agency for Higher Education (2001), who stated that midwifery knowledge and practice are dynamic and should be responsive to the changing needs of society. Acknowledgement of the nature and significance of knowledge to midwifery practice is important if the changing needs of women are to be met.

Now undertake Activity 12.3.

ACTIVITY 12.3 ■

Think of an aspect relating to student learning or midwifery practice that you feel requires being more evidence based (e.g. defining a rationale for introducing peer-mentors to facilitate student learning of biological sciences or a practice issue that could be more woman centred).
- Using the research process of Rees (2011), work through the stages, outlining detail that would be appropriate for each stage of the process.
- What would you consider to be the benefits and/or limitations of using such a framework when compiling a research proposal?

Future: Research Mindedness

In contemporary midwifery practice, midwives still face many challenges in providing care that is evidence based. Whilst it is universally considered as a cornerstone of women-centred maternity care, EBP has to counterattack the rapidly developing technologies which place more emphasis on high-risk obstetric-led care versus the drive towards natural physiological childbirth.

However, midwifery is unique, and midwives have a perspective that is different from that of obstetricians. This allows a close relationship with the woman throughout her pregnancy and childbirth. The midwifery view of birth is essentially *normal*, with interventions only if needed in an emergency. This view is different from medicalized birth and has led to midwives defining and seeking answers to different research questions, which can present them with a challenge of their own.

Education and practice are the elements that form the link to midwifery research and EBP. The foundations of acquiring good knowledge and a good understanding of the value of all aspects of midwifery research and EBP, including the importance of nurturing an inquiring mind, begins with the student midwife and consequently develops through life-long learning as a practising midwife (see Chapter 15). Critical reflection is part of the NMC (2019) revalidation process by which midwives examine their current practice to ensure it remains contemporary and their knowledge is up to date as detailed more fully in Chapter 2. To protect the childbearing woman from any harm, it is no longer acceptable to undertake ritualistic procedures and allow outdated practices to continue without any challenge (NMC 2018). It is vital that midwifery research capacity continues to develop *within* the profession so that first and foremost midwifery research is undertaken by midwives. Student elective placements with a university research team could be the way forward for those considering a career as a researcher to gain an insight into the role. Taking advantage of schemes such as the National Institute for Health Research fellowships enables early-career midwives to develop a role as a midwifery researcher (UK Clinical Research Collaboration 2008).

Now undertake Activity 12.4.

ACTIVITY 12.4 ■

You have just read a very interesting article about a study in midwifery education or practice that you are very passionate about and are enthused to use the findings in your practice as either a midwifery lecturer or a clinical midwife.
- With reference to transferring research knowledge into practice, consider what may be the barriers and/or the drivers within your organization to affect such a transfer and ultimately improve the experiences of either the student or the childbearing woman.

Conclusion

This chapter has provided an insight into the importance of the evolution of the application of EBP to maternity care. The debate on whether midwifery practice is either an *art* or a *science* is no longer valid. A shift of culture has occurred, which has accepted the compatibility of research and practice, and the integral role of both in the delivery of high-quality evidence-based midwifery. To make meaningful changes to practice and to pursue and provide evidence-based care, midwives have a professional responsibility to generate knowledge. To truly embrace the ongoing development of EBP, midwives must be thinking, questioning, reflective lifelong learners, receptive to new ideas and ways of working. The journey that the midwives began to positively embrace EBP, which ultimately supported women-centred care, must continue. However, midwives are accountable to always ensure their knowledge of contemporary scientific evidence is applied to their practice when making judgements and decisions about maternal and neonatal care.

KEY POINTS

- It is important for newly qualified midwives to value evidence from the full range of research methods, encompassing qualitative and quantitative studies.
- To truly embrace the ongoing development of EBP, midwives must be thinking, questioning, reflective lifelong learners, receptive to new ideas and ways of working.
- It is vital that midwifery research capacity continues to develop *within* the profession so that first and foremost midwifery research is undertaken by midwives, with the woman, her baby and her family at the centre.
- Caution needs to be taken when information has originated from various multimedia sources as the accuracy, reliability and validity cannot necessarily be guaranteed as the best available evidence to inform clinical decision-making.
- Student elective placements with a university- or practice-based research team could be the way forward for those considering a career as a researcher to gain an insight into the role.

References

Albers, L. L. (2001). Evidence and midwifery practice. *The Journal of Midwifery and Women's Health, 46*, 130–136.

Aveyard, H. (2014). *Doing a literature review in health and social care: A practical guide* (3rd ed.). Maidenhead: Open University Press/McGraw-Hill Education.

Carfoot, S., Williamson, P., & Dixon, R. (2005). A randomised controlled trial in the north of England examining the effects of skin-to-skin care on breast feeding. *Midwifery, 21*(1), 71–79.

Chalmers, I., Enkin, M., & Keirse, M. J. N. C. (1989). *Effective care in pregnancy and childbirth*. Oxford: Oxford University Press.

Chief Nursing Officers of England, Northern Ireland, Scotland and Wales. (2010). *Midwifery 2020: Delivering expectations*. London: Department of Health.

Cluett, E. R. (2006). Evidence-based practice (2nd ed.). In Cluett, E., R., & Bluff, R. (Eds.), *Principles and practice of research in midwifery* (pp. 33–56). Edinburgh: Churchill Livingstone.

Davis-Floyd, B. (1992). *Birth as an American rite of passage*. California: University of California Press.

Department of Health. (1993). *Changing childbirth: Report of the Expert Maternity Group*. London: HMSO.

Downe, S., Finlayson, K., Melvin, C., Spiby, H., Ali, S., Diggle, P., et al. (2015). Self-hypnosis for intrapartum pain management (SHIP) in pregnant nulliparous women: a randomised controlled trial of clinical effectiveness. *BJOG, 122*(9), 1226–1234.

Erickson-Owens, D. A., & Kennedy, H. P. (2001). Fostering evidence-based care in clinical teaching. *The Journal of Midwifery and Women's Health, 46*(3), 137–145.

Hoope-Bender, P., & Renfrew, M. J. (2014). Midwifery – a vital path to quality maternal and newborn care: The story of the Lancet series on midwifery. *Midwifery, 30*, 1105–1106.

Horton, R., & Astudillo, O. (2014). The power of Midwifery. *The Lancet, 384*(9948), 1075–1076.

International Confederation of Midwives. (2017). International definition of the midwife. Available at: https://www.internationalmidwives.org/assets/files/definitions-files/2018/06/eng-definition_of_the_midwife-2017.pdf.

Jones, K., Warren, A., & Davies, A. (2015). *Mind the gap: Exploring the needs of early career nurses and midwives in the workplace: Summary report from Birmingham and Solihull Local Education and Training Council Every Student Counts project*. NHS Health Education England.

Kennedy, H. P., & Lowe, N. K. (2001). Science and midwifery: paradigms and paradoxes. *The Journal of Midwifery and Women's Health, 46*, 91–97.

Kline, W. (2010). *Bodies of knowledge: Sexuality, reproduction, and women's health in the second wave*. Chicago: University of Chicago Press.

Lavender, T., Edwards, G., & Alfirevic, Z. (2004). *Demystifying qualitative research in pregnancy and childbirth.* Salisbury: Quay Books.

Lomas, J., Culyer, T., McCutcheon, C., McAuley, L., & Law, S. (2005). *Conceptualizing and combining evidence for health system guidance.* Ottawa: Canadian Health Services Research Foundation.

Medical Research Council. (1948). Streptomycin treatment of pulmonary tuberculosis. *British Medical Journal, 2,* 769–782.

McCourt, C. (2005). Research and theory for nursing and midwifery: Rethinking the nature of evidence. *Worldviews on Evidence-Based Nursing, 2*(2), 75–83.

Morgen, S. (2002). *Into our own hands: The women's health movement in the United States, 1969–1990.* New Brunswick: Rutgers University Press.

Naughton, F., Cooper, S., Foster, K., Emery, J., Leonardi-Bee, J., Sutton, S., et al. (2017). A large multi-centre pilot randomized controlled trial testing a low cost, tailored, self-help smoking cessation text message intervention for pregnant smokers (MiQuit). *Addiction, 112*(7), 1238–1249.

NHS England. (2016). Better births: Improving outcomes of maternity services in England. A five year forward view for maternity care. Available at: https://www.england.nhs.uk/wp-content/uploads/2016/02/national-maternity-review-report.pdf.

Nursing and Midwifery Council. (2017). *Enabling professionalism in nursing and midwifery practice framework.* London: Nursing and Midwifery Council. Available at: https://www.nmc.org.uk/globalassets/sitedocuments/other-publications/enabling-professionalism.pdf.

Nursing and Midwifery Council. (2018). *The Code: Professional standards of practice and behaviour for nurses, midwives and nursing associates.* London: Nursing and Midwifery Council.

Nursing and Midwifery Council. (2019). How to revalidate with the NMC. Available at: www.nmc.org.uk/revalidation.

Oakley, A. (1984). *The captured womb: A history of the medical care of pregnant women.* Oxford: Basil Blackwell.

Page, L. (1996). The backlash against evidence-based care. *Birth, 23,* 191–192.

Parahoo, K. (2006). *Nursing research: Principles, process and issues* (2nd ed.). London: Macmillan.

Polit, D., & Beck, C. (2014). *Essentials of nursing research: Appraising evidence for nursing practice* (8th ed.). Philadelphia: Wolters Kluwer/Lippincott Williams and Wilkins.

Power, A. (2015). Contemporary midwifery practice: art, science or both. *British Journal of Midwifery, 23*(9), 654–657.

Quality Assurance Agency for Higher Education. (2001). *Midwifery: Subject benchmark statement.* Gloucester: Quality Assurance Agency for Higher Education.

Rees, C. (2011). *An introduction to research for midwives* (3rd ed.). Edinburgh: Churchill Livingstone.

Renfrew, M. J., McFadden, A., Bastos, M. H., Campbell, J., Channon, A. A., Cheung, N. F., et al. (2014). Midwifery and quality care: findings from a new evidence-informed framework for maternal and newborn care. *The Lancet, 384*(9948), 1129–1145.

Roberts, J. (2012). *The visualised foetus: A cultural and political analysis of ultrasound.* Farnham: Ashgate.

Romney, M. L. (1981). Pre-delivery shaving: an unjustified assault? *Journal of Obstetrics and Gynaecology, 1,* 33–35.

Sackett, D. (1996). Evidence based medicine: What it is and what it isn't? *British Medical Journal, 312,* 71–72.

Simkin, P. (1991). Just another day in a woman's Life? Women's long-term perceptions of their first birth experience. Part 1. *Birth, 18,* 203–210.

Sleep, J., Grant, A., Garcia, J., Elbourne, D., Spence, J., & Chalmers, D. (1984). The West Berkshire perineal management trial. *British Medical Journal, 289,* 587–590.

Spiby, H., & Munro, J. (Eds.). (2010). *Evidence based midwifery applications in context.* Chichester: Wiley-Blackwell.

Trumble, W. ,R., & Brown, L. (2004). *Shorter Oxford English dictionary* (5th ed.). Oxford: Oxford University Press.

UK Clinical Research Collaboration. (2008). *Developing the best research professionals. Qualified graduate nurses: Recommendations for preparing and supporting clinical academic nurses in the future.* London: UK Clinical Research Collaboration.

Van Teijlingen, E. (2005). A Critical analysis of the medical model as used in the study of pregnancy and childbirth. *Sociological Research Online, 10*(2). http://www.socresonline.org.uk/10/2/teijlingen.html.

Further Reading

Gough, D., Oliver, S., & Thomas, J. (2012). *An introduction to systematic reviews*. London: Sage.

This text provides an overview of the nature, logic and process of undertaking a systematic review, covering statistical meta-analysis to meta-ethnography and is ideal for anyone undertaking their own systematic review. It provides all the necessary conceptual and technical background required to begin the process.

Rees, C. (2011). *An introduction to research for midwives* (3rd ed.). Edinburgh: Churchill Livingstone.

This text explains in simple language the world of research from the perspectives of those who use research findings in practice to those undertaking research. Its student-friendly approach provides clear guidelines in critiquing research articles and producing successful literature reviews.

Silverman, D. (2011). *Qualitative research* (4th ed.). London: Sage.

This text introduces the reader to qualitative research and the process of undertaking studies. Each chapter is written by an expert in qualitative research methodologies, with examples providing the reader with the application of the theory in context.

Useful Websites

American College of Nurse-Midwives Evidence Based Practice: Pearls of Midwifery. http://www.midwife.org/Evidence-Based-Practice-Pearls-of-Midwifery

Cochrane Library and reviews: https://www.cochrane.org

Joanna Briggs Institute: http://joannabriggs.org

INVOLVE (resource centre): http://www.invo.org.uk/resource-centre

The Lancet series on midwifery: http://www.thelancet.com/series/midwifery

National Institute for Health Research: https://www.nihr.ac.uk

Royal College of Midwives' Better Births Initiative: https://www.rcm.org.uk/better-births-initiative

Royal College of Obstetricians and Gynaecologists: https://www.rcog.org.uk

UK Clinical Research Collaboration: http://www.ukcrc.org

CHAPTER 13

Leadership and Management in Midwifery

Jayne E. Marshall ▪ Lesley Kay

CONTENTS

LEARNING OUTCOMES

By the end of this chapter the reader will be able to:

- appreciate the difference between the concepts of leadership and management
- compare and contrast different leadership theories
- recognize different styles of leadership and their impact on others working within the organization
- determine the role and qualities of the midwifery leader
- understand the value of developing strong and effective leadership within all aspects of the midwifery profession

- consider the value of talent management in developing future midwife leaders during initial pre-registration midwifery education programmes
- appreciate the range of leadership development opportunities available to students, early career midwives and more experienced midwives to support their own career aspirations, be it in clinical practice, education or research.

Overview

In this chapter leadership theories and styles will be explored within the context of contemporary midwifery education and practice. Examples of leadership frameworks and the range of opportunities available to midwives that can enable them to further develop their leadership knowledge and skills are included. The introduction of talent management as a strategy to nurture and develop aspiring leaders in their midwifery careers is essential for succession planning and sustaining the future of the midwifery profession, and is everyone's business. Throughout the chapter there are reflective exercises that enable the reader to apply the theory to practice whilst also considering their own leadership potential and the impact on others who follow.

Introduction

There has been much interest in leadership throughout human history, but only recently have a number of formal leadership theories emerged which aim to explain the reason why and the process by which certain individuals become leaders. Such theories often focus on the characteristics of leaders, although others attempt to identify the behaviours that individuals can adopt/develop to improve their leadership abilities in a variety of situations. Early debates on the psychology of leadership often suggested that leadership skills were simply abilities that an individual was born with, whereas more recent theories have purported that possessing certain traits may contribute towards creating a natural leader and that experience and situational variables also play an essential role.

Leadership and Management Theories

To understand leadership, it is necessary to first distinguish between leadership and management. Kotter (1990) compares the two concepts in that *management* is about coping with complexity and *leadership* is about coping with change. Management is not an activity that exists in isolation but is a variety of activities carried out by individuals within an organization whose role is that of a manager. Bowles and Bowles (2000) suggest that leadership is the product of personal characteristics rather than the mere occupation of managerial positions, arguing that it is these characteristics which draw, inspire and motivate followers towards achieving organizational goals. Furthermore, Girvin (1998: 1) purports that defining leadership is extraordinarily complex such that

> *when we come into contact with good leadership, whether it is our own or someone else's, we are able to recognise it immediately, but ask us to describe it and our terms are nebulous and subjective.*

A LEADER OR A MANAGER?

Leadership and management, however, go hand in hand, but they are not the same thing. They are necessarily linked and complementary, with the *leader* focusing on people, whereas the *manager* focuses on systems and structure. A useful distinction between managers and leaders is drawn by Watson (1983) in the '*seven S's framework*', which indicates managers use *strategy*, *structure* and *systems* and leaders use *their style, staff, skills* and *shared goals* in fulfilling their role.

WHAT IS A LEADER?

The word *leader* originates from an old Viking term and was the name given to a person who stood at the front of the boat and directed it through the 'leads' or gaps in the ice (i.e. going before and preparing the way for those following). It was a role that required immense judgement as well as the ultimate trust of their colleagues to follow wherever they judged it appropriate to lead the boat. The leader's role is to inspire and motivate. Bednash (2009) supports this image and refers to the leader as being an individual who is at the front, moving things forward, taking risks and challenging the status quo, consequently influencing and guiding direction, opinion and course of action within a group or organization.

WHAT IS A MANAGER?

A manager may be considered to be someone in the organization who has a position of authority with formal responsibility for the work carried out by other workers. Bednash (2009) refers to the manager as a person who brings things about, being one who accomplishes, has the responsibility, and conducts. *To manage* means *to handle*, which implies a high degree of direct involvement. The activities of a manager are generally grouped together and described under the auspices of a process of management that includes:

- planning
- organizing
- coordinating.

Put simply, the difference between leaders and managers is that leaders have people who follow them, whilst managers have people who work for them. Bennis (2009) composed a list of the differences between leaders and managers that has been adapted and is shown in Table 13.1.

A great manager would be considered to possess leadership skills and the ability to create a vision within the overall goals of the organization and encourage employees to work together as a group to reach that vision. However, whilst great managers may have leadership skills, this does not mean that all leaders are in a management role. An individual can be both a manager and a leader, or one or the other. In *management mode*, a midwife would be working towards the short-term goals and objectives of their organization, such as ensuring there is an adequate skill mix within the maternity services, whereas in *leadership mode*, the midwife would be laying out the foundations of

TABLE 13.1 ■ **Differences Between a Leader and a Manager**

Leader	Manager
Creates a vision	Creates goals
Innovates	Administers
Is unique	Is a copy
Develops	Maintains
Coaches	Directs
Focuses on people: builds relationships	Focuses on systems and structure
Inspires trust	Relies on control
Takes risks	Controls risk
Has a long-range perspective	Has a short-range view
Questions the *what* and *why*	Questions the *how* and *when*
Has their eye on the horizon	Has their eye on the bottom line
Originates	Imitates
Challenges the status quo: a change agent	Accepts the status quo
Is their own person	Is the classic good soldier
Does the right thing	Does things right
Creates followers/fans	Has employees/subordinates

Adapted from Bennis (2009).

influencing others in heading towards their future vision, which may include involving maternity service users *and* current student midwives in the selection and recruitment of future students.

Now undertake Activity 13.1.

ACTIVITY 13.1 ■

Consider a midwife in each of the following roles with whom you have contact in the university and clinical setting:

- personal tutor/academic assessor
- programme lead
- lead midwife for education/head of midwifery education
- mentor/practice supervisor/practice assessor
- ward manager
- consultant midwife
- head/director of maternity (and neonatal/children's) services.

Do you think of them as a *midwife*, *leader* or *manager*?
What factors led you to these conclusions?

Whilst many different leadership theories have emerged, most can be classified as one of seven major types as shown in Box 13.1. Midwives need to be aware of the various approaches to leadership theory and their benefits and challenges so as to adopt the most appropriate model to best advantage for the circumstances.

THE *GREAT MAN* THEORY

Many leadership theories have been developed in an attempt to understand how behaviour can best be influenced. According to Bednash (2009), the *great man theory* was the starting point for most leadership research until the mid-1940s, inspired by the study of influential heroes, and as its name suggests, only a man could possess the characteristics of a great leader. This theory believes that leaders are born and not made and that they possess certain innate qualities or characteristics, such that a leader is one who, by virtue of their birth, is destined to be a great leader, rising to that position when confronted with the appropriate situation. It has been argued, however, that these *heroes/great men* are simply the product of their times and their actions are the results of social conditions.

TRAIT THEORY

Similar to the *great man* leadership theory, *trait* *l*eadership theory believes that people are either born or made with certain qualities, such as intelligence, creativity and a sense of responsibility, that will make them excel in leadership roles. This approach to leadership, however, extended to analysing mental, physical and social characteristics to gain a better understanding of those traits

BOX 13.1 ■ Types of Leadership Theory

The *great man* theory
Trait theory
Behavioural theory
Contingency theory
Situational theory
Transactional theory
Transformational theory

that are common among leaders. Handy (2007) describes a major flaw of the trait theories in that they disregard the influence of others or the situation on the leadership role.

BEHAVIOURAL THEORY

This type of leadership theory focuses on identification of different behaviours that are exhibited by effective leaders. Stogdill and Coons (1957) identified two broad groupings of behaviours – those relating to *task* and those relating to *people and relationships* – which Bowers and Seashore (1966) further expanded to four dimensions of behaviour:

1. supportive behaviour; enhancing the self-esteem of the follower
2. interactive facilitation; group and team building
3. goal emphasis
4. work facilitation; planning, co-ordinating and organization.

Anyone with the right conditioning, according to the focus of this theory, has the potential to become a leader: that is, leaders are made, not born. *Adair's action-centred* leadership model (Thomas and Adair 2011) incorporates a range of three work behaviours relating to *task*, *team* and *the individual*, suggesting that a balance of activities in each of the three groupings is required to achieve effective leadership. In situations where a leader concentrates on one area at the exclusion of others, the leader is less likely to be effective in their role. Furthermore, a criticism of this leadership approach is that it fails to give due regard to the environment in which the leading takes place.

CONTINGENCY THEORY

To some extent *contingency* leadership theories are an extension of the trait theory, in that human traits are related to the situation in which leaders exercise their leadership skills. This affirms that whilst there is no single way of leading others, a leader's effectiveness is dependent/contingent on how well their style matches a specific setting or situation. This indicates that there are certain people who perform at their best in certain situations, but at the minimum level when taken out of their comfort zone. The leader is more likely to express their leadership when they believe their followers will be responsive. In *contingency theory*, effective leadership *depends on the degree of fit* between a leader's qualities and style and the specific situation or context rather than *adaptation* to the situation, which is the focus of *situational theory*.

SITUATIONAL THEORY

The *situational leadership theory* approach was developed by Hersey and Blanchard (1977) and draws on *contingency theory*, considering that different situations require a different style of leadership, and to be effective, the leader has to be able to *adapt* or *adjust* their style to the circumstances of the situation. As tasks are different, each type of task will require a different leadership approach. The key factor that determines how the leader should adapt is the assessment of the competence and commitment of their followers, which will determine to what extent they are required to use a more *directive* or *supportive* approach, the process of which Hersey and Blanchard (1977) demonstrated in their model (Fig. 13.1). The dimensions of the model are as follows:

For the leader: *Leadership style*
Amount of *direction* given *(task focused)*
Amount of *support given (relationship focused)*

For the follower: *Maturity level*
Amount of competence/ability
Amount of commitment/motivation

The implication of this approach is that anyone can become an effective leader provided they behave in a way appropriate to the situation. There is no one right style, and it is up to the leader

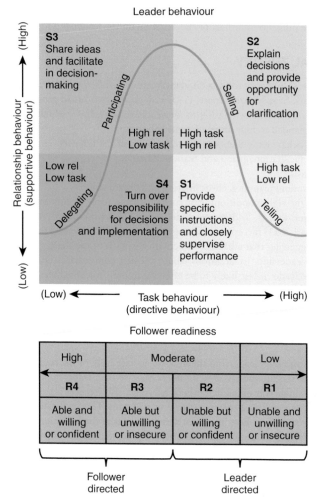

Fig. 13.1   Hersey and Blanchard's (1977) situational leadership model.

to gauge this by judging the readiness of the followers. Hersey and Blanchard (1977) state that the leadership style (S1–S4) must correspond to the development level of the follower (D1–D4) and it is the leader who should adapt. D1-D4 follows the arc (Fig. 13.1) from right to left with D1 denoting the least developed follower who requires the most direction and support from the leader to D4 representing a follower who has sufficiently developed to undertake tasks requiring little if any, support from the leader, By the leader adopting the right style to suit the follower's development level, work gets done, relationships are built and the follower's development level rises to everyone's benefit. The main failing of this theory, however, is that a leader does not materialize in every crisis, and even if they did, this would not necessarily ensure effective leadership, as the leader could be effective in one situation or organization and not in another. Nevertheless, a positive criticism of this model is that in addition to addressing the qualities of the leader, it also focuses on the maturity and competence of the group followers; factors that are often overlooked in good leadership.

TRANSACTIONAL/MANAGERIAL THEORY

Transactional theory, also referred to as *exchange leadership theory*, is characterized by a transaction made between the leader and the followers, valuing a positive and mutually beneficial relationship (Burns 1998). The foundation of transactional leadership is in the *bottom line* of an organizational structure, based on the need to complete a task and be rewarded, and therefore has some resonance with management theory. Consequently, this approach recognizes positional power, with rewards being exchanged between the leader and followers when the followers have made good effort and performed well. Transactional leaders are most efficient when they develop a mutual reinforcing environment, for which the individual and the organizational goals are in harmony and the environment is stable. However, it can be argued that although there are positive followers' attitudes and behaviours attributed to successful transactional leadership, the followers may not necessarily exceed their performance beyond what is expected and rewarded (Boseman 2008).

TRANSFORMATIONAL THEORY

The leadership approach increasingly advocated throughout the health care literature is that based on the *transformational* model. This is a mutually stimulating relationship between leaders and followers that raises each to higher levels of motivation and morality. That individuals can be lifted into their better selves is the essence of transforming leadership and the moral and practical theme of this work. Rules and regulations are flexible, guided by group norms. Such attributes provide a sense of belonging for the followers as they can easily identify with the leader and their purpose. Bass and Bass (2008) purport that the leader in this model transforms followers through a number of crucial processes:

- *idealized behaviours*: living one's ideals
- *inspirational motivation*: inspiring others
- *intellectual stimulation*: stimulating others
- *individualized consideration*: coaching and development opportunities
- *idealized attributes*: respect, trust and faith.

Through these processes, leaders act to raise awareness of what is appropriate and important, increase motivational maturity and encourage followers to go beyond their own interests for the benefit of the wider organization. Consequently, as followers are provided with a sense of purpose, transformational leadership extends beyond the simple exchange of rewards for effort, as is apparent in the transactional leadership model. According to Leach (2005: 228) transformational leadership is a suitable approach in organizations requiring '*change, development, initiative, and creativity in turbulent and uncertain environments*'; see Chapter 14. Northouse (2018) points out that as the leadership process incorporates the needs of both leader and follower, leadership emerges as an interaction between the two, as opposed to being the sole responsibility of the leader.

Deckard (2010) argues that as the transformational leader is required to possess a particular type of trait or characteristics, for example charisma, such a model would suggest a return to a trait-based approach to leadership. However, others such as Bass (1990) claim that such characteristics (e.g. self-confidence, determination and good interpersonal skills) can be taught. When transformational leadership is successfully used within an organization, Boseman (2008) explains that followers appear more satisfied, more optimistic, less likely to leave the organization and more likely to trust the leader and exert more effort in their work, with consequential higher performance levels.

Leadership Frameworks

In recent years within the National Health Service (NHS) there has been a move towards identifying and nurturing talent in leadership skill development through the introduction of the concept of *talent management*. This is a systematic process of attracting, identifying, developing, engaging/retaining and deploying individuals who show high potential and who can be of particular value to the organization (Chartered Institute of Personnel and Development 2017). It therefore serves a dual purpose in supporting individuals' career development and organizational succession planning, especially with the demographic challenges of an ageing senior workforce and increasing recognition of the value of a diverse workforce (NHS Employers 2009). A whole organizational approach is optimal, with senior and line managers and human resource departments being ideally placed to take responsibility for developing individuals throughout the organization. Consequently, as Blass (2007) affirms, the development of a *talent culture* that is dependent on all members understanding the importance of investing in a talent management strategy is essential to the organization's future success and direction.

The emergence of leadership frameworks offers a more structured approach to developing leadership potential, and departure from the totally unstructured approach of the past where individuals had little or no formal career development before taking on midwifery leadership roles in clinical practice, education and research. The following sections discuss such frameworks.

NHS LEADERSHIP ACADEMY HEALTHCARE LEADERSHIP MODEL

The Healthcare Leadership Model was developed by the NHS Leadership Academy in 2013, working with the Hay Group and the Open University. It is an evidence-based research model that reflects:
- the values of the NHS
- what is known about effective leadership
- lessons learned from the leadership framework (NHS Leadership Academy 2011)
- feedback from patients and communities on what they want from health care leaders.

The Healthcare Leadership Model (NHS Leadership Academy 2013) is used to assist those who work in health and care to become better leaders and is useful for everyone, regardless of the extent of their leadership responsibility, regardless of the service setting and regardless of the size of the team. The comprehensive detail contained within the model describes the activities leaders undertake and is organized in such a way that enables everyone to see how they can develop as a leader. It can be applied to the whole variety of roles and care settings that exist within health and care.

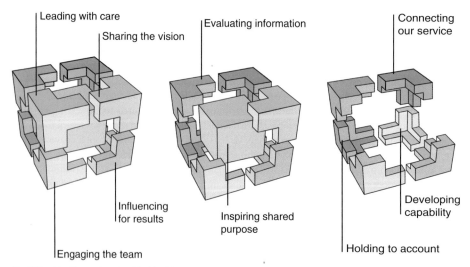

Fig. 13.2   Healthcare Leadership Model: nine dimensions of leadership behaviour. (NHS Leadership Academy 2013).

There are nine dimensions to the model as shown in Fig. 13.2, with each being made up of a brief description of what the dimension is about and why it is important, along with a section that says '*what it is not*' to provide further clarity. There are also behavioural indicators which are presented as a series of questions to guide leaders' thoughts and result in effective leadership behaviour. These questions provide an opportunity to reflect on personal intentions and motivations to see where strengths and areas for development may lie rather than providing a simple *yes* or *no* answer. Furthermore, providing evidence to support the responses given is noted to be good practice.

The nine dimensions of the Healthcare Leadership Model are:

- inspiring shared purpose
- leading with care
- evaluating information
- connecting our service
- sharing the vision
- engaging the team
- holding to account
- developing capability
- influencing for results.

For each dimension, leadership behaviours are shown on a four-part scale which ranges from *essential* through *proficient* and *strong* to *exemplary*. Although the complexity and sophistication of the behaviours increase as the leader moves up the scale, this is *not* assigned to particular job roles or levels. Individuals in junior roles may find themselves to be within the *strong* or *exemplary* parts of the scale, and senior staff may find themselves on the *essential* or *proficient* part of the scale. Similarly, where a midwife judges themselves may vary depending on the dimension itself: the midwife may be mostly *strong* in a few dimensions, *exemplary* in one, and *essential* or *proficient* in others. This may be appropriate depending on the nature of the midwife's role or may show that there are areas that need some development or that are a particular strength.

Research has shown that all nine dimensions of the model are important in an individual's leadership role. However, the type of job they have, the needs of the people they work with and the context of their role within their organization will all affect which dimensions are most important for them to use and develop. It is also important to realize that areas identified for development within the model may be as much about how the individual manages themselves as about how they manage their behaviour and relate to other people.

ROYAL COLLEGE OF MIDWIVES MIDWIFERY LEADERSHIP COMPETENCY FRAMEWORK

The Royal College of Midwives (RCM) (2012) *Midwifery Leadership Competency Framework* as shown in Fig. 13.3 was derived from both the *NHS Leadership Qualities Framework* (NHS Institute for Innovation and Improvement 2003) and the *Clinical Leadership Competency Framework* (NHS Leadership Academy 2011). It describes the leadership competencies that midwives are required to demonstrate to become more actively involved in the planning, delivery and transformation of the health services offered to childbearing women, their babies and their families. The central core of the Midwifery Leadership Competency Framework applies to all health care workers engaged in clinical practice and is built on the concept of *shared* leadership. This indicates that leadership is not restricted to individuals who hold designated leadership roles, but is where there is a shared sense of responsibility for the success of the organization and its services. As acts of leadership can come from anyone in the organization, they should be focused on the *achievement of the group* rather than of an individual.

The framework consists of seven leadership domains, with each domain consisting of four subsections. Domains 1–5 address core leadership skills that all health care workers who are engaged

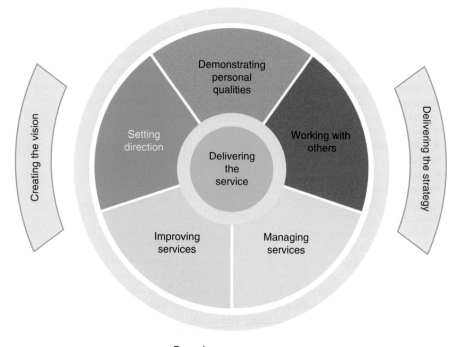

Domains

1. Demonstrating personal qualities
2. Working with others
3. Managing services
4. Improving services
5. Setting direction

6. Creating the vision
7. Delivering the strategy

Fig. 13.3   Midwifery Leadership Competency Framework. (Adapted from Royal College of Midwives 2012).

in the provision of maternity care, by planning and implementing care at the clinical level working directly with childbearing women, their babies and their families, should be competent in, through to the heads or directors of maternity services, who apply the domains at a more strategic level. Domains 6 and 7 are more applicable to senior midwives as they address service leadership from a strategic approach. However, they should not be overlooked as they can be valuable to all midwives in enabling them to explore practice from a strategic perspective and offer support to midwifery leaders.

The framework document includes examples from practice, some of which are quite general. Student midwives may find they are confident in some of the more complex issues of the framework if they have been exposed to them, whereas more experienced midwives may find there is a benefit in reflecting on certain elements of practice from earlier in their careers. The two strategic domains that surround the core domains not only apply to heads or directors of maternity services and professionals in general management roles but can also be used in an inspirational way to support the identification and development of future senior leaders for the midwifery profession. The framework is structured in such a way that it enables midwives to develop the competencies throughout a midwifery career to become the leaders who will be better equipped to make a difference to the women, babies and families for whom they provide care. This makes the framework directly relevant to the context in which the midwifery profession works to deliver a safe, high-quality and women-focused service.

Now undertake Activity 13.2.

ACTIVITY 13.2 ■

Consider a high-performing and successful team (inside or outside of work) that you are/have been part of (e.g. midwife-led team, university midwifery society, hockey team).

- What does/did it feel like to be part of this team and its success?
- What is/was significant about the behaviours and nature of the relationships within the team?
- What style of leader do you perceive you are? Do the perceptions of others agree with your own?
- How could you use this knowledge and experience to be an effective leader within the team you are currently working with or may be planning to work with in the future?

Leadership Styles and Power

Style theory succeeded both trait theory and situational theory, and is based on the belief that employees will work harder and more effectively for managers who use certain styles of leadership. Leadership style concerns the behaviours of leaders and focuses on what leaders do and how they act, including their actions towards subordinates in a variety of contexts. As a result, any leadership style can exhibit a mix of *directive* and *supportive* behaviours. In their influential leadership decision experiments, Lewin et al (1939) identified three different styles of leadership: *autocratic*, *democratic* and *laissez-faire*. According to Ralston (2005), the major differences in the three styles is in the focus of power.

AUTOCRATIC/AUTHORITARIAN LEADERSHIP STYLE/DIRECTING: THE DRIVER

In the autocratic style the leader takes decisions without consulting others and consequently causes the most level of discontent. This particular style strongly resembles *Theory X*, described by McGregor (1960), where it is assumed people lack ambition, prefer to be directed and controlled and want security rather than any responsibility. Ralston (2005) also describes this type of style as *authoritarian*, stating that communication is top-down and that staff are not expected or encouraged to take any initiative. It is a useful style to use in the short term, such as in an emergency, but can foster dependence, submissiveness and a loss of individuality that can in time affect the creativity and personal growth of staff. This results in individuals losing interest in their work and so they become dissatisfied, such that autocratic leadership ultimately can create discontent, hostility and in some cases aggression.

DEMOCRATIC LEADERSHIP STYLE/SUPPORTING: THE DEMOCRAT

In *Theory Y* (McGregor 1960), a democratic style of leadership, the leader involves members of the team in the decision-making, and this style is often described as *participative*, assuming that the average individual is inherently resourceful, self-motivated and will take on responsibility when given the opportunity. The democratic leader treats individuals as fully capable of working on their own, which is usually appreciated by others and improves staff morale and ownership. However, this type of leadership can require more time and commitment from the leader, and although work is accomplished, it is acknowledged that it may not always be achieved as efficiently as in the case where the leader adopts an autocratic and directive style. Furthermore, a wide range of opinions may arise, and there may not necessarily be a clear way of reaching an equitable decision.

LAISSEZ-FAIRE LEADERSHIP STYLE

The laissez-faire leadership style minimizes the leader's involvement in the decision-making. It neither attempts to control individuals as Theory X/autocratic leaders nor does it try and nurture and guide them as would Theory Y. The laissez-faire leader is a nominal leader, by virtue of their position in the organization and does not necessarily display leadership skills (Ralston 2005). They engage in minimal influence, and whilst they recognize others, they are very laid back and make no attempt to influence their subordinates' activities or appraise/regulate their progress. Very little is therefore accomplished under a laissez-faire leader as team members have complete freedom that often creates an environment of chaos. Without a sense of purpose and direction, these individuals will have difficulty finding meaning in their work, becoming unmotivated and disheartened, which often results in a reduction in productivity. The laissez-faire leadership style works best when team members are capable of and motivated in making their own decisions and where there is no requirement for any central coordination.

Qualities of the Leader and Emotional Intelligence

When the qualities of a *perfect leader* are considered, the picture that may come to mind is some-one who never loses their temper, no matter what challenges they are facing, or someone who has the complete trust of their team, listens to their followers, is approachable, is a good communicator and always makes careful, informed decisions (see Chapters 3 and 14). These are qualities of someone with a high degree of *emotional intelligence*. *Emotional intelligence* refers to an individual's ability to understand and manage their own emotions and those of the people around them. People with a high degree of emotional intelligence are self-aware of what they are feeling, what their emotions mean, and how these emotions can affect other people.

For leaders, having emotional intelligence is essential for success. A successful leader is one who when under stress stays in control and calmly assesses the situation, in contrast to the leader who shouts at their team of followers when in a similar situation. Goleman (1996) claims there are

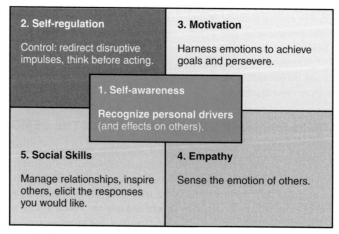

Fig. 13.4   Key elements of emotional intelligence. (Goleman 1996).

five key elements of emotional intelligence that the leader should possess, as shown in Fig. 13.4. The more the leader addresses each of these elements, the higher their emotional intelligence.

Individuals with high emotional intelligence tend to have better mental health, job performance, and leadership skills, and although no causal relationships have been shown, such findings are likely to be attributable to general intelligence and specific personality traits rather than emotional intelligence as a construct.

Now undertake Activity 13.3.

ACTIVITY 13.3 ■

As a leader, in what ways can you improve each element?

Element	Provide details of the sources you could use to evidence your development in each element.
Self–awareness	
Self-regulation	
Motivation	
Empathy	
Social skills	

The Future Leader in Midwifery

From recent reports into the failings of health care in the United Kingdom (UK), a recurrent theme that has emerged was the inefficient management structures and lack of leadership (Francis 2013; Kirkup 2015; Knight et al 2018). As a consequence, NHS England (2016) and Warwick (2015) have advocated increased representation of midwives in senior leadership roles at local and national level, such that their contribution as leaders can improve the quality of maternity/neonatal care. Warwick (2015) further reaffirms that leaders need to be innovative, enabling different midwives to work in different ways throughout their careers, such that traditional hierarchies are abandoned and opportunities are given to *all* midwives, playing to their enthusiasms and strengths. To transform the future of the maternity services, midwifery leadership has to be transformed.

INITIATIVES TO DEVELOP THE FUTURE MIDWIFERY LEADER

To improve leadership development opportunities available to midwives, a range of initiatives are available and are presented in the following sections, addressing the diversity of roles midwives may occupy, including those in clinical practice and in higher education. Furthermore, opportunities to talent-spot and develop the leadership potential of student midwives and practising midwives in low- to middle-income countries are also discussed.

Council of Deans of Health Student Leadership Programme

In 2017, the Council of Deans of Health, supported by the Burdett Trust for Nursing, launched its *Student Leadership Programme*, which offers innovative ways for developing leadership skills in future health care professionals from midwifery, nursing and the allied health professions. The programme is targeted at 150 first- and second-year students across the UK, and offers exposure to leadership training, networking and mentoring. The programme has been co-designed with students based on a student survey and the input of students on the project advisory group to ensure it focuses on areas not covered in pre-registration curricula. Each student is mentored by a

---

CASE STUDY 13.1   **Pre-registration Midwifery Curriculum Leadership Development**

The University of Leicester is at the vanguard of developing the next generation of leaders of the midwifery profession by offering an innovative 4-year undergraduate pre-registration Master in Science (MSci) Midwifery with Leadership programme through an income-share business venture with the local National Health Service (NHS) trust providers in Leicestershire.

The focus on leadership runs throughout the programme, with the students undertaking a specific leadership module every year of the 4-year programme. In addition to their clinical midwife mentor/practice supervisor, every student has a leadership mentor (an experienced NHS clinician/midwifery expert/leader) as part of a leadership learning set. The midwives are also educated by academic subject specialists from the university's School of Business to optimize their learning experience.

The development of short elective placements/internships that embrace all aspects of midwifery leadership roles (e.g. in clinical practice, education and research departments) where the students work alongside effective role models and are nurtured in developing their leadership potential is also a key feature of the programme.

As part of the business case, the University Hospitals of Leicester NHS Trust will offer all successful midwife graduates from the programme, who demonstrate the NHS values and behaviours, the opportunity of employment and the potential for fast-track career opportunities that use their leadership skills and knowledge. http://www2.le.ac.uk/departments/ahp/midwifery

---

leader from within the health and higher education sectors and from an online community to support their leadership journey following a 2-day residential programme that includes workshops, scenario-building activities and self-reflection activities.

It is vital for the future of the midwifery profession that it is led by enthusiastic, visionary and innovative midwives, and as discussed earlier, talent-spotting student midwives and those early in their career who show leadership potential must be a priority so they can be nurtured and mentored to fulfil such an aspiration (Marshall and Furber 2017). Case Study 13.1 provides one example of an innovative pre-registration midwifery curriculum development that aims to prepare the future leaders of the profession from the start of their career journey as a student midwife.

The NHS Leadership Academy

In 2013, the largest ever leadership development programme, aimed at changing the culture of the NHS, was developed through the NHS Leadership Academy. This organization provides a range of resources and programmes to support individuals, organizations and local academies to develop leaders, sharing and celebrating where outstanding leadership has made a real difference. There are a wide range of programmes available that combine successful leadership strategies from international health care, private sector organizations and academic expert content, and consequently they aim to meet the learning development needs of every leader at all stages of their career, from aspiring leader to executive directors. Programme delivery ranges from online to face-to face/regional workshop attendance, leading to a recognizable award from the NHS Leadership Academy. Whilst there is a cost for the programmes (except the *Edward Jenner programme*, which is free), bursaries may be available for under-represented groups across leadership levels. For those midwives new to leadership or aspiring to a leadership role, the following programmes are available:

- the *Edward Jenner programme*, for participants who are new to leadership by assisting them to gain a fresh perspective on the delivery of services and impact on service user experience
- the *Mary Secole programme*, for participants looking to move into their first formal leadership role, or those new to first time leadership

- *the NHS Graduate Management Training Scheme,* for graduates to become future leaders in the NHS
- *the Ready Now programme,* for aspiring black, Asian and minority ethnic leaders (available to Band 8a staff).

The Royal College of Midwives

The RCM recognizes that leadership is a significant and important role of all midwives, albeit for midwives to have the time and access to appropriate education and training to support leadership development can be challenging (RCM 2012). As a result and evolving from the *Midwifery Leadership Competency Framework* (RCM 2012), the RCM has developed a range of resources, including courses and workshops, for its members to access. The online learning platform *i-learn* provides *leadership modules* that reflect the NHS Leadership Academy Leadership Framework and focuses on activities that will develop and improve the midwife's leadership skills. The RCM also facilitates a *strategic leadership programme* as well as bespoke leadership programmes for midwives in the UK and abroad.

Florence Nightingale Foundation Leadership Scholarships

Midwives in clinical practice, education and research may wish to consider applying for a leadership scholarship with the Florence Nightingale Foundation. However, these scholarships tend to be for those who have some degree of experience from band 7 or equivalent and above, but could be worth considering in the future, one example being the *Emerging Leaders Scholarship* (of up to £10,000), which is available to band 7 and band 8 midwives and nurses who have already completed a front-line leadership development programme before the start of the scholarship. The scholar undertakes a core development programme in addition to a bespoke programme geared to their individual needs relating to their leadership potential.

International Confederation of Midwives: Young Midwives in the Lead

In collaboration with the United Nations Population Fund, Jhpiego, Johnson & Johnson and the World Health Organization, the International Confederation of Midwives organizes workshops that highlight leadership principles and effective communication with symposia. These activities showcase how investments in early-career midwives (Young Midwives in the Lead) can improve quality care within midwifery worldwide, especially in low- to middle-income countries, and emphasize the importance of investments in research, advocacy, mentorship and leadership skills of Young Midwives in the Lead.

The Leadership Foundation for Higher Education

As a registered charity, the Leadership Foundation for Higher Education (now part of Advance HE), which was established by Universities UK and Guild Higher Education, is committed to developing and improving the management, governance and leadership skills of existing and future leaders within the higher education sector. Leadership programmes are facilitated around the UK and Ireland to meet the needs of higher education employees at all stages of their careers, ranging from the *Transition to Leadership* programme (new leaders) to the *Vice Chancellors/Principals* programme, some of which are offered as an online programme. Since 2013, the Leadership Foundation for Higher Education has offered women-only programmes, notably the *Aurora* programme, which aims to take positive action to address the under-representation of women in leadership positions in the higher education sector. Furthermore, the foundation also offers the *Research Team Leadership* programme for both research professionals and academics.

Conclusion

Effective and visionary leadership is vital within the midwifery profession to ensure it is steered in the right direction, continuing to be responsive to the dynamic and complex nature of 21st century maternity care. It is essential that midwifery education and practice reflect leadership approaches that are distributed, collective and transformational to optimize effect at all levels, particularly the impact on the education of the future midwife and the care childbearing women, their babies and their families receive. An understanding of leadership and management theory is also crucial and should be integral in all pre-registration midwifery curricula to ensure that midwives develop their knowledge and skills from a much earlier stage in their career. This would provide midwives with increased confidence not only to lead midwifery care provision on an individual level within their own organization but also to lead teams and drive forward the profession on a wider scale. This chapter has presented a number of key leadership theories, styles and frameworks that midwives can use to develop their own leadership knowledge and skills. A range of leadership development opportunities and activities have been presented to inspire midwives to consider their own leadership career trajectory and ongoing continuing professional development.

KEY POINTS

- Reports into the failings of health care in the UK have advocated for more efficient management structures and improved leadership at all levels in the organization.
- Having an understanding of the benefits and challenges of leadership theories and styles is essential so the most appropriate model is adopted to optimal effect within the organization.
- Over recent years, leadership theory has evolved from leader-centric approaches to those that are distributed, collective and transformational, as reflected in health care leadership developments.
- Leaders need to be visionary and innovative, working in different ways throughout their careers, such that traditional hierarchies are abandoned and opportunities are given to all midwives, playing to their strengths.
- The *perfect* leader is someone who has a high degree of *emotional intelligence:* who understands and manages their own emotions and those of the people around them.
- Leadership theory and skills must become integral within initial midwifery education for student midwives to better understand the principles and subsequently influence the future direction of the midwifery profession.
- Talent-spotting student midwives and early-career midwives who demonstrate leadership potential and developing a strategy to nurture and mentor them is vital to succession planning and sustaining midwifery as a profession.

References

Bass, B. M. (1990). From transactional to transformational leadership: Learning to share the vision. *Organizational Dynamics, 18*(3), 19–31.

Bass, B. M., & Bass, R. (2008). *The Bass handbook of leadership: Theory, research and managerial applications* (4th ed.). New York: The Free Press.

Bednash, G. (2009). Developing leadership. In Marquis, B., & Huston, C. (Eds.), *Leadership roles and management functions in nursing: Theory and application* (4th ed.). Philadelphia: Lippincott, Williams and Wilkins.

Bennis, W. G. (2009). *On becoming a leader.* New York: Basic Books.

Blass, E. (2007). *Talent management: Maximising talent for business performance (executive summary).* London: Chartered Management Institute and Ashridge Consulting.

Boseman, G. (2008). Effective leadership in a changing world. *Journal of Financial Service Professionals, 62*(3), 36–38.

Bowers, D. G., & Seashore, S. E. (1966). Predicting organizational effectiveness with a four-factor theory of leadership. *Administrative Science Quarterly, 11*(2), 238–263.

Bowles, A., & Bowles, N. B. (2000). A comparative study of transformational leadership in nursing development units and conventional clinical settings. *Journal of Nursing Management, 8*, 69–76.

Burns, J. M. (1998). Transactional and transforming leadership. In Robinson Hickman, G. (Ed.), *Leading organizations: Perspectives for a new era* (pp. 133–135). London: Sage Publications.

Chartered Institute of Personnel and Development. (2017). *Research insight: Talent management*. Available at: https://www.cipd.co.uk/knowledge/strategy/resourcing/talent-factsheet.

Deckard, G. J. (2010). Contemporary leadership theories. In Borkowski, N. (Ed.), *Organizational behaviour in health care* (pp. 209–230). Sudbury: Jones and Bartlett.

Francis, R. (2013). *Report of the Mid Staffordshire NHS Foundation Trust Public Inquiry*. London: The Stationery Office. Available at: https://www.gov.uk/government/publications/report-of-the-mid-staffordshire-nhs-foundation-trust-public-inquiry.

Girvin, J. (1998). *Leadership and nursing: Essentials of nursing management*. Basingstoke: Macmillan Press.

Goleman, D. (1996). *Emotional intelligence*. London: Bloomsbury.

Handy, C. (2007). *Understanding organisations* (4th ed.). London: Penguin.

Hersey, P., & Blanchard, K. H. (1977). *Management of organizational behavior: Utilizing human resources* (3rd ed.). Englewood Cliffs: Prentice Hall.

Kirkup, B. (2015). *The Report of the Morecambe Bay Investigation*. Preston: The Stationery Office. Available at: https://www.gov.uk/government/uploads/system/uploads/attachment_data/file/408480/47487_MBI_Accessible_v0.1.pdf.

Knight, M., Bunch, K., Tufnell, D., Jayakody, H., Shakespeare, J., Kotnis, R., Kenyon, S., & Kurinczuk, J. J. (Eds.), on behalf of MBRRACE-UK, (2018). *Saving Lives, Improving Mothers' Care- Lessons learned to inform maternity care from the UK and Ireland Confidential Enquiries into Maternal Deaths and Morbidity 2014-16*. Oxford: National Perinatal Epidemiology Unit, University of Oxford.

Kotter, J. P. (1990). What leaders really do. *Harvard Business Review, 68*(3), 103–111.

Leach, L. (2005). Nurse executive transformational leadership and organizational commitment. *Journal of Nursing Administration, 35*, 228–237.

Lewin, K., Lippit, R., & White, R. K. (1939). Patterns of aggressive behavior in experimentally created social climates. *Journal of Social Psychology, 10*, 271–301.

Marshall, J. E., & Furber, C. (2017). Who will educate and prepare the midwives of the future? The crisis in midwifery education in the UK. *MIDIRS Midwifery Digest, 27*(3), 277–280.

McGregor, D. (1960). *The human side of enterprise*. New York: McGraw–Hill.

NHS Employers. (2009). *Talent for tough times: How to identify, attract and retain the talent you need. Briefing 65*. Available at: http://www.nhsemployers.org/~/media/Employers/Publications/Talent_for_tough_times-Briefing_65.PDF?dl=1.

NHS England. (2016). *Better births: Improving outcomes of maternity services in England. A five year forward view for maternity care*. Available at: https://www.england.nhs.uk/wp-content/uploads/2016/02/national-maternity-review-report.pdf.

NHS Institute for Innovation and Improvement. (2003). *NHS Leadership Qualities Framework: The full technical research paper*. Available at: http://nhsleadershipframework.rightmanagement.co.uk/assets/x/50130.

NHS Leadership Academy. (2011). Leadership framework – a summary. Available at: http://www.leadershipacademy.nhs.uk/develop-your-leadership-skills/leadershipframework/supporting-tools-and-documents/documents-to-download.

NHS Leadership Academy. (2013). *Healthcare leadership model: The nine dimensions of leadership behaviour*. Leeds: NHS Leadership Academy. Available at: https://www.leadershipacademy.nhs.uk/wp-content/uploads/2014/10/NHSLeadership-LeadershipModel-colour.pdf.

Northouse, P. G. (2018). *Leadership theory and practice* (8th ed.). Thousand Oaks: Sage.

Ralston, R. (2005). Transformational leadership: Leading the way for midwives in the 21st century. *RCM Midwives Journal, 8*, 34–47.

Royal College of Midwives. (2012). *Midwifery leadership competency framework*. London: RCM Trust.

Stogdill, R. M., & Coons, A. E. (1957). *Leader behavior: Its description and measurement*. Columbus: Ohio State University Press.

Thomas, N., & Adair, J. (2011). *The John Adair handbook of leadership and management*. Claremont: Viva Books.

Warwick, C. (2015). *Leadership in maternity services*. London: The Health Foundation. Available at: http://patientsafety.health.org.uk/sites/default/files/resources/6.leadership_in_maternity_services-v2.pdf.

Watson, C. (1983). Leadership, management and the seven keys. *Business Horizons, March–April*, 8–13.

Further Reading

Ashton, D., Ripman, J., & Williams, P. (Eds.). (2017). *How to be a nurse or midwife leader*. Chichester: Wiley-Blackwell.

    This is a useful concise guide for all midwives and nurses who wish to develop and improve their practice as leaders. It was written in collaboration with the NHS Leadership Academy and draws on the experience of more than 10,000 nurses and midwives, bringing leadership dilemmas to life in specific situations. In addition, exercises and reflective questions assist the reader in applying theory to leadership practice.

Martin, M., & Whiting, F. (2017). *Human resource practice* (7th ed.). London: Chartered Institute of Personnel Development.

    This fully updated edition written by two renowned experts in the field explores the application of models within the practice of human resources. The inclusion of international case studies, examples and activities enables the reader to engage with the key areas of practical human resource management, such as the legal background to employment, learning and development; changes in organization and employee relations (for example, recruitment and selection, performance management and reward and well-being in the workplace) are explored in more detail.

Northouse, P. G. (2018). *Leadership theory and practice* (8th ed.). Thousand Oaks: Sage.

    This market-leading text used at more than 1600 institutions in 89 countries and translated into 13 different languages provides an academically robust account of the major theories and models of leadership. New to this edition are chapters on Followership that explores the characteristics of effective and ineffective followers in the leadership process and new coverage on destructive leadership, the dark side of leadership and pseudo-transformational leadership is included. Case studies, questionnaires and a video (via the interactive eBook version) provide students with practical examples and opportunities to deepen their personal understanding of their own leadership style.

Schedlitzki, D., & Edwards, G. (2017). *Studying leadership: Traditional and critical approaches*. (2nd ed.). London: Sage.

    This text provides a comprehensive overview of the key theories, topics, research debates and major developments in the field of leadership studies.

    Split into three parts, the text covers the traditional and mainstream theories on leadership; leadership research, and the recent trends in leadership studies such as gender and diversity, ethics, sustainability, language and identity.

    A new chapter on "Researching Leadership" with extended case studies is included to enhance learning and support students with their dissertations and research projects.

    The text is complemented by a companion website featuring a range of tools and resources for lecturers and students, that includes multiple-choice questions, case studies, videos with critical thinking and discussion questions.

Useful Websites

Burdett Trust for Nursing: http://www.btfn.org.uk

Business Balls: https://www.businessballs.com

Chartered Institute of Personnel and Development: https://www.cipd.co.uk

Council of Deans of Health: https://www.councilofdeans.org.uk

Florence Nightingale Foundation: https://www.florence-nightingale-foundation.org.uk

International Confederation of Midwives: https://www.internationalmidwives.org

Jhpiego: https://www.jhpiego.org

Leadership Foundation for Higher Education: https://www.lfhe.ac.uk (now part of Advance HE [https://www.advance-he.ac.uk] as a result of the merger with the Equality Challenge Unit and the Higher Education Academy).

Mind Tools: https://www.mindtools.com

NHS Leadership Academy: https://www.leadershipacademy.nhs.uk

Royal College of Midwives: https://www.rcm.org.uk

TED Talks: https://www.ted.com/talks

United Nations Population Fund: https://www.unfpa.org

CHAPTER 14

Change and Innovation in Midwifery Education and Practice

Lai Yen Polenz ▪ Jane Forman ▪ Jayne E. Marshall

CONTENTS

LEARNING OUTCOMES

By the end of the chapter the reader will:

• understand the concept of change management
• appreciate the various models and tools used to facilitate change
• recognize the qualities required to be an effective change agent in midwifery
• appreciate the value of entrepreneurialism in midwifery
• understand how innovations in midwifery can advance midwifery education and practice.

Overview

In this chapter change management theories will be explored and the models and tools that can facilitate change will be discussed. These will be applied to contemporary midwifery education and practice, with examples of innovation and entrepreneurialism from within the profession being explored through case studies and reflective exercises.

Introduction

The pace of change has increased dramatically globally, enabled by the World-Wide-Web, such that a state of continuous change can appear to be the norm (Luecke 2003). A number of events have had and are continuing to have an impact on the way we all live, work and play. Such global changes include the global economic recession, social networking, climate change and the impact of an increasing fragile earth, the growth of China, India and the Pacific Rim economies and an increasing movement towards moral and social responsibility in leadership and change (McCalman et al 2016). All these, to varying degrees, and how they are addressed within local contexts, have an impact on the way midwives work in the international context.

It is well evidenced that there are many challenges facing the midwifery profession that need to be borne in mind by educators when they are designing new curricula to ensure that the future workforce consists of midwives who are fit for practice and purpose in all aspects of the profession, be it in clinical practice, education or research. The effects of the increasing diversity of backgrounds and complex health care needs of childbearing women, their babies and their families (Knight et al 2018), the consequences of an ageing midwifery workforce and high attrition among midwives in the United Kingdom (Royal College of Midwives 2016) and the ongoing reviews into midwifery practice and education (Scottish Government 2014; Kirkup 2015; Department of Health 2016) support a change in how midwives should be educated and maternity and neonatal care should be delivered so as to address these challenges.

Midwives are at the heart of midwifery practice and are key to improving the lives of childbearing women and their babies worldwide (Renfrew et al 2014), and so it is essential each midwife possesses the knowledge and understanding of change theory in order to influence advancements in practice based on the best available evidence. Furthermore, change management theory should be a key feature within all midwifery curricula to provide students with the foundation upon which to build confidence within their subsequent midwifery career. Without midwives being bold and advocating changes to support women-focused care in whatever setting they work, it could be argued they are doing a disservice to women. However, the reality is that organizational culture can indeed affect how midwives practise, and for some they can become just as entrenched in the medical model as their obstetric colleagues (Scamell 2011; Einion 2017). It therefore requires an understanding of the culture of a profession and the organization as well as the theories of change for any innovation to be successful.

Change Management Theory

For change to be successful in an organization, many aspects are involved, including the organization itself as well as the individuals working within it. According to Steiner (2001), overly bureaucratic and hierarchical organizations traditionally do not fare well when faced with change as they are less amenable to change, less flexible, and less likely to empower staff. Directing change by a top-down approach without any staff engagement is unlikely to effect change and effective working practices (Steiner 2001) (see Chapter 13). Hence it is pertinent to understand the organizational structure and culture one works within, examining the internal and external factors that can influence its performance before initiating any change.

DEFINING CHANGE MANAGEMENT

There are many different definitions of *change management* from both business and academia. Change management is essentially about how to transform or modify something to improve its effectiveness (Hayes 2018). It is questionable as to how much difference a leader or manager can actually make and effect change within an organization without a robust understanding of change management and the support of the organization and the people within it.

Hughes (2010) distinguishes between *determinism* and *voluntarism*. *Determinism* refers to a situation where change is determined by the environment and is in the main a direct response to the operating environment. Determinism seems overly fatalistic, with the belief that outside uncontrollable sources will influence the outcome and is not great leadership and change management. Because of this, most modern change management advice is based on *voluntarism*. This concept, in contrast, provides a role for the managerial decisions and actions in influencing the change process and tends to be the approach taken in managing change in health care. Others refer to *planned* change, describing a situation where the conscious decisions and deeds of the management have a central role in the change process (Marrow 1969). Robbins et al (2010) separate *planned change* from unintended change, focusing on change events as intentional, proactive and goal orientated.

Models to Facilitate Change

It is essential that midwives understand the culture within their organization so they can work to its strengths to create a productive and satisfying workplace. Key to this is having an appreciation of management styles to use as a framework when they are considering introducing an innovation or facilitating a change in practice.

HANDY'S GODS OF MANAGEMENT

Handy (2009) describes a model of culture based on the way in which organizations are structured, using four Greek gods as metaphors for his cultural types: gods of *Management* (Fig. 14.1).

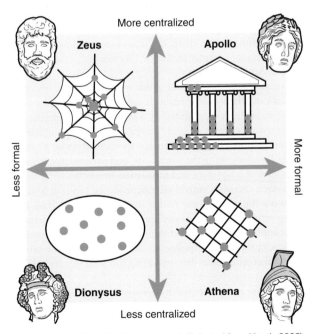

Fig. 14.1   Handy's gods of management. (Adapted from Handy 2009)

It is worth acknowledging that a single organization may have more than one of these cultures as parts of the organization may be structured differently and also comprise different occupations or professional cultures. Each of the four Greek gods *Zeus*, *Apollo*, *Athena* and *Dionysus* represents a particular trait or set of values and they are equal in value.

Power/club culture is represented by *Zeus*, a dynamic strong entrepreneurial leader who uses power and is graphically depicted by a spider's web. All lines of communication lead to the leader/ the spider at the centre of the web. Organizations with this type of culture are usually small and informal, where personal contact is more important than formal liaison. They consist of like-minded people who generally make snap decisions and respond quickly to change. The success of the organization depends on the luck or judgment of key individuals. However, if power is held by one person, the very same person can destroy the organization they have created. Zeus the leader tends to communicate on a personal, face-to-face basis or via telephone. Costs to the organization are reduced by there being less documentation. This leadership style has been criticized for nepotism and being paternalistic. The dependence on the powerful individual and contact networks may become redundant as the situation changes. However, Handy (2009) argues that they are very effective in the right situation, where trust based on personal contact to get things done is not necessarily a bad thing. Typical organizations with this type of culture include investment banks and brokerage firms.

Role culture is personified by *Apollo*, the god of order and rules and represented by a Greek temple, signifying a bureaucratic organization. This form of organization is predicated on individuals being rational beings, and the environment being one of stability and predictability where individuals are defined through their job descriptions and not personality. It suits individuals who like conformity, routine and clearly defined roles determining lines of authority and responsibility of individual managers. It is important for individuals to fulfil their job descriptions and not step out of the boundaries of their authority, and consequently the organization is hierarchical, where decision-making occurs at the top. The Apollo approach works well for large organizations with predictable work in a stable environment. However, Apollo organizations tend to be inflexible and slow to adapt to change. According to Handy (2009), in the face of change, this type of organization could either ignore the changes or set up 'cross-functional liaison groups' to support the current structure. Life insurance companies, the civil service and local government organizations are likely to resemble an Apollonian culture.

Task culture is associated with *Athena*, the goddess of knowledge, who recognizes expertise. It is found in organizations where management is focused on completing a series of projects or solving problems. The structure is represented by a net, denoting bringing people together and capturing all available resources from around the organization to complete the tasks. Working parties, subcommittees, taskforces and study groups are formed on an ad hoc basis to deal with problems. The principal goal is getting the work done, and performance is judged by results. Task culture fosters a high level of adaptation and innovation by emphasizing talent, youth and team problem solving. However, excessive individual independence can lead to irresponsibility. There can be a conflict between the desire to see results in meeting targets (task culture) and the way accountability is being enforced through procedures, returns, etc. (bureaucracy). The leader's role is to ensure there is an appropriate balance between these competing demands. In some instances, the organization may adopt a greater Apollonian work mode, and as a result, task cultures are often short-lived. Typical organizations demonstrating this structure include advertising agencies and consultancies.

Existential/person culture is represented by *Dionysus*, the god of wine and song. Organizations characterized by these cultures are those where the organization exists to serve the individual, where individuals are in charge of their destiny, are not instruments of others and owe little allegiance to a manager. They consist of groups or clusters of professionals (e.g. doctors, lawyers) with no 'boss'. Coordination may be provided by a committee of peers. Such organizational structures may appear disorganized but are becoming more common as more conventional organizations increasingly contract out work to professionals and specialists whose services are used only as and when required. Management can happen only with the consent of the managed, and the success of the organization depends on the talent of the individuals. However, Handy (2009) warns that a Dionysian culture can lead to toxic, ideological tensions among its professionals.

Handy (2009) advocates that the most effective organizations have an appropriate fit between the individuals, the type of work, the environment and the culture. Changes in the work or the environment may also lead to a requirement for cultural change, and thus midwives should have an understanding of organizational culture frameworks when considering issues around decision-making and change management. An effective organization learns to build bridges between different forces. Handy's (2009) framework helps to decide the scope and composition of an effective set of interventions to effect change and can be used at an organizational, group and individual level. However, it is important to remember that whilst the model provides insight, organizations do not stick to one culture.

LEWIN'S THREE-STAGE APPROACH TO CHANGE

Lewin (1947) presented a three-stage approach to implementing change, and although this was more than 70 years ago, the model remains relevant to contemporary practice. These three stages comprise the following elements:

1. *Unfreezing:* preparing for change, weighing up the pros and cons, overcoming the inertia, and dismantling the existing mindset. This is the basis of Lewin's (1951) force field analysis (discussed later in this chapter).
2. *Change:* transition. It can take time for individuals to learn about and understand the changes. Support in the form of training, coaching and expecting errors as part of the process is essential.
3. *Freezing/refreezing:* crystallizing the new mindset and establishing stability once the change has been made and becomes the norm.

Lewin (1947) argued that change does not happen in a stationary environment but is rather like a river which is flowing in a certain direction. Influencing individuals within an organization to change their behaviour is like changing the direction of the river. Use of force without unlocking the existing behaviour is not likely to be successful because all behaviour is governed by a subtle interaction between different interests and forces, and resistance will just increase. Most modern change theories are based around this original idea of a three-stage process (Hayes 2018), which Fig. 14.2 illustrates through the changing of an ice cube into a sphere.

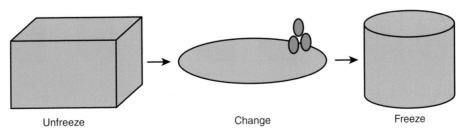

Unfreeze   Change   Freeze

Fig. 14.2   Lewin's (1947) Three-stage approach to change.

Now undertake Activity 14.1.

ACTIVITY 14.1 ■

Consider a successful change that has taken place in your organization or that you have implemented in your personal life.

Using Lewin's model, work through each stage of the process to determine how the change was achieved.

Is there any other approach that could have been used?

KOTTER'S EIGHT-STEP PROCESS FOR CHANGE MODEL

Kotter (1996) examined the activities that individuals undertake to successfully transform their organizations and developed an eight-step change model for assisting others to deal with transformational change (Fig. 14.3). The first three steps are very similar to many models in that they involve initially creating an environment where change can flourish. The next focus is on engaging and enabling others to move towards the change within the organization, with the final two stages geared to implementing and sustaining the change for the long term. Barr and Dowding (2012) affirm that any change must be perceived to have a purpose/be necessary for it to be implemented successfully.

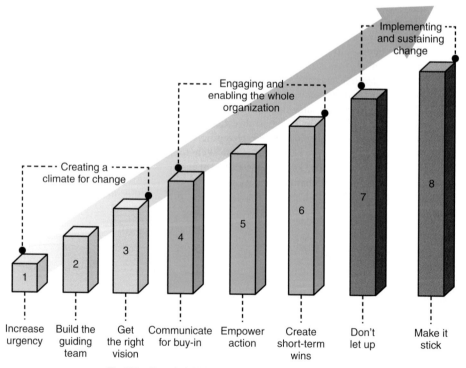

Fig. 14.3   Kotter's (1996) Eight steps to successful change.

Tools to Plan and Facilitate Change

In addition to using the structure of a model to support a change, there are a number of tools that midwives can use to effect the change (e.g. *PEST analysis, SWOT analysis* and *force field analysis*). Each of these tools identifies specific areas where more effort may need to be focused to successfully implement the change.

PEST ANALYSIS

A PEST (an acronym for *political, economic, social* and *technological*) analysis, as shown in Table 14.1, can be used to assess the market for change in an organization from a macro perspective; that is, *the big picture* (Heery and Nitton 2017). This tool is useful for a number of reasons:

- It assists in the identification of business or personal opportunities, providing advanced warning of any possible threats.
- It reveals the direction of change to assist in shaping the change, working *with* the change rather than *against* it.
- It assists in avoiding starting projects that are likely to fail for reasons beyond the individual's control.
- It assists in developing an objective view of the *new* environment, breaking free of any unconscious assumptions.

This form of analysis can be undertaken by review of the external environment. PEST analysis is a useful tool for understanding the wider implications and the opportunities that may be present. By understanding the environment, one can use opportunities for change and innovation and minimize barriers to change. There are also variations of PEST analysis that bring other factors into consideration, such as *demographic, environmental, ethical, international* and *legal* factors, as shown in Table 14.2, and the variations can be selected according to each specific situation, such as understanding change in multinational organizations.

A PEST analysis is often linked with a SWOT analysis; however, whilst the former explores the macro perspective/external factors, the latter focuses more on the micro/personal perspective/internal factors from the product line or product level.

TABLE 14.1 ▪ **Pest Analysis**

Categories	Midwifery Education	Maternity Services
Political factors	Current Nursing and Midwifery Council standards and European Union directives	Provision of maternity care. Models of midwifery care
Economic influences	Tuition fees and change of funding	Lack of real-time increase in money to fund the National Health Service (NHS). Social enterprise.
Sociocultural implications	Demographics of students. Part-time courses. Increasing popularity of midwifery as a career through media exposure	Health inequalities Continuity of care(r). Place of birth
Technological innovations	Virtual learning and online learning, e-portfolios	Telemedicine, pregnancy apps, electronic maternity records, accessibility to intranet

TABLE 14.2 ■ Variations of Pest Analysis

Acronym	Factors
PESTLE/PESTEL	Political, economic, sociocultural, technological, legal, environmental
PESTLIED	Political, economic, sociocultural, technological, legal, international, environmental, demographic
LONGPESTLE	Local, national, global versions of PESTLE: use when understanding change in multinational organizations
STEEPLE	Social/demographic, technological, economic, environmental, political, legal, ethical

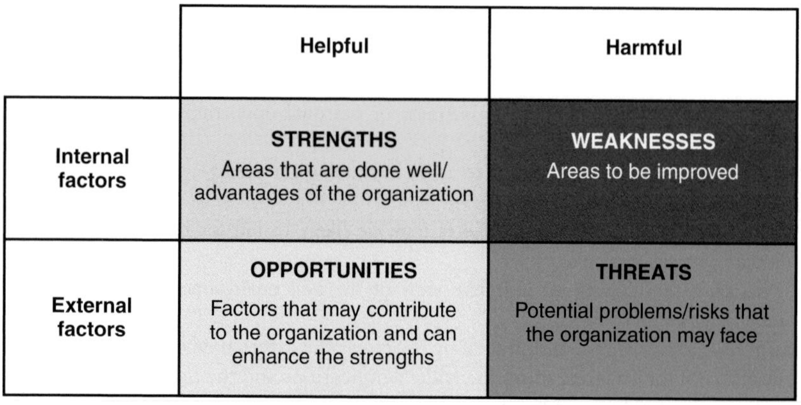

	Helpful	Harmful
Internal factors	**STRENGTHS** Areas that are done well/ advantages of the organization	**WEAKNESSES** Areas to be improved
External factors	**OPPORTUNITIES** Factors that may contribute to the organization and can enhance the strengths	**THREATS** Potential problems/risks that the organization may face

Fig. 14.4 SWOT analysis.

SWOT ANALYSIS

The actual origin of *SWOT analysis* or the *SWOT matrix* as shown in Fig. 14.4 is unclear but it is a simple structured planning method that can effectively evaluate the *strengths, weaknesses, opportunities* and *threats* of an organization, enabling achievable objectives to be set to effect change and development (Panagiotou 2003). It is particularly powerful in that with little consideration it can help individuals to uncover opportunities that they are well placed to exploit at both an organizational level and a personal level. However, as it involves subjective decision-making at each stage, it should be used as a guide rather than as a prescription. Nevertheless, by understanding weaknesses of the organization, one can manage and eliminate any threats that otherwise would have gone unnoticed. A SWOT analysis is an iterative process as it is often the first step in a more complex and in-depth analysis of an organization that can lead to initiation of a strategy formulation at a higher level.

FORCE FIELD ANALYSIS

The NHS Institute for Innovation and Improvement (2008) highlights a further tool for managing change, namely *force field analysis*, which was adapted from Lewin (1951). It is a framework for listing, discussing and assessing the various forces for and against a proposed change. Once these are identified, strategies can be developed to reduce the impact of the opposing (*restraining*) forces and to strengthen the supporting (*driving*) forces. It is a particularly effective tool when one is attempting to overcome resistance to change. A weighting is given to each force, where a

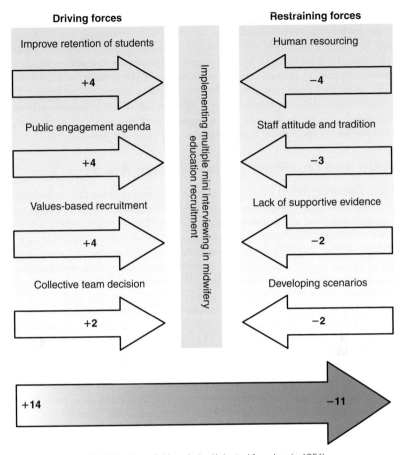

Fig. 14.5   Force field analysis. (Adapted from Lewin 1951)

score of 1 is considered weak and 5 is strong. These are charted with the driving forces on the left and the restraining forces on the right. The results of the force field analysis will determine how to improve the probability of success by either: reducing the strength of the restraining forces opposing the change or increasing the strength of the forces driving the change.

For change to occur, the driving forces should outweigh the restraining forces, otherwise there will remain a status quo where the forces balance each other out. Lewin (1951) suggested that change tends to be easier and longer lasting if the restraining forces are reduced and the forces that maintain the status quo are modified, rather than the driving forces being increased. Figure 14.5 provides an example of how a force field analysis can be used to effect change in the higher education setting. The example chosen is the change from unstructured face-to-face interviews to the use of multiple mini interviews in health recruitment that includes service user involvement. The driving factors outweigh the restraining forces by a weight of 3, which indicates the change is likely to be successful.

Following the publication of the Mid Staffordshire NHS Foundation Trust Public Inquiry report (Francis 2013), which identified substandard care and failings from many staff in exhibiting core values such as care and compassion, Health Education England (2016) developed a national values-based recruitment framework. This framework (initially published in 2014) aims to encourage higher education institutions to complement their existing recruitment processes with values-based recruitment, and ensure that successful candidates to health care programmes, such as pre-registration midwifery education programmes, have the appropriate values as well as the intellectual capacity to become compassionate midwives (Department of Health and Social Care 2015). To identify these values, multiple mini interview scenarios were devised. These are scenarios not usually related to health that test different values and behaviours expected of all individuals working in the health care setting: namely *working together for patients*, *respect and dignity*, *everyone counts*, *commitment to quality of care*, *compassion* and *improving lives*.

The Role and Qualities of the Change Agent

According to Lunenburg (2010) a change agent is an individual or group that undertakes the task of initiating and managing change in an organization. The characteristics of change agents are often associated with those of effective leaders (see Chapter 13). The exploratory study by van der Heijden et al (2015) into the characteristics of teachers as change agents found that most of them matched those of Stogdill's (1974) leadership characteristics, such as positivity, commitment, self-assurance, and being creative/innovative. An effective change agent is one with purpose and vision, the ability to manage people through difficult situations, the ability to take accountability and responsibility and the ability to motivate people to achieve respective goals.

Lippit and Lippit (1975) purport that the behaviour of the change agent runs along a continuum of eight different roles depending on whether they are being *directive* or *non-directive*. These roles are not mutually exclusive but may vary according to the stage that the change or innovation has reached. They range from *advocate, technical specialist, trainer* or *educator* on the directive side to *collaborator in problem solving, alternative identifier, fact finder, process specialist* and *reflector* on the non-directive side. Lippit and Lippit (1975) further emphasize the multiple-role nature of the change agent, the situational focus that determines these roles and the need to work in close collaboration with those within the organization, regardless of what role is being used.

It has been argued that it is difficult for an individual to be skilled in all these roles (Tearle 2007). For those who are, they have a number of attributes which classify them as *change masters*. However, Carnell (2003) believes that change management should not be a specialist skill possessed by experts, but should be an increasingly important part of every manager's role. The change master according to Tearle (2007) would possess the following attributes:

- common sense and the courage to use it
- credibility and trust: the ability to work at all levels in the organization
- a wide range of business knowledge (e.g. an MBA degree or general management experience)
- knowledge of change management
- the ability to work with teams of people both inside and outside the organization and across all departments
- the ability to do very unstructured work
- creativity and design skills: the ability to customize design processes to meet the goals of the organization
- self-confidence offset by humility
- facilitation skills
- coaching skills
- a passion for innovation and new ways of doing things
- a sense of humour and sense of fun
- a spirit of caring
- the ability to inspire others: to bring out the magic within every individual and every team.

When an individual is taking on the role of change agent, Margulies and Raia (1978: 113) affirm that the individual needs to be mindful of a number of key principles to be effective in their role:

1. The change agent needs to define the problem and work with the organization to verify this.
2. The relationship between the change agent and the client organization is crucial to developing the change process and needs to be nurtured and developed.
3. The change agent's focus of attention is on helping the client organization discover and implement solutions to the problem.
4. The change agent's expertise is in diagnosing and facilitating the process of change: steering the organization through the change.
5. The change agent supports the organization to a position where it can manage change itself.

Early in the process the change agent will take on the role of information seeker, and as the process develops and solutions emerge, the role becomes more directive in terms of moving the organization through learning to the accomplishment of new procedures that solve the particular problem/improve the situation. The role(s) that the change agent occupies during the process of change should be facilitative in assisting the organization in every way.

LEADING AND MANAGING CHANGE

Effective change agents have to carefully consider how to manage change and engage participants if the change is to be successful. Balfour and Clarke (2001) showed how it is tempting to revert to familiar ways of working once those instigating pressure to adopt changes have moved on. Public sector organizations, often large and bureaucratic, need to look at their organizational requirements and use an approach that best matches these requirements (Coram and Burnes 2001). All successful organizations need to be dynamic, and an understanding of the change process by managers and leaders will help with this. Leaders should assist employees to structure and build effective teams by developing an organizational structure that embraces a shared vision for the change. Such inspiring leadership is critical and essential for organizations to be successful in achieving change, which can be very challenging for any change agent.

Managing change requires the change agent to have the qualities that can inspire and motivate people (Barr and Dowding 2008). Chapter 13 explores the various leadership styles, but those that would be effective as a change agent would be similar to the style of a *transformational* leader (Burns 1978), or the *democratic* leader who encourages everyone to have a voice can be effective in driving forward change, as opposed to an *autocratic/coercive* leader, where all the power and control rest with the self-elected leader (Lewin 1947). Although the autocratic leader can be useful in swiftly driving forward a change in challenging situations, the change is unlikely to be sustained. Barr and Dowding (2012) suggest that a democratic leader also effects an improvement in communication and team interaction, but a leader who is both *charismatic* and passionate about the change is indeed a great influence in persuading others to follow and embrace the change.

Within organizations are individuals who are stakeholders: people who will be affected by the change. Hence Tinsley (2005) created a *commitment chart* which identifies stakeholders who may support or hinder change. The individual wishing to influence a change will identify the people who may assist/hinder the achievement of change so as to channel positive participation in assisting the 'leader' work out the strategy/action plan. However, as Tinsley (2005) emphasizes, the action plan can be fulfilled only if the stakeholders approve it and consent to it. The use of a commitment chart anticipates the change agent is knowledgeable of the interests of all the people within the organization, which can be questionable. Furthermore, human relationships, including respect for the change agent to lead the change, are vital for success.

Now undertake Activity 14.2.

ACTIVITY 14.2 ■

Think of a midwife from the following areas of practice who has implemented a change or introduced an innovation that has influenced local/national/international midwifery practices:
- clinical practice
- education/university
- research.

What qualities to these midwives have in common?

What qualities do they have that makes them effective change agents and different from other midwives?

Innovations in Midwifery

The term *innovation* simply refers to developing a *new idea*, *product* or *method of doing something*, and about *doing things differently* or *doing different things to achieve large gains in performance*. Consequently over time, innovation has developed into meaning *change for success* in organizations. Innovation is also associated with business and the concept of *entrepreneurship*.

Historically, the principal driver of innovation and improvement in maternity services has been safety (see Chapter 9). A more recent driver of change has been the desire to increase choice for women throughout pregnancy and childbirth and in postnatal care (Department of Health 1993, 2016). Public sector innovation is often initiated by frontline staff and middle managers, although the established culture and systems in place often do not work to support innovation. Other barriers are that staff do not feel that innovation is part of their day-to-day job, and successive change initiatives can lead to change fatigue, particularly if change initiatives are *owned* by and led from the top of the organization. Public sector innovation must be assessed on the basis of a range of social as well as economic value indicators. Drivers for innovation may include political pushes, the capacity and desires of the workforce, financial and non-financial support, technology, and the presence or involvement of third-sector and private sector organizations.

The level of autonomy individuals and organizations have can affects their ability to develop and test new ideas, and to implement change. Clearly, the accountability and ownership structures of the public sector affect levels of autonomy. Human capital is also a key factor in innovation, and the skills necessary for innovation, such as creativity, team working and cognitive skills, are increasingly important.

MIDWIFERY EDUCATION

In midwifery education, innovations in facilitating learning are vital so that midwifery curricula can be exciting and interesting to engage students and maximize their learning, such as including art and drama to explore theory and practice (see Chapter 11) as well as keeping up with the increasing demands and change within the maternity services. With the advancements in telecommunications, various educational technologies have been incorporated into midwifery education. An example of this was reported by Carr (2003), where midwifery educators within the American College of Nurse-Midwives have continued to innovate with distance-learning and Web-enhanced curricula to increase access to midwifery education and degree programmes. Marshall (2012) developed a ground-breaking, work-based learning/distance learning module that introduced authentic assessment within a degree pathway for practising midwives where the

CASE STUDY 14.1 | **Innovation in Midwifery Education**

INTRODUCING SERVICE USERS IN MULTIPLE MINI INTERVIEWING WITHIN MIDWIFERY EDUCATION

The emphasis on the inclusion of patients and the public in the design and delivery of health care is an international phenomenon (Davis and McIntosh 2005; Brown and Macintosh 2006). In the United Kingdom specifically, there have been several drivers that have placed patients/service users and the public at the centre of the design and delivery of services (e.g. Department of Health 1999, 2016; General Medical Council 2009, 2011; Chambers and Hickey 2012; Nursing and Midwifery Council 2018).

In the Department of Midwifery at Kingston University and St George's, University of London, the admissions tutors wanted to embed maternity service user involvement in the selection and recruitment of student midwives.

Support was obtained from the Head of Midwifery Education and the faculty's Centre for Public Engagement. The local *Healthwatch* charities were contacted to ascertain interest and recruit service users. A number of small focus groups with interested childbearing women were convened to explore their expectations and involvement and revise existing scenarios and develop additional scenarios to be used in the multiple mini interview process. These service users were invited to attend the interview days to observe the process, before participating in the process themselves.

The change in interviewing process was introduced gradually to department and administrative staff through a series of team meetings to ensure they were clear about the purpose of the change and the role of the service users, including the training they required. Following evaluation of service user involvement, this innovation is now embedded in the midwifery curricula and has influenced a change in other health and social care programmes throughout the faculty.

students undertook project work. The students' innovative projects included the development of clinical guidelines, the development of teaching packages for staff and students, virtual maternity unit tours for parents and the development information of booklets/leaflets for parents and health professionals, all of which contributed to bringing about positive change in their workplace, which was reward in itself for the midwives.

Innovations and creativity in midwifery education must continue so as to prepare midwives for their future practice and should be developed in partnership with service providers and service users. Case Study 14.1 shows one such innovation, which involves services users in the selection and recruitment of future midwives. Furthermore, including opportunities within the midwifery curricula for students to undertake project work that involves creativity in designing an innovation to influence change in an aspect of practice should be considered as a means of inspiring confidence to effect change in their future midwifery careers.

MIDWIFERY PRACTICE

In 2012, the Royal College of Midwives produced the guide *Innovation and Improvement in Maternity Services* in association with the Involvement and Participation Association (Royal College of Midwives and Involvement and Participation Association 2012). This guide provides examples of ways in which midwives have taken the lead within maternity services and through innovations have made improvements to the care that women and their families receive, within specific budgets or even generating efficiency savings. The Involvement and Participation Association selected the following case studies: *the South Central Strategic Health Authority maternity network, productive maternity at Nottingham, maternity support worker apprenticeships at Basildon,* and *modernising maternity at East Cheshire NHS Trust.* These case studies are all quite different in terms of scale, objectives and methods. They all demonstrate that it *is* possible to develop new and more effective ways of working, and in doing so to improve maternity outcomes and women's experience of care.

Innovations in Midwifery Practice

PREGNANCY APPS

The Department of Health (2016) National Maternity Review advocated that National Health Service providers should invest in technological solutions that include all women having access to a comprehensive digital tool that provides them with all the information they require throughout pregnancy and childbirth. Such a digital tool has much greater value if it enables the personalization of information, and therefore should provide an interface with the woman's electronic maternity record so that she can access her own record and receive information that is tailored to her needs.

A number of websites and apps have been developed by public, private and third-sector organizations to help women manage their pregnancy and childcare, such as *Baby Buddy* by the charity Best Beginnings and *Pocket Midwife* by midwives in Nottingham.

NORTH BRISTOL NHS TRUST: PROMPT – A FRAMEWORK FOR MULTIPROFESSIONAL LEARNING

The maternity team at Southmead Hospital in Bristol initiated by an obstetrician and midwife, have designed an evidence-based multiprofessional training programme (*PRactical Obstetric Multi-Professional Training, PROMPT*) to improve outcomes for women and babies. The training takes place locally in clinical areas and a homebirth setting and is attended annually by all maternity staff: midwives, maternity theatre staff, maternity support workers, obstetricians and anaesthetists.

Using practice-based tools, workshops and emergency drills with simple props, high-fidelity mannequins and service user actors, PROMPT aims to optimize management of maternity emergencies. Since the implementation of PROMPT at Southmead, there have been significant improvements in birth outcomes, such as a 70% reduction in brachial plexus injuries, a 50% reduction in encephalopathy and a 50% reduction in the time taken to expedite birth in potentially life-threatening cases of umbilical cord prolapse and a significant reduction in litigation claims (Draycott 2013). PROMPT is now used throughout the United Kingdom and has been introduced in other countries – including Australia, New Zealand, Zimbabwe, Hong Kong, China, the United States of America, Mongolia and Singapore – with similar improvements in perinatal outcomes.

In 2016, NHS England introduced the framework *Leading Change, Adding Value* that enables all nursing, midwifery and care staff to lead change and add value, wherever they work, whatever their role (NHS England 2016). To reduce unwarranted variation and improve outcomes for individuals and populations, nursing, midwifery and care staff all have a vital role in leading change, no matter how big or small. Case Study 14.2 provides examples of some of the innovations that midwives have developed and successfully implemented in practice. Now undertake Activity 14.3.

ACTIVITY 14.3 ■

Consider an innovation or change you would like to make in midwifery education or midwifery practice.
- Identify the key players, their relationship and their anticipated reaction to your innovation or change.
- Identity the primary aim/rationale for implementing the innovation or change and identify a valid measure of success.
- Identify any constraints related to the development and implementation of the innovation or change.

Develop what you have identified by conducting further environmental tests using tools such as force field analysis, PEST analysis or SWOT analysis to identify where your energies would need to be specifically focused to ensure the successful implementation of your innovation or change. Briefly detail how you would proceed.
- Who would be involved?
- How will your innovation/change be evaluated?

Entrepreneurship in Midwifery

Entrepreneurship is the process by which either an individual or a team identifies a business opportunity and acquires and deploys the necessary resources required for its exploitation: shifting economic resources out of an area of lower productivity into an area of higher productivity and greater yield. Consequently, entrepreneurs create something new, something different and change or transform values (Drucker 1993). To become an entrepreneur, Shane (2003) identifies the following four criteria:

1. There must be opportunities/situations to recombine resources to generate profit.
2. Entrepreneurship requires differences between people, such as the ability to recognize information about opportunities.
3. Taking on risk is necessary.
4. The entrepreneurship process requires the organization of people and resources.

An *entrepreneur* is a person who is willing and able to convert a new idea or invention into a successful innovation. The role of the entrepreneur in the economy has been viewed as *creative destruction*: launching innovations that simultaneously destroy old industries while ushering in new industries and approaches. However, such *dynamic disequilibrium* brought on by the entrepreneur has been viewed as the norm of a healthy economy (Schumpeter 1950). Entrepreneurs generally have strong beliefs about market opportunities and willingly accept a high level of personal, professional and financial risk. They possess different characteristics that provide a skill set for achieving success and a high level of reward. Such characteristics associated with entrepreneurs include:

- independence
- self-discipline
- persistence
- creativity
- hard working
- motivation
- confidence
- willingness to take risks
- good communication skills.

Becoming an entrepreneur can be an option for midwives who identify a need and create a service/product to meet that need. Midwife entrepreneurs enjoy the autonomy derived from operating their own maternity business. There is global evidence of midwives who have been bold enough to take up the challenge and create their own business or community-based social enterprises to provide individualized continuity-of-care packages to childbearing women, as shown in Case Study 14.3. A social enterprise is a business where society benefits from any profits made and where the entrepreneurs are self-employed. Other midwives own and operate their own publishing company, management consultancies, etc.

As with any endeavour, there can be disadvantages with running a small business, such as losing the financial investment if the business is unsuccessful. In particular, there can be fluctuations in income in the early days, and there can be great pressure in meeting deadlines and paying bills, taxes and salaries or wages, but there are also great opportunities (Tiran 2018). The intangible rewards such as the autonomy and freedom to be in control of their own practice for some is incentive enough to compensate for the increased pressure and initial uncertainty.

| CASE STUDY 14.3 | **Social Enterprise in Midwifery** |

INTERNATIONAL NURSING AND MIDWIFERY SOCIAL ENTERPRISES (NMEs)

These are community-level health services delivered through provider practices owned and/or operated by nurses and midwives, often working in collaboration with community health workers and other predominately female frontline workers. Examples of NMEs can be found in countries across income levels, one example being *Jacaranda Health*, which is a social venture combining business and clinical innovations that targets women living in periurban areas in Nairobi, Kenya. It provides high-quality, friendly and affordable maternal care through a set of self-sustaining and scalable clinics. The programme has a dual focus of addressing the needs of the women it serves and improving the standard of care.

NMEs have various corporate structures, including both for profit and not for profit, and often serve remote or underserved populations. Payment for services differs, including contracting with governments for service delivery, insurance or self-pay arrangements. NMEs are often organized through cooperatives, networks or franchises, as well as individual, free-standing arrangements. Many NMEs have characteristics that are well aligned with empowerment of women that extend beyond service delivery.

ONE TO ONE MIDWIVES

One to One Midwives was founded by a midwife and is a social enterprise community caseloading midwifery service, commissioned by the National Health Service (NHS) in six areas of the United Kingdom. One to One Midwives provides a *free* personalized service that places women and their families at the heart and is delivered by teams of passionate, highly motivated midwives who are experts in all aspects of midwifery-led care. The midwives work in partnership with multiple organizations, including GPs and the local hospitals, should women require specialist input from other services, such as an obstetrician or a neonatologist. The service does not replace local National Health Service services but complements local provision by offering women a choice with an alternative model of community midwifery care. Consequently, most women receive care from their dedicated midwife for more than 90% of their care package.

One to One Midwives has professional indemnity insurance through the Clinical Negligence Scheme for Trusts and is regulated by the Care Quality Commission.

To date, One to One Midwives has achieved safe, excellent outcomes evidenced by the high normal birth rate, low caesarean section rate, low premature birth rate and low neonatal admission rate. Women rate the service very highly, and some have provided birth stories on the One to One Midwives website.

Conclusion

Change is a constant factor in life and can proceed at a fast pace. Such immense change can in fact provide great opportunities for midwives who are creative and have initiative and business savvy to influence future practice. It is vital that midwifery education and practice respond to changes that occur in the profession and the maternity services worldwide and incorporate them in the education of the future midwife and the care childbearing women and their babies and families receive. Furthermore, an understanding of organizational culture and change management theory should be a key component in pre-registration midwifery curricula to ensure that midwives continue to drive innovations and change within the profession. The chapter has presented a number of key frameworks that midwives can use when considering implementing an innovation or change in practice. Examples of successful innovations, entrepreneurship and social enterprise schemes where midwives have been the spearhead have been presented to inspire midwives to consider becoming a change agent. However, to effect change, the midwife change agent needs to have confidence and have the support of colleagues and the organization.

KEY POINTS

- Midwives are at the heart of midwifery practice, and it is essential they possess the knowledge and understanding of change theory to influence advancements in practice, based on the best available evidence.
- Change management theory should be a key feature within all midwifery curricula to provide students with the foundation upon which to build confidence and influence developments within their subsequent midwifery career.
- Midwives should be cognizant of the culture of the organization in which they work to appreciate how this may impact on the implementation of innovation and change.
- The use of frameworks that include change management models and tools supports a logical planning, development and implementation process for the change or innovation that is more likely to be successful.
- An effective change agent is one with purpose and vision, the ability to manage people through difficult situations, the ability to take accountability and responsibility and the ability to motivate people to achieve respective goals.
- As a result of the rapid changes occurring in the maternity services, there are new and exciting opportunities for midwives who possess creativity, initiative and business savvy to exploit these opportunities and become innovative entrepreneurs.
- Becoming an entrepreneur and running their own business or social enterprise can be an option for midwives, but because of the potential risks, many are reluctant to make such a choice.

References

Balfour, M., & Clarke, C. (2001). Searching for sustainable change. *Journal of Clinical Nursing, 10*(1), 44–50.

Barr, J., & Dowding, L. (2012). *Leadership in health care*. London: Sage Publications.

Brown, I., & Macintosh, M. J. (2006). Involving patients with coronary heart disease in developing e-learning assets for primary care nurses. *Nurse Education in Practice, 6*(4), 237–242.

Burns, J. M. (1978). *Leadership*. New York: Harper Row.

Carnell, C. A. (2003). *Managing change in organizations*. Harlow: Pearson Education.

Carr, K. C. (2003). Innovations in midwifery education. *Journal of Midwifery and Women's Health, 48*(6), 393–397.

Chambers, M., & Hickey, G. (2012). *Service user involvement in the design and delivery of education and training programmes leading to registration with the Health Professions Council*. Available at: https://www.hcpc-uk.org/globalassets/resources/reports/service-user-involvement-in-the-design-and-delivery-of-education-and-training-programmes.pdf.

Coram, R., & Burnes, B. (2001). Managing organisational change in the public sector: Lessons from the privatisation of the Property Service Agency. *International Journal of Public Sector Management, 14*(2), 94–110.

Davis, D., & McIntosh, C. (2005). Partnership in education: The involvement of service users in one midwifery programme in New Zealand. *Nurse Education in Practice, 5*(5), 274–280.

Department of Health. (1993). *Changing childbirth: Report of the Expert Maternity Group*. London: HMSO.

Department of Health. (1999). *Patient and public involvement in the new NHS*. London: The Stationery Office.

Department of Health. (2016). Better births: Improving outcomes of maternity services in England. A five year forward review for maternity care. Available at: https://www.england.nhs.uk/wp-content/uploads/2016/02/national-maternity-review-report.pdf.

Department of Health and Social Care. (2015). *2010 to 2015 Government Policy: Compassionate Care in the NHS*. London: HMSO. Available at: https://www.gov.uk/government/publications/2010-to-2015-government-policy-compassionate-care-in-the-nhs/2010-to-2015-government-policy-compassionate-care-in-the-nhs.

Draycott, T. (2013). *Practical Obstetric Multi-Professional Training –PROMPT*. Bristol: The Health Foundation.

Drucker, P. F. (1993). *Innovation and entrepreneurship: Practice and principles*. New York: HarperBusiness.

Einion, A. (2017). The medicalization of childbirth. In Squire, C., (Ed.), *The Social Context of Birth* (3rd ed.). Abingdon: CRC Press.

Francis, R. (2013). *Report of the Mid Staffordshire NHS Foundation Trust Public Inquiry*. London: The Stationery Office. Available at: https://www.gov.uk/government/publications/report-of-the-mid-staffordshire-nhs-foundation-trust-public-inquiry.

General Medical Council. (2009). *Tomorrows doctors: Outcomes and standards for undergraduate medical education*. London: General Medical Council.

General Medical Council. (2011). *Patient and public involvement in undergraduate medical education advice supplementary to tomorrow's doctors (2009)*. London: General Medical Council.

Handy, C. (2009). *Gods of management: The changing work of organisations*. London: Souvenir.

Hayes, J. (2018). *The theory and practice of change management* (5th ed.). London: Palgrave Macmillan.

Health Education England. (2016). *Values based recruitment*. London: Health Education England. Available at: https://www.hee.nhs.uk/our-work/values-based-recruitment.

Heery, E., & Nitton, M. (2017). *A dictionary of human resource management* (3rd ed.). Oxford: Oxford University Press. Available at. http://www.oxfordreference.com/view/10.1093/acref/9780191827822.001.0001/acref-9780191827822.

Hughes, M. (2010). *Managing change: A critical perspective*. London: Chartered Institute of Personnel and Development.

Kirkup, B. (2015). *The Report of the Morecambe Bay Investigation*. Preston: The Stationery Office. Available at: https://www.gov.uk/government/uploads/system/uploads/attachment_data/file/408480/47487_MBI_Accessible_v0.1.pdf.

Knight, M., Bunch, K., Tufnell, D., Jayakody, H., Shakespeare, J., Kotnis, R., Kenyon, S., & Kurinczuk, J. J., (Eds) on behalf of MBRRACE-UK. (2018). *Saving Lives, Improving Mothers' Care- Lessons learned to inform maternity care from the UK and Ireland Confidential Enquiries into Maternal Deaths and Morbidity 2014-16*. Oxford: National Perinatal Epidemiology Unit, University of Oxford.

Kotter, J. P. (1996). *Leading change*. Boston: Harvard Business School Press.

Lewin, K. (1947). Frontiers in group dynamics. In Cartwright, D., (Ed.), *Field theory in social science*. London: Social Science Paperbacks.

Lewin, K. (1951). *Field theory in social science*. New York: Harper and Row.

Lippit, R., & Lippit, G. (1975). Consulting process in action. *Training and Development Journal, 29*(5), 48–54 29(6), 38–44.

Luecke, R. (2003). *Managing change and transition: Harvard business essentials* (Vol. 3). Boston: Harvard Business School Publishing.

Lunenburg, F. C. (2010). Managing change: the role of the change agent. *International Journal of Management, Business and Administration, 13*(1), 1–6.

Margulies, N., & Raia, A. (1978). *Conceptual foundations of organizational development*. New York: McGraw–Hill.

Marrow, A. J. (1969). *The practical theorist: The life and work of Kurt Lewin*. New York: Teachers' College Press.

Marshall, J. E. (2012). Developing midwifery practice through work-based learning: an exploratory study. *Nurse Education in Practice, 12*(5), 273–278.

McCalman, J., Paton, R., & Siebert, S. (2016). *Change management: A guide to effective implementation* (4th ed.). London: Sage Publications.

NHS England. (2016). *Leading change, adding value: A framework for nursing, midwifery and care staff*. London: NHS England. Available at: https://www.england.nhs.uk/wp-content/uploads/2016/05/nursing-framework.pdf.

NHS Institute for Innovation and Improvement. (2008). *The handbook of quality and service improvement tools*. Available at: http://webarchive.nationalarchives.gov.uk/20160805122939/http://www.nhsiq.nhs.uk/media/2760650/the_handbook_of_quality_and_service_improvement_tools_2010.pdf.

Nursing and Midwifery Council. (2018). *Quality assurance framework for nursing, midwifery and nursing associate education*. London: Nursing and Midwifery Council. Available at: https://www.nmc.org.uk/globalassets/sitedocuments/edandqa/nmc-quality-assurance-framework.pdf.

Panagiotou, G. (2003). Bringing SWOT into focus. *Business Strategy Review, 14*(2), 8–10.

Renfrew, M. J., Homer, C. S. E., Downe, S., McFadden, A., Muir, N., Prentice, T., et al. (2014). *Midwifery: An executive summary for the lancet series*. Available at: http://www.thelancet.com/series/midwifery.

Robbins, S. P., Judge, T. A., & Campbell, T. T. (2010). *Organizational Behaviour*. Harlow: Pearson Education.

Royal College of Midwives. (2016). *Why midwives leave revisited.* London: Royal College of Midwives. Available at: https://www.rcm.org.uk/sites/default/files/Why%20Midwives%20Leave%20Revisted%20 -%20October%202016.pdf.

Royal College of Midwives & Involvement and Participation Association. (2012). *Innovation and improve- ment in maternity services.* London: Royal College of Midwives and Involvement and Participation Asso- ciation. Available at: https://www.rcm.org.uk/sites/default/files/Innovation%20and%20Improvement%20 in%20Midwifery.pdf.

Scamell, M. (2011). The swan effect in midwifery talk and practice: a tension between normality and the language of risk. *Social Health and Illness, 33*(7), 987–1001.

Schumpeter, J. A. (1950). *Capitalism, socialism and democracy* (3rd ed.). New York: Harper and Row.

Scottish Government. (2014). *Setting the direction for nursing and midwifery education in Scotland. The strategic aims from the chief nursing officer's education review.* Edinburgh: Scottish Government. Available at: http:// www.gov.scot/Publications/2014/02/4112/downloads.

Shane, S. A. (2003). *A general theory of entrepreneurship: The individual-opportunity nexus.* Northampton: E. Elgar.

Steiner, C. (2001). A role for individuality and mystery in managing change. *Journal of Organizational Change Management, 14,* 150–167.

Stogdill, R. (1974). *Handbook of Leadership.* New York: Free Press.

Tearle, R. (2007). The role of a change master. Available at: https://changedesignsportal.worldsecuresystems. com/public/organisation/change/Roles-in-change-management.html.

Tinsley, V. (2005). Making management decisions. In Raynor, M. D., Marshall, J. E., & Sullivan, A., (Eds.), *Decision making in midwifery practice* (pp. 113–126). Edinburgh: Churchill Livingstone.

Tiran, D. (2018). *The business of maternity care: A guide for midwives and doulas setting up private prac- tice.* London: Singing Dragon.

van der Heijden, H. R. M. A., Geldens, J. J. M., Beijaard, D., & Popeijus, H. L. (2015). Characteristics of teachers as change agents. *Teachers and teaching: Theory and practice, 21*(6), 681–699.

Further Reading

Hayes, J. (2018). *The theory and practice of change management* (5th ed.). London: Palgrave Macmillan.

This bestselling textbook, now in its fifth edition, provides the reader with all the skills they will need to success- fully identify the need for change and implement change. It covers all the key theories, tools and techniques for or- ganizational change and includes examples based on real-life organizations and video interviews with experienced change practitioners, case studies and change tools for the reader to apply the theory to authentic scenarios.

McCalman, J., Paton, R., & Siebert, S. (2016). *Change management: A guide to effective implementation* (4th ed.). London: Sage Publications.

This revised text guides readers through the technological, organizational and human-oriented strategies that managers use to implement change, including International and cross-cultural case studies. Frameworks for apply- ing different models of change to various scenarios assist the reader to place change management theory in context and gain a greater understanding of how to best effect change..

Tiran, D. (2018). *The business of maternity care: A guide for midwives and doulas setting up private practice.* London: Singing Dragon.

This book guides the reader through the process and challenges of establishing themselves in a maternity-related busi- ness. The content covers the legal, and financial aspects of setting up a business including marketing and pricing. There is debate around the professional, legal and ethical issues for midwives and doulas with an interesting section on avoiding conflicts and maintaining professional integrity. Throughout the book are activities and exercises for the reader to complete with real-life case studies of successful business to help place the detail in context.

Useful Websites

American College of Nurse Midwives: http://www.midwife.org
General Medical Council: https://www.gmc-uk.org
Health and Care Professions Council: https://www.hcpc-uk.org/
Jacaranda Health Kenya: https://healthmarketinnovations.org/program/jacaranda-health
NHS England: https://www.england.nhs.uk

NHS England Sustainable Improvement Team: https://www.england.nhs.uk/sustainableimprovement (replaced NHS Improving Quality in 2016, which had replaced the earlier NHS Institute for Innovation and Improvements in 2013)

Nursing and Midwifery Council: https://www.nmc.org.uk

One to One Midwives: http://www.onetoonemidwives.org

Royal College of Midwives: https://www.rcm.org.uk

CHAPTER 15

Continuing Professional Development and Midwifery Career Pathways

Jayne E. Marshall ▪ Michelle Knight ▪ Lynne Cornford-Wood

CONTENTS

LEARNING OUTCOMES

By the end of this chapter the reader will be able to:

- appreciate the importance of continuing professional development and the concept of lifelong learning
- determine their professional education and development needs and consider how these might be met
- use a framework with which to guide their future career pathway
- understand the requirements of professional regulation and the process of revalidation.

Overview

This chapter explores a range of continuing professional development (CPD) opportunities that can assist in framing a newly qualified midwife's career trajectory. The National Health Service (NHS) Career Framework and the NHS Knowledge and Skills Framework (Department of Health [DH] 2004) provides direction and guidance that midwives can use when contemplating their CPD. The discussion extends beyond the clinical area into developing a career in midwifery education, leadership and research as it is vital that *all* areas of the midwifery profession continue to flourish, with midwives always at the helm. Included is the Circle of Care Career Midwifery Development Pathway (Courtesy Michelle Knight), which can support a midwife's professional development and be used in discussion with their line manager/employer at the annual appraisal. This model can also complement the revalidation process that each midwife must to undergo to renew their registration every 3 years. Opportunities for midwives to work overseas and further advance their own development as well as contribute to improving the health and well-being of others, particularly in low- and middle-income countries (LMICs), are also explored. Within the chapter there are activities for the reader to engage with as well as a comprehensive reference list, annotated further reading and appropriate website links to encourage further enquiry and study.

Introduction

As presented in other chapters, the International Confederation of Midwives (ICM) *Global Standards for Midwifery Education* (ICM 2013) were developed as a consistent approach to strengthen midwifery within the global context by preparing fully qualified midwives to provide childbearing women, their babies and their families with high-quality, evidence-based health care. These standards represent the *minimum* expected from a quality midwifery programme that focuses on *competency*-based education rather than high academic attainment, such as degrees, and is detailed in *Essential Competencies for Basic Midwifery Practice* (ICM 2018). The minimum academic level of pre-registration midwifery education programmes in the United Kingdom (UK) has been degree level since 2008 (Nursing and Midwifery Council [NMC] 2007). It is also expected that all midwifery education programmes should comply with the standards for pre-registration midwifery education endorsed by the recognized professional and statutory regulatory body (PSRB) of the country in which the programme is undertaken, which should be guided by the international definition of the midwife (ICM 2017). Furthermore, midwives educated within the European Union are required to fulfil the training requirements of the Professional Qualifications Directive (2005/36/EC; amended by Directive 2013/55/EU), which under European Union Law determine the theoretical and clinical components and the professional activities that each student midwife should undertake during their programme of study.

In the UK, once a student midwife has successfully completed the requirements of a pre-registration midwifery education programme as laid down by the NMC and has been confirmed as being of good character and good health, they are then eligible to apply for entry to the midwives' part of the professional register, for which they are required to pay a registration fee. They will then acquire a unique personal identification number that corresponds to their entry on the professional register and to which they should refer whenever they contact the NMC or provide it to women for authenticity if they are working independently/self-employed. Following initial registration, the midwife has to pay a retention fee to the NMC each year, and every third year has to comply with the requirements of the revalidation process (NMC 2019). At the point of registration, the knowledge, skills and professional attitude that a midwife has acquired during their pre-registration education programme need to continue to support lifelong learning, CPD, including career advancement, and the NMC's revalidation process. Registration should be viewed as the beginning of more meaningful learning, when things learned in the pre-registration period fall into place.

Lifelong Learning and Continuing Professional Development

Lifelong learning is about creating and maintaining a positive attitude to learning for both personal and professional development. Lifelong learners are motivated to assimilate knowledge and develop because they have the desire to: it is therefore a deliberate and voluntary act. From the point of registration, all midwifery registrants embark on a journey of lifelong learning. Lifelong learning is the process and provision of both formal and informal learning opportunities throughout a midwife's life and career that nurtures the continuous development and improvement of the knowledge and skills required for employment and personal fulfilment. However, the organization in which a midwife practises should be creative and encouraging towards learning, whereby positive events and any errors are reflected on in order to provide high-quality care to women, their babies and their families.

The Code (NMC 2018) upholds the notion of lifelong learning, with the responsibility lying with the individual registrant. It is essential that midwives continually keep up to date with changes in the maternity services and develop their knowledge and skills accordingly so they are able to deliver safe, competent and effective care. The concept of CPD contributes to upholding public safety, the maintenance of clinical competence and compliance with professional registration requirements (Munro 2008). The focus is on the individual as a professional, developing differing job profiles and career pathways, as well as the organization. Figure 15.1 provides an overview of the range of CPD activities available to midwives.

In recent years there has been an increase in mandatory *in-house* training required for midwives to keep pace with the complexities associated with maternal and neonatal health and well-being as well as technological advances in reproductive health. Furthermore, the reductions in funding to universities to facilitate CPD activities for NHS employees and the challenges midwives may face in acquiring study leave from the workplace to attend courses have called for a rethink in the way lifelong learning should be accessed and delivered. Consequently, and by exploitation

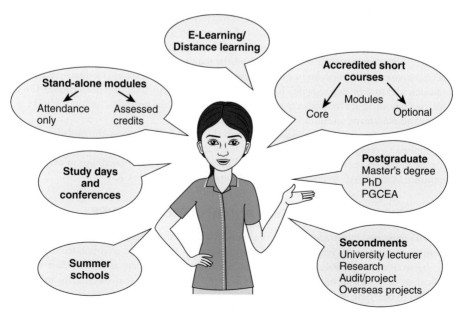

Fig. 15.1 The range of continuing professional development activities.

of the advances in digital technology, there has been an increase in e-learning, such as through the i-Learn platform of the Royal College of Midwives (RCM) and through the Mum and Baby Academy, part of the Health Professional Academy.

Professional Revalidation

The process of revalidation has developed from the principles established by the postregistration education and practice standards (NMC 2011) and has been effective since April 2016. Revalidation has replaced the postregistration education and practice standards and the annual meeting with the supervisor of midwives, following the disestablishment of statutory supervision in 2017, where midwives were accustomed to discuss their practice and CPD needs, including their own practice development plans. Professional revalidation is a process which all midwives and nurses must complete every 3 years to maintain their registration with the NMC (NMC 2019). It embraces the principles of *The Code* (NMC 2018) as the guide for registrants to reflect on and demonstrate that their practice is up to date, safe and effective. Failure to comply with the triennial revalidation requirement will result in a midwife or nurse being removed from the register.

The NMC (2019) requirements for revalidation include:

- 450 practice hours (or 900 practice hours if the registrant is renewing as both a midwife and nurse)
- 35 hours of CPD, including 20 hours of participatory learning
- five pieces of practice-related feedback
- five written reflective accounts
- reflective discussion with a fellow registrant
- health and character declaration
- professional indemnity arrangement
- confirmation.

The revalidation process does not assess a registrant's fitness to practise as its purpose is to ensure midwives and nurses are conversant with *The Code* (NMC 2018) and ultimately raise professional standards. It is also worth noting that revalidation is for *all* midwives, not just those working in clinical practice. Those midwives who are in leadership, education or research roles are legitimately practising midwifery in their respective fields and are also registered with and regulated by the NMC. In these situations, *peer review* with a fellow registrant rather than *clinical supervision* is the more appropriate means for them to meet the requirements of revalidation. The midwife is expected to maintain a portfolio of evidence (see Chapter 5), which should be discussed with the confirmer, who may be the midwife's line manager or another registrant (but not a friend). On the NMC website there are templates that can be used to format the portfolio, such as a CPD log, a reflective account form, a feedback log and a practice hours log.

As there is some degree of self-certification in the revalidation process, the midwife is therefore required to provide an honest account of their activities in practice. Failure to do so would place the midwife's registration at risk. A small number of registrant's portfolios of evidence are scrutinized by the NMC to ensure quality and consistency across the UK.

PROFESSIONAL REVALIDATION AND STUDENT MIDWIVES

All nurses registered in the adult field who are undertaking a shortened pre-registration midwifery education programme are responsible for ensuring they pay their annual retention fee to maintain their registration during their studies. For a proportion of these student midwives, their triennial revalidation may also fall within this time. It is therefore important that the student midwife is supported to complete the process successfully by their personal tutor/academic assessor and midwife mentor/practice supervisor (both of whom could act as the student's *registrant confirmer*).

However, at this stage, the evidence should reflect only *nursing* activities as this is the part of the register on which the student midwife is registered and for which they will be undertaking the re-validation process.

Now undertake Activity 15.1.

ACTIVITY 15.1 ∎

- What are the three main goals you wish to achieve in the first year of employment as a midwife?
- How can your preceptor help you in your new role to achieve them?
- In what ways will you use these experiences to guide your continuing professional development and the triennial revalidation process?

Midwifery Career Pathways

Recruitment of newly qualified midwives is facilitated in the UK through NHS trust processes and procedures. The NHS is usually the first employing organization for each midwife beginning their midwifery career, and it is important for them to be prepared for this process. The unique partnership between the university and its NHS practice partners ensures that student midwives are not only ready for registration but are also fully equipped for a career in midwifery as lifelong learners. It is good practice to include opportunities for student midwives to practise interview techniques and develop skill and confidence within their education programme in readiness for their employment interviews. Furthermore, their understanding of and commitment to the philosophy of lifelong learning should be explored at interview when long-term career aspirations are discussed. Many student midwives may have considered their own midwifery career pathway as early as their third year during their education programme, with some developing an interest for a particular specialist role (e.g. perinatal mental health, breastfeeding, teenage pregnancy) and which subsequently can lead and transform a midwife's career over time.

KNIGHT'S CIRCLE OF CARE MIDWIFERY CAREER DEVELOPMENT PATHWAY

Developed by a clinical midwife, the Circle of Care Midwifery Development Pathway can be used to support midwives in directing the annual appraisal process, preparing them for the triennial revalidation process and in guiding them in actualizing their career aspirations by following a specific pathway (Fig. 15.2). Midwives should be nurtured through this process, and the idea of their pathway being embedded within a *circle of care* with support at every stage (depicted by the embracing arms of the arrows), be it in clinical practice, management, education or research, is paramount. Construction of a personal/practice development plan that identifies where additional knowledge and skills are required to achieve their career goals is a useful exercise for midwives to undertake.

CLINICAL MIDWIFERY CAREER PATHWAYS

In the UK, the NHS Career Framework has been designed to improve career development and job satisfaction for NHS employees and encourages individuals to learn new skills and take on responsibilities that enable them to progress within the organization. It is based on an *outcomes approach* to competence that is favoured by *Skills for Health* and the NHS Knowledge and Skills Framework (DH 2004). Midwives are placed within a nine-band pay structure through

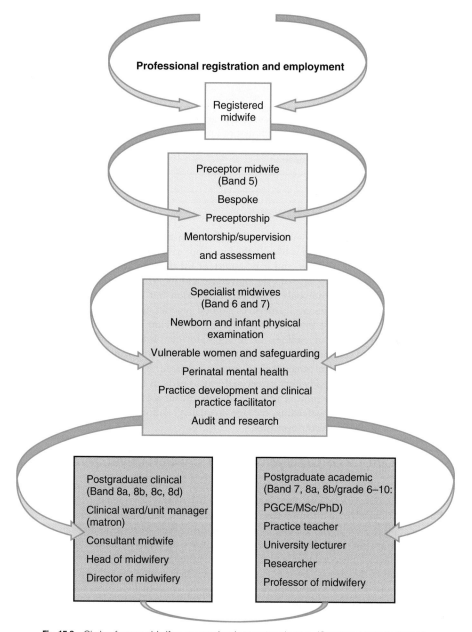

Fig. 15.2 Circle of care: midwifery career development pathways. (Courtesy Michelle Knight).

the *Agenda for Change* (AfC) system that reflects the level of knowledge and skills they have acquired and are working towards within their career trajectory. This pay system is designed to deliver fair pay for non-medical staff on the basis of the principle of equal pay for work of equal value and to provide better links between pay and career progression using the Knowledge and Skills Framework (DH 2004).

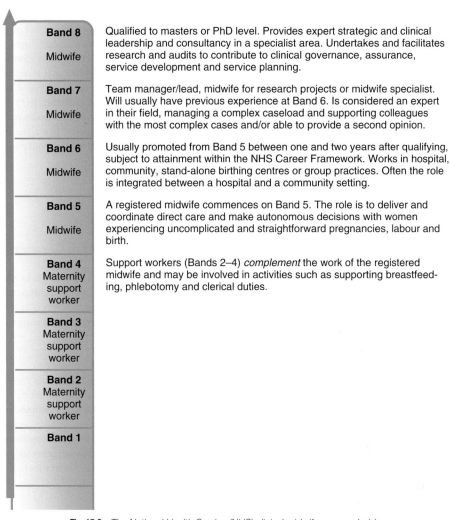

Fig. 15.3   The National Health Service (NHS) clinical midwifery career ladder.

Each band of the career ladder represents an expected set of competencies in the domains of clinical leadership, management, education and practice (Fig. 15.3). Movement up the career ladder is merit based and is dependent on the midwife being able to show that they have the required knowledge, skills and attitudes. So, for example, if two midwives applied for a Band 6 role, it would be offered to the one who can demonstrate that they have the required competencies – knowledge, skills and attitudes – regardless of age or years of service, which could mean a younger midwife may be employed in a more senior position than an older midwife. The following sections discuss these career pathways for midwives with reference to the AfC banding structure and the requirements to reach the next gateway to the following band.

Agenda for Change: Band 5 Midwives

A robust preceptorship programme offers the newly qualified midwife a layer of support and protection in the transition from student midwife to practising midwife, and is fundamentally important for consolidating knowledge and skills as well as empowering the midwife with confidence. Each newly qualified midwife should be assigned an experienced midwife known as a *preceptor* (see Chapter 11) to help them in this process and further develop competence in additional skills that expand their scope of practice (see Chapter 8) by planning a programme pertinent to their needs. Depending on the midwife's contractual working hours, the preceptorship programme may last from 12 to 18 months. The range of competencies a midwife would be expected to acquire to succeed in moving through the gateway to Band 6 can differ according to NHS Trust policy and clinical context, but may consist of:

- intravenous cannulation
- intravenous injection administration
- perineal suturing
- epidural analgesia/care (top-ups and patient-controlled analgesia pumps)
- water births
- operating department scrubbing skills (in settings where midwives scrub for caesarean sections)

The completion of the preceptorship programme is a precursor for the midwife to move to the second gateway – Band 6 – by which time they would be expected to be acquiring more advanced competencies. It is essential that the midwife is not only competent in the clinical aspects of the role but also has the professional qualities, accountability and frontline managerial skills required that are associated with the role.

Agenda for Change: Band 6 Midwives

Most midwives develop their careers through a clinical route. As midwives move up the career ladder, they take on more specialist roles, for example promoting physiological birth working in midwife-led settings or in high-dependency care practising in high-risk labour ward settings. In most cases, these midwives will have undergone additional education and training to take on the specialist advisory roles in areas where there are specific health needs, such as smoking cessation, teenage pregnancies, substance misuse and diabetes. Although most specialist midwives are working at Band 6, a small number practise at Band 7. The range of competencies for Band 6 may include:

- mentorship/supervision and assessment
- newborn and infant physical examination
- high-dependency care
- leadership.

The accomplishment of reaching AfC Band 6 is where the pathway for some midwives ends. However, many midwives consider undertaking further practice and educational development to gain experience and acquire specialist skills that subsequently develop into specialist roles. Band 6 midwives would usually be educated to degree level (academic level 6), with some having achieved a master's degree or can provide evidence that they have studied at academic level 7.

CLINICAL MIDWIFERY LEADERSHIP AND MANAGEMENT CAREER PATHWAYS

Midwives may develop their careers through a management route and gain the position of birth centre manager or ward manager. They could be promoted to the role of matron, with management responsibility for hospital services or community services. The Head/Director of Midwifery has responsibility for maternity services in the entire locality of an NHS Trust, which will incorporate hospital and community maternity care and may cover a considerable geographical area.

Specific managerial competencies using the Knowledge and Skills Framework (DH 2004) criteria help clinicians to focus on developing clear mentorship skills and knowledge to a more advanced level of competence in preparation for progression from Band 6 to Band 7. Specialist degrees and master-level education also incorporate fundamental competencies to enable midwives to follow career pathways (e.g. public health, management and business administration). The AfC pay bands detail clear expectations and components that midwives must demonstrate within a clinical management and leadership framework, such as time management and the ability to work autonomously and cooperatively whilst managing others efficiently.

Agenda for Change: Band 7 Midwives

The value of supporting midwives to undertake leadership and managerial programmes is to equip them with the organizational, financial, educational and team-building skills within a culture of sound practice development and subsequently progress to Band 7 and more dedicated specialist roles, such as:

- leadership and management (people management)
- labour ward coordinating role
- specific specialist roles (e.g. perinatal mental health, female genital mutilation)
- team leadership in community, antenatal and postnatal care (matron)
- clinical specialist, practice development, clinical governance and risk management.

Agenda for Change: Band 8 Midwives

Senior managerial roles, namely Band 8a and 8b roles, encompass a range of interpersonal skills and personal attributes that include advanced leadership, people management, organizational planning and development of a strategic philosophy. The Knowledge and Skills Framework (DH 2004) details that Bands 8a, 8b, 8c and 8d staff must demonstrate clinical expertise and knowledge within their own clinical field. Consultant midwives, academics and researchers are within this midwifery career framework, which states such clinical specialists must have or be working towards a master's degree or even a doctorate. It is expected that these midwives would contribute at a national and international level as their body of knowledge is expert within their speciality.

THE ACADEMIC MIDWIFE: EDUCATION

Evidence clearly indicates that midwifery care is crucial in maintaining high-quality maternity and neonatal services, with midwifery education being fundamental to sustaining the profession (Renfrew et al 2014) and future workforce (West et al 2017). Midwives may also develop a career in education, where they facilitate the learning of midwives and other health professionals at all academic levels: undergraduate, postgraduate and doctoral. At each university in the UK, there is a lead midwife for education (LME), who is the conduit between the university and the PSRB, the NMC, and is responsible for the quality assurance of all midwifery education programmes in their employing university, in that they meet the PSRB standards. Midwifery education is an attractive and rewarding career for those midwives who are enthusiastic in preparing dynamic, innovative and high-quality midwives of the future, capable of providing safe, competent and holistic evidence-based care to childbearing women, their babies and their families in a diversity of contexts.

There are a range of roles the midwife can undertake in midwifery education:

- *lecturers in midwifery*, who work in a university setting with a focus on teaching and learning, research or practice learning
- *lecturer practitioners*, who work between the university and practice placement setting
- *practice educators/teachers/assessors*, who work predominantly in the practice placement setting.

Midwives wishing to develop a career in midwifery education should be registered on the midwives part of the professional register and have a degree. Many universities, however, require the midwife to have a doctorate (PhD degree or equivalent) or be able to demonstrate they have the equivalent knowledge and experience in midwifery or related subjects to be able to effectively contribute to the academic components of midwifery education. In addition, the university may require the midwife to have a teaching qualification and/or be a Fellow of Advance HE (formerly the Higher Education Academy). However, if the midwife shows an aptitude towards a career in midwifery education, the university may support them in acquiring a teaching qualification/Advance HE fellowship once they have commenced their employment and, in the long term, to undertake doctoral studies, which will enhance an academic career.

The challenge facing the midwifery profession of its ageing workforce is also reflected in midwifery education (RCM 2017), with concerns being expressed by Marshall and Furber (2017) as to how midwifery education capacity can be sustained and further developed so that midwives do not lose sight of educating future generations of midwives. The development of an *education-focused* clinical academic career pathway facilitated between health service providers and universities to reinforce and strengthen the link between education and practice while developing midwifery education capacity, similar to that developed for early-career researchers (UK Clinical Research Collaboration 2008), could be the way forward.

It has also been suggested that opportunities to explore a career in midwifery education should start during pre-registration education as an academic career is often a *second vocation* for clinical midwives, so plans to pursue this should be timely (Marshall and Furber 2017). This will enable *interested* students to plan their route into academia early in their career. Included in midwifery curricula should be short elective placements at another university for the *interested* student to shadow and observe the work of the midwifery lecturer and its different aspects (e.g. recruitment of future students, planning, developing and facilitating learning, assessment and optimizing the student experience). This type of experience will enable a student midwife to 'test out' midwifery education as a viable career option. The student midwife who shows aptitude, motivation and interest in a career in midwifery education should be talent-spotted by midwifery lecturers and provided with mentoring support by a registered midwife to enable them to develop the knowledge, skills and academic qualifications for entry to higher education. Similarly, opportunities for secondment to the university can provide practising midwives with insight into the role of the lecturer as well as higher-degree-level study, such as research degrees and doctoral programmes, which are essential if they wish to pursue an academic career in higher education. Secondments should have role descriptions with clear aims and outcomes to maximize the potential for recruitment to a future lecturer vacancy.

Clinical midwives can provide assistance on an ad hoc basis with targeted teaching sessions in the university setting and/or involvement with objective simulated clinical examinations. Such sessions are useful in providing insight into an academic career where secondments do not exist. It is important, however, that clinical midwives fulfilling these roles should be guided by the midwifery lecturer in preparing for new tasks, and provided with constructive feedback so that they can reflect on their performance and continue to develop professionally. Mentorship from midwifery lecturers for clinical midwives can also involve support with scholarly activities such as writing about their practice for professional journals. This will help to sustain motivation and increase confidence in their abilities to consider pursuing an academic career.

THE ACADEMIC MIDWIFE: RESEARCHER

The UK Clinical Research Collaboration subcommittee for nurses in clinical research (UK Clinical Research Collaboration 2008) established clinical academic career pathways between health service providers and universities to reinforce and strengthen the link between education provision and practice while developing research capacity. This led to the provision of a structured training programme for doctoral research students (including midwives), running in partnership between employers and local universities through the National Institute for Health Research. This enables the doctoral student to undertake CPD alongside a career in clinical practice.

A midwife may wish to embark on a career as a researcher undertaking project work in areas specifically related to childbirth and maternity care in order to make a difference to the childbearing experience. There are many progressive joint-funded NHS and university projects that may interest midwives and those aspiring towards a career in research. Final-year student midwives can apply to start a doctoral programme as soon as they are registered with the NMC as it is not necessary to have postgraduate experience. Furthermore, after award of a PhD degree, there are opportunities for the midwife to develop further their research skills through postdoctoral studies or enrol in a lectureship training scheme/undertake a teaching qualification and become an Advance HE fellow should they decide on an academic career.

Now undertake Activity 15.2.

ACTIVITY 15.2 ■

Find a job summary/role specification for a position you are aspiring to achieve in the next 5 years.
- Review the *essential* and *desirable* attributes associated with the role and identify those that you already possess, including how you can evidence these to a selection panel.
- For those attributes you have *little experience/no experience of*, formulate a personal development plan detailing how you intend to acquire the knowledge, skills and attitudes to be successful in being offered the new position.
- Define the specific support you would require from individuals within your employing organization to enable you to realize your long-term career aspiration (e.g. line manager, colleagues/peers, employer-led supervisor/professional midwife advocate).

Opportunities Overseas

It is well recognized that internationally midwives share a common aim to provide safe, quality and effective care to all childbearing women, their babies and their families. However, most maternal and neonatal deaths occur in LMICs and could easily be prevented if access to professional midwives equipped and resourced within effective health systems were improved. The impact of globalization, migration, the country's income status and the extent to which the health system is functional will pose various degrees of challenges to midwives. Furthermore, the role of the midwife in sexual, reproductive, maternal and newborn health will differ depending on the midwife's country of practice, whether a low-, middle- or high-income country and whether located in the north or south (World Health Organization 2015).

Building on the eight Millennium Development Goals (MDGs) of the United Nations (UN), further initiatives such as the UN Secretary General's *Global Strategy for Women's and Children's Health* (Ki-Moon 2010), the *Every Woman, Every Child* movement (United Nations Foundation 2016) and the Commission on Information and Accountability for Women's and Children's Health (COIA 2014), stimulated global reporting, oversight and accountability with regard to women's and children's health. In 2015, the UN General Assembly adopted 17 Sustainable Development Goals (SDGs) with 169 indicators that were constructed from the lessons of the MDGs and set the 2030 agenda for all countries and all regions of the world (United Nations General Assembly 2015) as shown in Fig. 15.4. There is one specific health-related goal (SDG 3) 'Ensure healthy lives and promote well-being for all at all ages', which has 13 targets, and SDG 5 relates to achieving gender equality and empowering all women and girls, which also

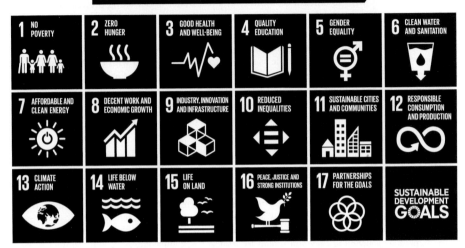

Fig. 15.4   Sustainable Development Goals. (From United Nations General Assembly 2015).

has implications for global midwifery. The SDGs create a broader, novel, transformative agenda, established for maternal mortality and call for acceleration of current progress to achieve the global targets, including reducing mortality rates among childbearing women (SDG 3.1), their babies and their children (SDG 3.2).

As part of CPD, some midwives may decide to enrol for a short- or long-term assignment overseas in LMICs to help specifically support SDG 3.1 and 3.2, whereas midwives from LMICs may travel to high-income countries for study tours or personal professional advancement. Midwives in these situations must adapt to vastly differing situations when practising in countries other than the one in which they were educated and trained. The following sections explore these learning opportunities further.

EXPERIENCE IN LOW- AND MIDDLE-INCOME COUNTRIES

When deciding to go and work in an LMIC, midwives would need to have considerable experience and be conversant with contemporary evidence-based practice. It may be useful for the midwife to acquire competence in additional skills (see Chapter 8), such as suturing vaginal and cervical lacerations, vacuum extraction, manual removal of placenta and insertion of intrauterine contraceptive devices, before travelling abroad to support their role overseas. Whilst it may not be policy or culturally accepted within the organization in which the midwife practises for such skills to be developed, discussion with an obstetrician and a senior midwife who are receptive, altruistic and understand the context of the LMIC in which they intend to be practised could lead to suitable learning opportunities being arranged for the midwife. In addition, undertaking a short course in tropical medicine can be useful to the midwife as can gaining better insight into the country from discussions with individuals who have worked there.

All midwives should be clinically competent, able to adapt to the local context and respectful of the differing culture and religion of the country they are to practise in. Knowledge of a second language is an advantage but is not essential when a midwife is applying to work overseas; however, a willingness to learn would be seen as positive. What midwives need to be mindful of when practising in LMICs is that their purpose is to provide external expertise supporting local colleagues who are working in very different situations, often with extremely limited resources, including less accessibility to information and resources that midwives from high-income countries so readily take for granted. Consequently, change is often hard to implement and it has to come from *within* a country for it to be sustainable (see Chapter 14): it is not a requirement of the midwife from the high-income country. A number of organizations support midwives working overseas, including Médecins Sans Frontières (MSF) and Voluntary Services Overseas (VSO), which are discussed in the following sections.

Médecins Sans Frontières (Doctors Without Borders)

MSF is a private international humanitarian association that provides emergency care to individuals in conflict zones, natural disasters and epidemics. It is mainly made up of doctors and health sector workers and is also open to all other professions that might help in achieving its aims. Officially created on 22 December 1971, MSF is based on the belief that all people have the right to medical care regardless of gender, race, religion, creed or political affiliation, and that the needs of these individuals outweigh respect for national boundaries. Members of MSF agree to honour the following principles:

- to provide assistance to populations in distress, to victims of natural or man-made disasters and to victims of armed conflict irrespective of gender, race, religion, creed or political convictions
- to observe neutrality and impartiality in the name of universal medical ethics and the right to humanitarian assistance and full and unhindered freedom in the exercise of its functions
- to respect their professional code of ethics and to maintain complete independence from all political, economic or religious powers
- to understand the risks and dangers of the missions they carry out and make no claim for themselves or their assigns for any form of compensation other than that which the association might be able to afford them.

If midwives are contemplating working for MSF, they require experience in both physiological and complicated births as their role is a vital part of most project teams, and regardless of context – whether working in natural disasters, conflicts or poverty-affected communities – babies will continue to be born and midwives will always be required. Midwives often work in health centres and conduct outreach work in the community, and consequently their role can be very diverse and challenging, ranging from visiting pregnant women deep in the jungle to undertaking antenatal examinations and training traditional birth attendants in busy maternity departments in large hospital settings. The role is, however, very rewarding as the midwife can learn from the women to whom they provide care and thus improve their understanding of cross-cultural issues surrounding childbirth.

Midwives working with MSF may be responsible for some or all of the following:

- pre- and post birth care
- births (often complicated)
- care of survivors of sexual violence
- setting up maternity/mother and child health departments in new rural health centres/hospitals
- working with community birth attendants to ensure safe community birthing practices
- running reproductive health care awareness programmes from mobile clinics in the community
- training local midwives/traditional birth attendants
- on-call care, often 24 hours.

The MSF website offers further details regarding the credentials required to work as a midwife in its organization, suggesting that it is *not* essential to be a nurse, but a tropical medicine course would be an asset as would knowledge of sexually acquired infections and family planning experience. Depending on the current nature of MSF's work, there may be specific language requirements that would prove advantageous to midwives being accepted onto the MSF register, such as French and Arabic skills for placing them on a mission in the Democratic Republic of the Congo, Chad or Yemen. In most MSF projects the living and working conditions are likely to be very stressful, without many of the things the midwife may take for granted and, more importantly, safety and security are taken very seriously by the organization. By the very nature of MSF's work, it is clear that staff need to be fully aware of the risks they may have to face and the lengths that MSF goes to keep them safe. These are very serious considerations the midwife must be aware of before considering applying to MSF.

Voluntary Services Overseas

VSO is an international development charity that has a vision for a *world without poverty* and a mission to *bring people together to fight poverty*. VSO recruits professionals to work as volunteers, living and working alongside local populations in developing countries in three areas: health care, education and everyday living. Consequently, volunteers are recruited from a range of backgrounds, such as medical and health care, teaching and education, business, management and information technology, engineering and technical services and agricultural and natural sciences. Since its foundation in 1958, VSO has sent more than 50 000 volunteers to work in 24 developing countries across Africa, Asia and the Pacific. However, VSO works only where local partners request its presence, which means that local knowledge is acquired in order to provide the most appropriate skills and training directly to communities in need.

Although the work is voluntary, VSO provides comprehensive financial, personal and professional support. The financial package includes a local living allowance, return flights, accommodation and insurance, including an extensive training programme before a volunteer takes up their placement. The local offices and partners in each of the countries in which VSO works also provide ongoing support for the time the volunteer is working overseas. A range of case scenarios are presented on the VSO website highlighting the range of activities volunteer midwives are engaged in. These can be seen at https://www.vsointernational.org/news/blog/call-the-midwife-six-inspiring-health-workers-saving-young-lives.

EXPERIENCE IN HIGH-INCOME COUNTRIES

Those midwives from LMICs who intend to work or study in high-income countries are likely to face the challenge of more advanced technology and the concept of the midwife–woman partnership, including informed choice/consent, which they may not experience in their home country. In addition, the emphasis on medico-legal issues and the impact of litigation on midwifery and obstetric practice may be far greater than they have been accustomed to. As part of their CPD, these midwives need to evaluate new practices in the context of the LMIC, the resources that are available and national priorities before they attempt to transfer their newly acquired knowledge and practice from one country to another. From another perspective, midwives from LMICs who have practised where resources are limited can share their skill at improvising as well as any innovations with colleagues in high-income countries, who face different, although significant, resource limitations. Those midwives who practise in remote areas no doubt will have a wealth of experience to share in managing complications that are rarely seen in developed countries.

Royal College of Midwives Global Midwifery Twinning Project

The Global Midwifery Twinning Project (GMTP) was a 3-year multicountry partnership in the Health Partnership Scheme (HPS) funded by the UK government and managed by the Tropical Health and Education Trust which ran from 2012 to 2015. The HPS was conceived to improve health outcomes for poor people in Department for International Development-priority and other low-income countries, aiming to strengthen health systems through transfer of health service skills and capacity development.

The RCM formed twinning partnerships with midwifery associations in Uganda, Cambodia and Nepal, which are all low-income countries with a high maternal mortality burden. The twinning relationships were as follows:

- England and Cambodia
- Scotland and Nepal
- Wales and Northern Ireland and Uganda.

The GMTP sent 67 volunteer midwives (including student midwives) on 75 placements over 3 years. The volunteers worked not only with the midwifery associations but also with key stakeholders and practising midwives to address the ICM's three pillars of midwifery: *education*, *regulation* and *association* (see Chapter 2). In addition, volunteers worked alongside midwives to support them in providing quality midwifery care, build individual leadership capacity and transfer skills and knowledge. This also extended to education providers, where volunteer midwives supported curricula developments to improve teaching standards and to support student midwives in their learning. Volunteer midwives worked with associations and regulatory bodies to build leadership and advocacy capacity, to develop strategic planning capacity, to build networks and connections to stakeholders and to role-model the potential of midwife associations to support a strong midwifery profession. Key achievements of the GMTP are shown in Table 15.1.

The GMTP ended in March 2015, and the RCM appointed an independent consultant to conduct an evaluation of the project. The summary report includes case studies from each country (RCM 2016). However, the RCM is committed to continuing its work with its GMTP twins and to developing new twinning relationships where opportunities arise in other countries. These would provide another volunteering opportunity for UK midwives that would be conducive to their CPD needs and to enhancing their long-term career prospects.

TABLE 15.1 ■ **Key Achievements of the Global Midwifery Twinning Project**

Cambodia	Nepal	Uganda
1. Creation of a 5-year strategic plan for the Cambodian Midwives Association.	1. Development of a 5-year strategic plan for the Midwifery Society of Nepal.	1. Development of the master's degree in midwifery curriculum at Uganda Christian University.
2. Formation of the Cambodian Midwives Council competency-based curriculum assessment tool for education providers.	2. Establishment of the Mangala Devi midwife-led birthing centre at Tribhuvan University Teaching Hospital in Kathmandu.	2. Establishment of a multiparty advocacy group and midwifery research interest group, demonstrating greater commitment to midwives working together across private, public, non-profit and faith-based sectors.
3. Increase in the membership of the Cambodian Midwives Association by 50% to more than 4000 members	3. Founding of the first national midwifery conference in Nepal, September 2013, with more than 300 participants	3. Strengthening of private midwife clinical practice sites and a pilot mentorship project with Kibuli School of Nursing and Midwifery

Conclusion

It is useful to have a framework that has clearly set parameters and appropriate tools to support the development of a midwife's career trajectory, such as the Circle of Care Development Pathway (Courtesy Michelle Knight) the NHS Career Framework and the NHS Knowledge and Skills Framework (DH 2004). Midwives who show an aptitude for a certain aspect of midwifery practice and who choose to follow a specific career pathway should be nurtured and guided by their employing organization to do so as well as being supported through the process of appraisal and revalidation. Lifelong learning for the new registrant midwife commences with preceptorship and should continue throughout their career. Midwifery career pathways covering the diversity of roles midwives occupy, be it a clinician, an educationalist, a manager/leader or a researcher, are not only useful in enabling midwives to fulfil their potential within their chosen field but are also vital to the future development of the profession as a whole. In addition to overseas electives that may inspire some student midwives to consider an international career or to be a volunteer midwife, placements for students and secondments to midwifery academic and research teams for early-career midwives must be the way forward to build midwifery education and research capacity for the future at local, national and international level.

KEY POINTS

- Lifelong learning and CPD are essential to the role of the midwife and fundamental to the requirements of professional regulation, including the process of revalidation.
- The organization in which a midwife practises should be creative and encouraging towards learning with the aim of providing high quality care to women, their babies and their families.
- Revalidation is a statutory requirement for *all* midwives, including those in leadership, education and research-focused roles.
- Student midwives who are also registered nurses (*adult field*) must continue to pay their annual retention fee during their studies to maintain their nursing registration and be supported to complete the triennial revalidation process (*nursing focused*) should it occur before the end of the midwifery education programme.
- Midwifery career pathways, a system of annual appraisal and professional development plans can enable midwives to plan their career trajectory and CPD requirements more effectively, aspiring to specific roles in a more timely fashion.
- Providing elective placements, internships and secondments for students and early-career midwives to experience working alongside leaders and academics (lecturers and researchers) is vital to ensure the midwifery profession continues to flourish with midwives *always* at the helm.
- Overseas opportunities may inspire students and midwives towards an international career or to be a volunteer midwife: such contributions to global midwifery practice are vital in helping to achieve the Sustainable Development Goals of improving the health and well-being of women, their babies and their families throughout the world.

References

Commission on Information and Accountability for Women's and Children's Health. (2014). *Implementing the commission on information and accountability recommendations.* Available at: https://www.who.int/woman_child_accountability/news/background_progress_report_jan2014.pdf.

Department of Health. (2004). *The NHS knowledge and skills framework and the development review process.* London: Department of Health.

Directive 2013/55/EU of the European Parliament and of the Council of 20 November 2013 amending Directive 2005/36/EC on the recognition of professional qualifications and Regulation (EU) No 1024/2012 on administrative cooperation through the Internal Market Information System ('the IMI Regulation').

International Confederation of Midwives. (2013). *Global standards for midwifery education*. Available at: https://www.internationalmidwives.org/assets/files/general-files/2018/04/icm-standards-guidelines_ammended2013.pdf.

International Confederation of Midwives. (2017). *International definition of the midwife*. Available at: https://www.internationalmidwives.org/assets/files/definitions-files/2018/06/eng-definition_of_the_midwife-2017.pdf.

International Confederation of Midwives. (2018). *Essential competencies for basic midwifery practice*. Available at:https://www.internationalmidwives.org/our-work/policy-and-practice/essential-competencies-for-midwifery-practice.html.

Ki-Moon, B. (2010). *Global strategy for women's and children's health: Every woman, every child*. Available at: http://www.everywomaneverychild.org/global-strategy.

Marshall, J. E., & Furber, C. (2017). Who will educate and prepare the midwives of the future? The crisis in midwifery education in the UK. *MIDIRS Midwifery Digest*, 27(3), 277–280.

Munro, K. M. (2008). Continuing professional development and the charity paradigm: Interrelated individual, collective and organisational issues about professional development. *Nurse Education Today*, 28, 953–961.

Nursing and Midwifery Council. (2007). *Review of pre-registration midwifery education: Decisions made by the midwifery committee*. London: Nursing and Midwifery Council. NMC circular 14/2007.

Nursing and Midwifery Council. (2011). *The prep handbook*. London: Nursing and Midwifery Council.

Nursing Midwifery Council. (2018). *The code: Professional standards of practice and behaviour for nurses, midwives and nursing associates*. London: Nursing and Midwifery Council.

Nursing and Midwifery Council. (2019). *Revalidation: How to revalidate with the NMC*. London: Nursing and Midwifery Council.

Renfrew, M. J., McFadden, A., Bastos, M. H., Campbell, J., Channon, A. A., Cheung, N. F., et al. (2014). Midwifery and quality care: Findings from a new evidence-informed framework for maternal and newborn care. *The Lancet*, 384, 1129–1145.

Royal College of Midwives. (2016). *Supporting midwifery beyond our borders: Global midwifery twinning project*. London: Royal College of Midwives.

Royal College of Midwives. (2017). *RCM caring for you campaign. Survey results about the health, safety and wellbeing of midwives working in education*. London: Royal College of Midwives.

UK Clinical Research Collaboration. (2008). *Developing the best research professionals. Qualified graduate nurses: recommendations for preparing and supporting clinical academic nurses of the future*. London: UK Clinical Research Collaboration. Available at: http://www.ukcrc.org/wp-content/uploads/2014/07/Nurses-report-August-07-Web.pdf.

United Nations General Assembly. (2015). *Transforming our world: the 2030 Agenda for Sustainable Development (A/RES/70/1)*. Available at: https://sustainabledevelopment.un.org/content/documents/21252030%20Agenda%20for%20Sustainable%20Development%20web.pdf.

United Nations Foundation. (2016). *Every woman, every child*. Available at: http://www.everywomaneverychild.org.

West, F., Dawson, A., & Homer, C. S. E. (2017). Building midwifery educator capacity using international partnerships: Findings from a qualitative study. *Nurse Education in Practice*, 25, 66–73.

World Health Organization. (2015). *Trends in maternal mortality: 1990 to 2015. Estimates by WHO, UNICEF, UNFPA, World Bank Group and the United Nations Population Division*. Available at: www.who.int/reproductivehealth/publications/monitoring/maternal-mortality-2015/en/.

Further Reading

Maclean, G. D. (2013). *Electives and international midwifery consultancy: A resource for students*. London: Quay Books.
This is an informative text that would be of benefit to midwives or anyone with an interest in global maternal and neonatal health, particularly those wishing to volunteer overseas, or students undertaking electives or gap-year assignments. It provides practical, evidence-based guidance using reflective practice and the sharing of experience. Written before the Sustainable Development Goals were published, the emphasis on the former Millennium Development Goals (achievement target being 2015) highlights the importance of professionals sharing their experiences and skills cross-culturally.

Smoker, A. (2015). *Launching your career in nursing and midwifery: A practical guide.* London: Palgrave Macmillan.

This is a useful practical guide for any student or newly qualified midwife that provides a wealth of information on career planning, continuing professional development and the next steps in career progression. There is sound advice on interview planning, an overview of the selection process and authentic case scenarios for the reader to reflect on and use to identify their own strengths and weaknesses.

Useful Websites:

Advance HE (formed by a merger of the Equality Challenge Unit, the Higher Education Academy and the Leadership Foundation for Higher Education): https://www.advance-he.ac.uk

Department for International Development: https://www.gov.uk/government/organisations/department-for-international-development

Health Careers: https://www.healthcareers.nhs.uk

Health Professional Academy (Mum and Baby Academy): https://www.healthprofessionalacademy.co.uk/

International Confederation of Midwives, International Confederation of Midwives: https://www.internationalmidwives.org

Médecins Sans Frontières: https://www.msf.org.uk

National Institute for Health Research: https://www.nihr.ac.uk

NHS Employers: https://www.nhsemployers.org

Nursing and Midwifery Council: https://www.nmc.org.uk

Nursing and Midwifery Council revalidation: http://revalidation.nmc.org.uk

Royal College of Midwives: https://www.rcm.org.uk

Skills for Healtc: https://www.skillsforhealth.org.uk

Tropical Health and Education Trust: https://www.thet.org

United Nations Population Fund: https://www.unfpa.org

Voluntary Services Overseas: https://www.vsointernational.org

World Health Organization: http://www.who.int

INDEX

Note: Page numbers followed by "f" indicate figures, "t" indicate tables and "b" indicate boxes